CONCEPT DEVELOPMENT IN NURSING

CONCEPT DEVELOPMENT IN NURSING

Foundations, Techniques, and Applications

SECOND EDITION

Beth L. Rodgers, RN, PhD
Associate Professor
School of Nursing
University of Wisconsin–Milwaukee
Milwaukee, Wisconsin

Kathleen A. Knafl, PhD
Professor, College of Nursing
University of Illinois at Chicago
Chicago, Illinois

SAUNDERS
An Imprint of Elsevier

SAUNDERS
An Imprint of Elsevier
The Curtis Center
Independence Square West
Philadelphia, PA 19106

Library of Congress Cataloging-in-Publication Data

Concept development in nursing: foundations, techniques, and applications / [edited by] Beth L. Rodgers, Kathleen A. Knafl.—2nd ed.

p.   cm.

Includes bibliographical references and index.

ISBN-13: 978-0-7216-8243-3   ISBN-10: 0-7216-8243-X

1. Nursing—Philosophy.   2. Concepts.   I. Rodgers, Beth L.
   II. Knafl, Kathleen Astin.   [DNLM: 1. Nursing.   2. Concept Formation.
   WY 86 C7435 2000]
RT 84.5.C6624   2000   610.73'01—dc21

DNLM/DLC   99–31082

Editor: Thomas Eoyang
Designer: Paul Fry
Production Manager: Natalie Ware
Project Manager: Agnes Hunt Byrne
Illustration Coordinator: Rita Martello

CONCEPT DEVELOPMENT IN NURSING:
Foundations, Techniques, and Applications

Permissions may be sought directly from Elsevier's Health Sciences Rights Department in Philadelphia, PA, USA: phone: (+1) 215 239 3804, fax: (+1) 215 239 3805, e-mail: healthpermissions@elsevier.com. You may also complete your request on-line via the Elsevier homepage (http://www.elsevier.com), by selecting 'Customer Support' and then 'Obtaining Permissions'.

ISBN-13: 978-0-7216-8243-3
ISBN-10: 0-7216-8243-X

Printed in the United States of America.

Last digit is the print number: 9

Contributors

Cynthia Allen Abbott, RN, PhD, CNOR
Maj., Army Nurse Corps, Center for Healthcare Education and Studies, Fort Sam Houston, Texas
Wilsonian Concept Analysis: Applying the Technique

Kay C. Avant, RN, PhD, FAAN
Associate Professor, School of Nursing, University of Texas at Austin, Austin, Texas
The Wilson Method of Concept Analysis; Wilsonian Concept Analysis: Applying the Technique

Barbara J. Bowers, RN, PhD
Professor, School of Nursing, University of Wisconsin-Madison, Madison, Wisconsin
Methods and Application of Dimensional Analysis: A Contribution to Concept and Knowledge Development in Nursing

Teresa Britt, RN, MS
Assistant Professor, Samaritan College of Nursing, Grand Canyon University, Phoenix, Arizona
Simultaneous Concept Analysis: A Strategy for Developing Multiple Interrelated Concepts

Marion E. Broome, RN, PhD, FAAN
Professor and Associate Dean for Research, University of Alabama at Birmingham, Birmingham, Alabama
Integrative Literature Reviews for the Development of Concepts

Chantal D. Caron, RN, MS
Doctoral Student, University of Wisconsin-Madison, Madison, Wisconsin
Methods and Application of Dimensional Analysis: A Contribution to Concept and Knowledge Development in Nursing

Doris D. Coward, RN, PhD
Associate Professor, School of Nursing, University of Texas at Austin, Austin, Texas
Simultaneous Concept Analysis: A Strategy for Developing Multiple Interrelated Concepts

Kathleen V. Cowles, RN, PhD
Associate Professor, School of Nursing, University of Wisconsin-Milwaukee, Milwaukee, Wisconsin
The Concept of Grief: An Evolutionary Perspective; Grief in a Cultural Context: Expanding Concept Analysis Beyond the Professional Literature

Janet A. Deatrick, RN, PhD, FAAN
Associate Professor, School of Nursing, University of Pennsylvania, Philadelphia, Pennsylvania
Knowledge Synthesis and Concept Development in Nursing; Research Careers and Concept Development: The Case of Normalization

Geraldine DeNuccio, RN, MS
Assistant Professor of Nursing, Rhode Island College, Providence, Rhode Island
A Concept Analysis of Withdrawal: Application of the Hybrid Model

Joan E. Haase, RN, PhD
Associate Professor, College of Nursing, University of Arizona, Tucson, Arizona
Simultaneous Concept Analysis: A Strategy for Developing Multiple Interrelated Concepts

Marion L. Johnson, RN, PhD
Professor and Director, Graduate Programs, College of Nursing, University of Iowa, Iowa City, Iowa
Concept Development of Nursing-Sensitive Patient Outcomes

Hesook Suzie Kim, RN, PhD
Professor, College of Nursing, University of Rhode Island, Kingston, Rhode Island; Professor, Institute of Nursing Science, Faculty of Medicine, University of Oslo, Oslo, Norway
An Expansion and Elaboration of the Hybrid Model of Concept Development

Kathleen A. Knafl, PhD
Professor, College of Nursing, University of Illinois at Chicago, Chicago, Illinois
Introduction to Concept Development in Nursing; Knowledge Synthesis and Concept Development in Nursing; Research Careers and Concept Development: The Case of

Normalization; Applications and Future Directions for Concept Development in Nursing

Nancy R. Lackey, RN, PhD
Professor, School of Nursing, University of Missouri–Kansas City, Kansas City, Missouri
Concept Clarification: Using the Norris Method in Clinical Research

Nancy Kline Leidy, RN, PhD
Director and Senior Research Scientist, Center for Health Outcomes Research, MEDTAP International Inc., Bethesda; Adjunct Faculty, School of Nursing, Johns Hopkins University, Baltimore, Maryland
Simultaneous Concept Analysis: A Strategy for Developing Multiple Interrelated Concepts

Meridean L. Maas, RN, PhD, FAAN
Professor, College of Nursing, University of Iowa, Iowa City; Adjunct Executive in Nursing, Iowa Veterans Home, Marshalltown, Iowa
Concept Development of Nursing-Sensitive Patient Outcomes

Sue Moorhead, RN, PhD
Associate Professor, College of Nursing, University of Iowa, Iowa City, Iowa
Concept Development of Nursing-Sensitive Patient Outcomes

Janice M. Morse, RN, PhD(Nurs), PhD(Anthro), FAAN
Professor and Director, International Institute for Qualitative Methodology, University of Alberta, Edmonton, Alberta, Canada
Exploring Pragmatic Utility: Concept Analysis by Critically Appraising the Literature

Patricia E. Penn, PhD
Senior Research Specialist,

Department of Psychology, University of Arizona, Tucson; Research- and Clinical Psychologist, La Frontera Center, Tucson, Arizona
Simultaneous Concept Analysis: A Strategy for Multiple Interrelated Concepts

Beth L. Rodgers, RN, PhD
Associate Professor, School of Nursing, University of Wisconsin-Milwaukee, Milwaukee, Wisconsin
Introduction to Concept Development in Nursing; Philosophical Foundations of Concept Development; Concept Analysis: An Evolutionary View; The Concept of Grief: An Evolutionary Perspective; Beyond Analysis: Further Adventures in Concept Development; Applications and Future Directions for Concept Development in Nursing

Judith J. Sadler, RN, PhD
Assistant Professor, School of Nursing, Western Michigan University, Kalamazoo, Michigan
A Multiphase Approach to Concept Analysis and Development

Deborah Perry Schoenfelder, RN, PhD
Clinical Assistant Professor, College of Nursing, University of Iowa, Iowa City, Iowa
Concept Development of Nursing-Sensitive Patient Outcomes

Donna Schwartz-Barcott, RN, PhD
Professor and Director of Graduate Studies in Nursing,
College of Nursing, University of Rhode Island, Kingston, Rhode Island
An Expansion and Elaboration of the Hybrid Model of Concept Development; A Concept Analysis of Withdrawal: Application of the Hybrid Model

Janet P. Specht, RN, PhD
Associate Clinical Professor, Adult and Gerontology, College of Nursing, University of Iowa, Iowa City, Iowa
Concept Development of Nursing-Sensitive Patient Outcomes

Elizabeth A. Swanson, RN, PhD
Associate Professor, College of Nursing, University of Iowa, Iowa City, Iowa
Concept Development of Nursing-Sensitive Patient Outcomes

Bonnie L. Westra, RN, PhD
Adjunct Faculty, School of Nursing, University of Minnesota, Minneapolis; Vice President, Clinical Services, CareFacts Information Systems, Inc., St. Paul, Minnesota
Concept Development of Nursing-Sensitive Patient Outcomes

Judith Wuest, RN, PhD
Professor and Director of Graduate Studies, Faculty of Nursing, University of New Brunswick, Fredericton, New Brunswick, Canada
Concept Development Situated in the Critical Paradigm

Preface

Beginnings and endings (like concepts) can be elusive to pinpoint. Although we can identify the time when we first discussed the possibility of collaborating on a book on concept development, the origins of our individual and shared interests in concept analysis and concept development in general are considerably less clear. The idea for the book was first broached in 1990 at a research conference. We had been speakers at a symposium on concept analysis, and following the symposium a mutual friend suggested that we collaborate on a book on the subject. Rodgers had mulled over the idea of such a project for some time, and the prospect of working with Knafl, of sharing ideas and enthusiasm, as well as expertise, was an added impetus. The idea of working together appealed to both of us, and over the course of several conversations and planning sessions we developed an outline and prospectus to show to possible publishers. Although that first meeting at the conference was the official beginning of the project, our individual interests in concept development go back much further.

Rodgers had a history of fondness for analytical pursuits, scholarly questioning, and the abstract. In the 1980s, during graduate study, this attraction was focused on the nature of nursing and the many issues and problems encountered in attempts to develop the knowledge base of nursing. Philosophical pursuits quickly made it clear that many of the problems confronted in nursing were conceptual. This observation led to further inquiry to seek credible means to resolve these barriers.

Concept analysis had been used with some frequency to address such problems in nursing. Yet in the nursing literature this method was limited to a few approaches that were nearly identical in orientation. Existing descriptions provided little insight into elements of rigor associated with analysis, how methodological decisions were made, or specifically how the use of a particular method could advance nursing knowledge. On close examination there also was reason for concern regarding potential conflict between the philosophical basis implicit in the literature of concept analysis and the contemporary philosophy and beliefs espoused in nursing. Ultimately this led Rodgers to investigate various nursing and philosophical positions on concepts in general, to consider a variety of means to resolve conceptual problems, and to explore the linkage between concepts and nursing knowledge.

In contrast to the philosophical groundings of Rodgers' interests, as a family researcher Knafl was interested in the potential inherent in concepts for increasing understanding of family response to illness. She also was aware of the conceptual ambiguity surrounding many of the concepts used in family research (e.g., family coping, enmeshment) but accepted this as a "fact of life." This acceptance changed rather abruptly after she read the concept analysis section of the first edition of Chinn and Jacobs' book on theory development in nursing. For Knafl, that book raised an intellectual challenge and presented a strategy for addressing some of the intellectual ambiguity in family research.

For several years, Knafl and her colleague Janet Deatrick had puzzled over the meaning of two concepts, normalization and denial, that often were used to describe parents' responses to their child's chronic illness. During the course of their work with families of children with chronic illnesses, Knafl and Deatrick had noted that occasionally families they described as normalizing their children's illnesses were described by providers as denying the seriousness of the situations. Knafl and Deatrick knew that they wanted to do something to clarify this conceptual confusion, but it was not until they read about concept analysis that they found an appropriate strategy to pursue. In 1984 they published their first concept analysis of normalization. A second analysis of the concept of family management style was published several years later. While completing these analyses and reading more on concept analysis, Knafl and Deatrick became aware of other approaches to concept analysis and development that raised numerous questions about the relative merits and appropriate use of these alternative strategies. Rodgers' philosophical interest in this field provided the ideal complement to Knafl's more applied interest in concept development.

This book reflects our complementary interests. In it, we address both the philosophical underpinnings of concept development and the practicality of various techniques for furthering understanding and progress in important areas of nursing science. We have included an encompassing range of concept development strategies and have sought to address the advantages, disadvantages, and, most importantly, the appropriate use of each. Our goal was to provide a menu of possibilities representing the "state of the art" of concept development. We hoped this text would be a vital resource for everyone in nursing who is interested in contributing to the further clarification and development of the many concepts pertinent to nursing practice, research, and education.

For the first edition of *Concept Development in Nursing*, we brainstormed, pursuing our own ideas about concept development and methods or viewpoints consistent with that general focus of inquiry. Although there was some work in nursing that addressed ideas associated with concept development, there certainly was not an abundance of literature and thinkers with that interest. More often than not, we would contact prospective authors and explain to them how we saw their work and potential chapter as a part of the broad rubric of concept development. We certainly did not meet any resistance with our solicitations and ideas; and yet there was a common response from many of the people we contacted, indicating that they simply had not thought of their work "that way."

The preparation of this second edition was a far different experience. Since the first edition was published, "that way"—the way of concept development—has become much more commonplace, perhaps even mainstream. The volume of literature in this area has increased exponentially, and a broad and expanding audience is familiar with the terminology of concept development. This time we were challenged to sort through a myriad of works and viewpoints to assemble a text that would capture the new and current scope of the subject with depth and significance, without creating a volume of such size that it could double aptly as a doorstop.

This growing interest in concept development, and recognition of the value of such inquiry, is due to some extent to changes in contemporary philosophy. The evolution of philosophy has given legitimacy to forms of inquiry other than the traditional (that is, the hypothetico-deductive model). In addition, attention has been drawn to areas that cannot be addressed adequately through the usual forms of inquiry, which is presumed to be focused on objects and "facts." Instead of the reality revealed by biophysiological measures and paper and pencil tests, the realities revealed through language and ideas and the existence of personal worlds and social contexts have been brought to light through contemporary philosophical movements. Scholars in nursing, as in other fields that address the content of the human sciences, recognize the complexity of the systems of symbols and meanings that make up human interaction. All of these are the important elements of concept formation and development.

In the search for truth, there now is room for the quest for understanding and, as a necessary part of understanding, the development of concepts. Perhaps the greatest change comes in the search for usefulness, although this revolution has barely begun. We are delighted to have been a part of that movement and growth in nursing and hope that this second and expanded edition of *Concept Development in Nursing* will stimulate readers to join in the dialogue about nursing and the role of concepts in the development of the knowledge base for the discipline.

Many people have influenced this work, both directly and indirectly, and continue to affect the development of our ideas. In a field such as nursing in which inquiry easily becomes focused primarily on the empirical realm, we are grateful for those thinkers and authors in the past who recognized the importance of conceptual concerns in the advancement of nursing. Their works helped set the stage for this text, which we expect to represent the current state of the science of concept development.

We also want to acknowledge the contributing authors, who enthusiastically shared their expertise for this project and thus provided the support essential to make our plans and ideas for this book a reality. Kathleen Cowles provided much of the initial impetus for this work through her unfaltering belief that it was, indeed, a worthwhile pursuit. Janet Deatrick contributed her valuable insights and spirit of adventure to Knafl's initial forays into the realm of concept analysis. Finally, we wish to acknowledge and express our gratitude to the staff of W. B. Saunders Company, all of whom were nothing short of terrific to work with. Mr. Thomas Eoyang, Vice-President and Editor-in-Chief, Nursing Books, and Ms. Gina Hopf, Assistant Developmental Editor, deserve special recognition for their roles in this project.

We want to point out here that any reference to this book as a "finished" product must be considered again in regard to the elusiveness of beginnings and endings, as we noted at the opening of this preface. There is good reason to argue whether scholarly work and inquiry are ever truly "finished." Instead, it seems that we reach transition stages where it is worthwhile and important to share ideas and information garnered but equally important to stimulate further inquiry. Consequently, as we viewed the first edition as a beginning, we consider this second edition to represent another stage in development, rather than an end product. We hope that it can serve as the catalyst to stimulate further dialogue and work on concept development in nursing.

BETH L. RODGERS
KATHLEEN A. KNAFL

Contents

Introduction to Concept Development in Nursing

Beth L. Rodgers and Kathleen A. Knafl

S ome readers of this book, at first glance, may have the same type of reaction that many of our colleagues did when they heard of our first project in the early 1990s: "Hmmm. Sounds interesting." This is a classic, noncommittal response that, since it frequently is accompanied by a puzzled expression, conveys that the speakers really do not know what to think. Most likely, they really were wondering, "What is concept development, anyway, and what does it have to do with nursing (and why should anyone care)?" We had heard these questions many times before. Certainly, there were many people who responded to our ideas for the initial text with excitement and anticipation. This wide variety of reactions, which we both had encountered through our experiences with research, publishing, and giving presentations, provided much of the motivation for this work. We hope that it will answer at least some of the questions of the curious or puzzled, provide stimulation for those already excited about prospects for concept development for the advancement of nursing knowledge, and promote greater understanding of the depth and scope of concept development in nursing for all readers.

For the uninitiated, we aimed to provide information that would answer the "what is it?" (and, it is hoped, the "who cares?") question. We also wanted to stimulate interest in concept development methods as a part of the readers' own research programs or, at least, an appreciation of such inquiry. For the reader who has had some exposure to ideas related to concept development but lacks sufficient background to tackle this type of investigation, we have assembled a combination of how-to descriptions, along with practical examples and additional discussion on applications. The intent here also was to provide sufficient background information and rationale to promote investigations that

1

would be both rigorous and credible. Too often, concept development techniques seem to be relegated to the status of classroom learning exercises; thus, their place and contributions in the realm of nursing knowledge development may not be appreciated fully. Finally, for the advanced reader, we tried to create a text that is comprehensive, presenting views and discussions that were not available elsewhere, were available only in less depth or lesser states of development, or were more or less obscure by virtue of being scattered throughout existing literature. Assembling a wide variety of concept development approaches and applications in a single text makes the differences across methods and the opportunities for inquiry more apparent. An understanding of diverse approaches is necessary for the researcher to make informed choices in selecting a technique to employ in an investigation.

Concept development is not a new area or system of methods for inquiry. Books and articles on research methods and theory building are abundant, and occasionally include some attention to ideas related to concept development. Typically this attention is focused on concepts in general, particularly in texts related to theory or, in some cases, a discussion of concept analysis as a method. These efforts do not capture the scope or depth of the topic of concept development, nor do they adequately emphasize the contribution of concept development in the overall scientific enterprise of nursing.

The lack of concentrated attention to this topic is particularly troublesome in view of the importance of concepts in the development of knowledge. In the literature on research methods, the conceptual basis for a study often is discussed as the hallmark (or, in some cases, the primary failing point) of excellence in an investigation. In theory development literature, concepts are widely recognized as the "building blocks" from which theories are constructed. In philosophy, there is a lengthy history of discussions of science and knowledge, and psychologists have devoted immeasurable attention to how we learn and develop and communicate our ideas. Without variation, concepts are a major focus for the majority, if not all, of these writers.

This emphasis on concepts has increased somewhat in recent years. Prominent philosophers of science in the early twentieth century, particularly the logical positivists, confined conceptual problems to the realm of "nonsense." Later, however, philosophers such as Laudan (1977) gave considerable weight to both conceptual and empirical problems in scientific progress. For Laudan, progress consisted of achieving a balance between empirical advances and conceptual dilemmas; scientific progress was, in fact, viewed as the resolution of problems through developments based on "fact," without the addition of new conceptual troubles. Toulmin (1972) also emphasized the important role of concepts in the quest for knowledge, and gave them such prominence that he devoted an entire volume of his work to a discussion of progress and the maintenance of continuity in a discipline specifically through conceptual change and development. Thus, by improving or otherwise developing concepts, a discipline could make considerable advancements in achieving its intellectual goals (Toulmin, 1972).

More recently, philosophers associated with what commonly are called *postmodern* ideologies have provided even more foundation for exploring and developing concepts as a legitimate form of inquiry. Pointing out the individual, contextual, social, cultural, and authoritative influences on knowledge necessarily increases attention to concepts. It is in concepts that these forces become institutionalized. The concepts of pain, grief, suffering menopause, addiction, and so on do not reflect related objective "facts." Instead, they reflect all of the contextual forces that shape their development and variation, as well as their use in both daily life and in the development of a disciplinary knowledge base.

The emphasis on concept development in nursing also has increased in the last decade. Completed analyses, using a variety of methods, are common in the literature of nursing. Scholars and researchers in the discipline have increased attention to methodological concerns and underpinnings as well, as evidenced through the emergence of critiques of methodology and philosophically oriented writings. Overall, it is clear that concept development is supported widely as a significant form of inquiry to expand and develop the knowledge base of nursing and other scholarly disciplines.

In spite of the emphasis that philosophers, and a vast array of other scholars, have placed on concept development, we tend to know much more about how to tackle empirical concerns than we do about means to resolve conceptual barriers to progress. As a result, a substantial gap continues to exist in the literature concerning concept development and, consequently, in scientific activity as well. This book is an attempt to fill that gap, and to expand on the contributions made in the first edition. Actually, no single text could ever fill such a chasm, nor do the contents of this book exhaust the domain of knowledge that concerns concepts and concept development. Nevertheless, we do hope to call attention to conceptual problems and provide a basis for systematic and rigorous inquiry to address them. It is our wish to encourage additional work to develop new methods or to expand on the ones presented in this text.

It is not always clear to researchers how concept development techniques can be used appropriately. In some instances, certain features of an area of inquiry may be prominent and point to the need for such methods. Most common, perhaps, is a researcher's desire to operationalize or, at least, clarify a concept as a preliminary step in a formal investigation. However, we would argue that in many situations problems confronted in nursing knowledge may be primarily, if not strictly, conceptual in nature. Some of the more obvious conceptual problems include vague terminology, ambiguity regarding the definitions of important concepts in nursing, and inconsistencies among theories. For example, concepts such as self-care and coping are used extensively in nursing and are widely considered to be important. However, they also are defined and used in highly varying ways. This variation both is confusing and retards scientific advancement in these areas.

Concept development methods also may be appropriate in some less obvious instances: the classification of nursing phenomena, the need for new ways to address or describe a situation in nursing, or the synthesis of existing knowledge concerning a concept of interest. Sometimes concept development methods can be helpful to answer what-is-going-on-here type questions (for example, is a particular client experiencing *grief*?), and perhaps even some ethical problems can be illuminated by such techniques. For example, consider the new dimensions that might be added to discussions concerning the termination of life support in cases of persistent vegetative states if there were systematic efforts to identify various conceptions of "personhood" (Cowles, 1984). What constitutes personhood, as just one example, lies at the base of many ethical problems. It is not a question that can be answered empirically, but lends itself well to concept development techniques.

Fortunately, work on conceptual problems seems to have been increasing in recent years. Yet it still tends to be limited in terms of scope, depth, and methods. Concept development generally has been limited to the obviously abstract and is focused most often on concept analysis, especially adaptations of Wilson's (1963) work. Although such studies continue to make contributions to nursing knowledge development, they fail to address the broad range of problems, methods, and issues relevant to this type of inquiry. In short, the full potential of concept analysis, as well as other means to develop concepts, has yet to be tapped by nurse scholars.

Continuing and perhaps escalating the current pace of progress in nursing knowledge requires work on both the empirical and the conceptual matters that confront clinicians, educators, and researchers in nursing. We do not intend that this statement be misconstrued as yet another contribution to existing methods debates. The arguments about qualitative and quantitative research, a focus of much methodological debate (Duffy, 1985; Goodwin & Goodwin, 1984; Moccia, 1988), are tiresome enough (and frequently superficial) without our giving the impression of taking sides. Besides, the variety of concept development techniques, if taken as a separate class of methods, do not necessarily fit clearly within just one of these categorizations. Nor do we want to confuse the matter further by introducing a third category of research into the discussion. Instead, researchers need to be driven by the questions they pose or by the specific problem for which a solution is sought. Thus, we call attention to some different types of problems that may have received inadequate attention in the past, and provide some means to address these with quality inquiry.

As mentioned previously, the discussions and methods presented in this text do not exhaust the body of knowledge on concept development. We believe, however, that they are representative of the state of this art. In compiling this collection, we sought both well-established and less-developed approaches to concept development. Thus, this text contains a blend of "tried-and-true" methods, along with the most recent, innovative strategies.

In addition to the many other aims of this book, we also hoped to achieve balance in the discussions included. Doing so, however, proved to be a difficult task. Some of the methods presented are more complex, have a longer history, or are more developed than others. In such cases, the authors simply had more to contribute in discussing these approaches. Others could be described only in less complex or less specific ways by virtue of their state of development. Consequently, some discussions of methods are accompanied by example chapters to illustrate not only the results of completed research but the detailed procedures involved in a study using that particular method.

Equal treatment of approaches, then, could not be achieved relative to length or depth of discussion. Instead, the goal was to achieve a balanced overview of the various types and applications of methods available, and to balance the philosophical, methodological, and practical aspects of concept development as a whole. The book begins with a sort of intellectual history of the subject of concepts, focusing on the philosophical aspects and foundations of concepts and concept development. This chapter addresses our belief that the *how* of something (that is, the methods of concept development) must be associated with knowledge of *why* (the rationale) and what it *means* to use such methods. Where appropriate, some works are followed by an actual example of the method described for additional clarity.

Following these discussions is a section in which we captured some less-well-known or newer (or both) ideas and some unique applications. Ways to expand traditional analysis approaches through various forms of qualitative research and from critical perspectives are the focus of other chapters in this text, and Knafl and Deatrick share their story of their long-standing program of research. Rodgers' chapter, "Beyond Analysis: Further Adventures in Concept Development" points out how the work is merely starting, and the need for expansion of methods and methodology to meet the concept development needs of the discipline.

We conclude this text with additional discussion of the applications of concept development techniques. This reflects our belief not only that concept development is pursued too infrequently (for whatever reason) but also that the vast range of productive uses of such methods may not be recognized. Although concluding chapters in books often are used to bring closure to the text, we hope that this final chapter will open doors to increased recognition, use, and expansion of concept development techniques. Such an occurrence can only provide fuel for progress, whether through increasing awareness and discussion or—what would be the best outcome—by providing workable solutions to some perplexing and very real conceptual problems in nursing.

REFERENCES

Cowles, K. V. (1984). Life, death, and personhood. *Nursing Outlook, 32,* 169-172.

Duffy, M. E. (1985). Designing nursing research: The qualitative-quantitative debate. *Journal of Advanced Nursing, 10,* 225-232.

Goodwin, L. D., & Goodwin, W. L. (1984). Qualitative vs. quantitative research or qualitative and quantitative research? *Nursing Research, 33,* 378-380.

Laudan, L. (1977). *Progress and its problems.* Berkeley, CA: University of California Press.

Moccia, P. (1988). A critique of compromise: Beyond the methods debate. *Advances in Nursing Science, 10*(4), 1-9.

Toulmin, S. (1972). *Human understanding.* Princeton: Princeton University Press.

Wilson, J. (1963). *Thinking with concepts.* London: Cambridge University Press.

Philosophical Foundations of Concept Development

Beth L. Rodgers

What is a concept? Any researcher who desires to use or even understand concept development must grapple with this basic question and the philosophical foundations of inquiry if the investigations are to be meaningful and worthwhile. As with any form of research, this background has a tremendous influence on decisions concerning the design of a study, the interpretation of findings, and the eventual application of results.

Many scholars in nursing have pointed out that the development of concepts is important to expand nursing knowledge. Walker and Avant (1988, 1995), for example, include activities such as concept analysis, concept synthesis, and concept derivation as fundamental activities for theory development in nursing. Chinn and Kramer (1991) also address concept development in their text, and an expanded section on concept development is one of the more obvious additions to the most recent edition of the theory development text authored by Meleis (1997). Concept analysis is certainly the most familiar of these approaches as it has been used in attempts to resolve many significant conceptual problems in nursing (Beck, 1996; Bohlander, 1995; Boyd, 1985; Coyne, 1996; Duffy, 1987; Forsyth, 1980; Gibson, 1991; Haddock, 1996; Johns, 1996; Knafl & Deatrick, 1986; Matteson & Hawkins, 1990; Meize-Grochowski, 1984; Rawnsley, 1980; Rew, 1986; Simmons, 1989; also, see bibliography at end of this text). In spite of these efforts, however, relatively little attention has been directed toward uncovering the philosophical issues associated with concepts and existing techniques for concept analysis and development.

It is difficult, perhaps even naïve, for a researcher to merely accept such methods as legitimate or necessarily effective forms of inquiry. Scholars who write on the topic of concepts generally have failed to explain the philosophical basis of methods of concept analysis and development. Close examination of long-standing methods reveals that some important assumptions often are made, yet authors typically have not specified their assumptions nor discussed whether the assumptions are reasonable or defensible. As a result, researchers are left with several important questions that must be answered before proceeding with inquiry: What does it "mean" to use concept development methods? How do the products of concept development contribute to building the knowledge base of nursing? Even the question "what is a concept?" begs for an answer. Researchers cannot take it on faith that these procedures will work, but must understand how they work and how the results of inquiry can contribute to nursing knowledge if concept development methods are to be used effectively.

An incredible volume of literature is available on the subject of concepts. Although these writings are spread throughout several disciplines, there is a clear consensus that there is an important relationship between concepts and knowledge. There also are overwhelming debates regarding the nature of concepts, their role(s) in the development of knowledge, and a variety of implications for concept analysis and development. The notion of "concepts" had been the focus of much discussion and, perhaps, even abuse. It is easy to agree with Toulmin's (1972) poignant observation that "the term 'concept' is in danger becoming [sic] an irredeemably vague catch-all . . . it already carries as much intellectual load as it can safely bear and possibly more" (pp. 8-9). To proceed with our purpose here, then, it is necessary to return to the most fundamental question: What is a concept?

Nearly every writer who addresses the subject of knowledge must, at some point, grapple with the question of concepts—what they are, what role(s) they have, and how they relate to the development of knowledge. The mere volume of literature available on the subject makes it unreasonable, if not impossible, to accomplish an exhaustive review of existing thought regarding concepts and concept development. However, it is possible to gain insight into predominant issues associated with concept development by exploring the major philosophical schools of thought and the writings of the prominent individuals who represent these diverse viewpoints. Prior to beginning such a review, it is important to note that discussions relevant to concept development in nursing are not limited to the writings of philosophers and nurse scholars. The field of psychology, particularly, has offered a great many insights on the subject. A large volume of work in this discipline has been directed toward discussions of how an individual acquires or forms certain concepts and uses these concepts in the processes of learning and communicating. Recent advances in computer science, especially in regard to "artificial intelligence," have stimulated additional discussions of concept formation as well, and perhaps have even added to the confusion by approaching "concept formation" as a form of "machine learning" (Hadzikadic et al., 1996; Lebowitz, 1987). Examples from this body of literature are included in this chapter where appropriate to provide additional clarification and empirical evidence associated with major philosophical viewpoints. Such work is important in an attempt to understand the nature of concepts in general, although it is relevant to note that the views presented in other disciplines such as psychology are quite similar to, and are derived from, the major trends found in philosophy.

NURSING VIEWS OF CONCEPTS

A phrase familiar to anyone who has explored concepts, theories, and existing frameworks in nursing is that concepts are the "building blocks of theory." When the focus becomes more specific, however, the views of *concepts* presented by nurse authors reflect the diversity of approaches to this topic.

Concepts and Empirical Reality

Some authors have focused primarily on the relationship between concepts and empirical or observable reality, arguing that concepts essentially are symbols for objective elements in the world (Kim, 1983; Walker & Avant, 1988, 1995). Jacox (1974), for example, indicated that "words that describe objects, properties, events, and relations among these are called descriptive terms or concepts," and pointed out that "a major task in the definition of concepts is to specify the part of the empirical world that they are intended to represent" (p. 5). Hardy (1974) defined *concepts* in a similar way, stating they are "labels, categories, or selected properties of objects to be studied . . . concepts are the dimensions, aspects, or attributes of reality which interest the scientist" (p. 100). Becker (1983) also emphasized observation, and indicated that "concepts arise in the mind of an individual as a result of attempts to make order out of that which is observed" (p. 53). Also characteristic of such views of concepts was the definition provided by Keck (1986), in which concepts were referred to as "the subject matter of theory. They are symbolic representations of the things or events of which phenomena are composed. Concepts represent some aspect of reality that can be quantified" (p. 16). These views all have in common an emphasis on the external or observed world in reference to the formation and nature of concepts.

Concepts and Cognition

Other nurse authors have discussed concepts with an emphasis on the mind and human thought (King, 1988), a view exemplified by Watson's (1979) definition of *concept* as "a mental picture or a mental image, a word that symbolizes ideas and meanings and expresses an abstraction" (pp. 61-62). Meleis (1985) also focused on cognition in her discussion of concepts:

> Concepts evolve out of a complex constellation of impressions, perceptions, and experiences . . . concepts are a mental image of reality tinted with the theorist's perception, experience, and philosophical bent. They function as a reservoir and an organizational entity and bring order to observations and perceptions. They help to flag related ideas and perceptions without going into detailed descriptions. (p. 127)

Unlike other cognitively oriented definitions, in this definition Meleis gave particular emphasis to the role of individual perception in the formation of concepts. She continued this emphasis in her later work (Meleis, 1997) when she pointed out that "evolving concepts result from early experiences; their definitions and meanings reflect the theorists' educational background and the theoretical bases for their work" (p. 203). However, she often described a concept as a language entity, such as "a term or label" (Meleis, 1991, p. 12; see also Meleis, 1997). This association raises questions about the relationship between concepts and words, an association on which several other nurse authors focused their discussions of concepts.

Concepts and Language

A few nurse authors have addressed concepts specifically in reference to language by relating a concept to a particular word. Diers (1979), for example, described a concept as "simply a word to which meaning has been attached through formal definition or common usage . . ." (p. 69). Similarly, Tadd and Chadwick (1989) defined a concept as "the meaning of a word" (p. 156). Occasionally, "concept" is defined in regard to a general social aspect. Duldt and Giffin (1985), for example, noted that a concept is a "timeless, abstract, impersonal idea that serves as a norm" (p. 95), and thus pointed out, along with Diers, the possibility that concepts are shared or learned. Since language is social in nature, these authors indicated that personal interaction may be a significant factor in the formation or development of concepts, a view that was noticeably absent in other discussions of concepts.

It is obvious from all of these examples that there are numerous ways to approach the subject of concepts. The diversity of views expressed by these nurse authors raises questions about concepts in regard to processes of human thought, the relationship between concepts and empirical reality and between concepts and language, and the role of social contexts in concept development. An examination of major writings in philosophy provides insight into the generation and implications of such views for knowledge development in nursing. Investigators need to understand this foundation to ensure productive and meaningful contributions to the developing knowledge base.

PHILOSOPHICAL VIEWS OF CONCEPTS

The diversity of definitions of the term *concept* presented by nurse authors parallels the variety of viewpoints found in the literature of philosophy. Long-standing debates, focused on the nature and form(s) of concepts and the role of concepts in the development of knowledge, have resulted in the emergence of two principal philosophical schools of thought. These views are commonly referred to as the *entity* and *dispositional* theories of concepts. Entity theories of concepts are characterized by their primary emphasis on concepts as specific *things* or "entities." Typically, concepts are discussed as universal essences (Aristotle, 1947, 1984), abstract ideas in the mind (Descartes, 1644/1960; Kant, 1781/1965; Locke, 1690/1975), or words and their meanings (Frege, 1952a, 1952b; Wittgenstein, 1921/1981). These entities generally are considered to correspond with, or to match directly, actual elements of reality. For example, according to an entity view, the concept of health corresponds with some real and objective "thing," an abstract or concrete object, commonly referred to using the term *health*. Entity theories dominate much of the early literature in philosophy in some form; they still can be found in current writings as some of the examples from nursing indicate.

Dispositional theories, in contrast, present concepts as habits or *capacities* for certain behaviors. These behaviors include the ability to use language effectively as well as the performance of specific mental or physical acts relevant to the concept. For example, according to a dispositional viewpoint, a nurse could perform a technique "aseptically" only when the individual nurse has a grasp of the concept of asepsis. Similarly, acting in a "professional" manner is dependent upon the individual nurse's concept of professional. Consequently, whereas entity theories focus specifically on the concept itself as a "thing," dispositional theories emphasize the use of concepts and the behaviors that they make possible. Examples of dispositional theories are rarely found in a pure form in philosophy. However, British philosopher Ryle (1949, 1971a, 1971b, 1971c) and the later writings of Wittgenstein (1953/1968) made significant contributions to the overall development of such views and will be discussed later.

Although entity and dispositional theories of concepts are considerably different, there is no formal line of division between the two schools of thought. Philosophers, as well as nurses and others who write on the subject, cannot easily be categorized as clear advocates of one approach or the other. Often, there is considerable overlap, and characterization of a particular viewpoint can be based only on the author's primary emphasis. It is important to note as well that, if the development of views of concepts in philosophy is examined over time, there initially appears to be a smooth chronological progression. Certainly, philosophical thinking does exhibit some trends, but the transitions that have occurred throughout history do not necessarily demonstrate fluid shifts in thought. Exploration of the variety of viewpoints concerning what a concept is demonstrates the complex history of the subject and the influences that philosophical foundations have on current applications of concept development in nursing.

Concepts and Essentialism

One of the more familiar approaches to concept development is the method of concept analysis that is employed to "define" existing concepts (Chinn & Jacobs, 1987; Rodgers, 1989a; Walker & Avant, 1988; Wilson, 1963). The roots for this approach are traced easily to the writings of Aristotle in the fourth century BC and the subsequent development of what is commonly known as the classical approach to analysis. Aristotle (1947) pointed out that the purpose of scientific inquiry was to identify or demonstrate the "essence" of things; in other words, the attributes fundamental to their individual natures and that set each thing apart from all others. According to Aristotle (1947, 1984), the essences determined through analysis were "true universals"; they were thought to exist on a level removed from actual concrete objects and, consequently, to be unaffected by change and motion in the world.

In an approach typical of an entity theory, Aristotle described these concepts or essences as the special "objects" associated with thinking, and argued that they were formed in the mind through a process referred to as "successive generalization." In successive generalization, the mind moves from individual or particular objects or events to progressively broader categories of similar objects or events, focusing on the characteristics common to all objects in the categories. As Aristotle described it, this process eventually led to the identification of essences or attributes that applied universally to entire classes of objects. Based on these essences, the mind could effectively categorize various aspects of reality. Concepts, then, represent the essence of certain classes and are universally true of all members of a class.

This idea becomes clearer when it is viewed in reference to Aristotle's extensive background in biological studies and his interest in the development of taxonomies to definitively categorize various classes of biological species based on the essential features of each class. One class, for example, might be the category representing the concept of animal. When the essence of the concept of animal is clear, it is possible to accurately categorize an object as *animal*. A higher level, more inclusive category might concern all things that are organic, including *animal* and other organic things such as objects in the subordinate class of *plant*.

We can use as an example the concept of professional to see how this process might proceed with a concept of interest in nursing. To define the concept of professional, the nurse investigator first would observe and examine situations in which people are presumed to be, or are acting as, professionals. By examining these instances, the investigator could uncover the characteristics that are common to all the people or situations observed. The investigator might then continue the inquiry with other sets of "professionals," observing their situations and actions as well. As this process proceeds, continuing analysis of the data collected would reveal the characteristics of the concept of professional. The investigator would uncover the characteristics, or attributes, that make it possible to identify a *professional*—the defining characteristics of the concept that constitute the "essence" of *professional*.

This view is consistent with many subsequent developments in understanding concepts and methods of concept development, particularly concept analysis as it is usually presented in nursing. First, Aristotle established the process of definition as a fundamental scientific activity, and thus legitimized efforts to analyze and define concepts. In addition, he provided a foundation for methods of analysis by demonstrating that concepts are abstractions, comprised of the essential and unchanging features of elements or objects in the world. Ideas related to this view of essentialism emerged with new strength in the early twentieth century. However, the emphasis on concepts as special entities themselves, the objects of thought, gained a considerable following long before that time.

Concepts as Ideas

Rene Descartes

Entity theories began to flourish in Western philosophy in the mid-seventeenth century. Much of the stimulus for the further development of entity theories during that time can be attributed to Descartes (1644/1960). Particularly significant was Descartes' argument that the mind (soul) and body (physical reality) are distinctly different substances (the infamous Cartesian "dualism"). Descartes did not argue that the mind and body are totally separate; in fact, Descartes was careful to point out that they were intricately connected (although this connection was based in the pineal gland, according to Descartes). Instead, the dualism arose from his position that the mind and the body each had specific features that made them considerably unique. According to Descartes, "bodies" were "extended"; in other words, they occupied space in physical reality. The mind, in contrast, was an "unextended thinking substance" and formed the essence of human nature. According to Descartes, the central feature of the mind was the distinct group of entities referred to as "ideas," which served as the focus of all cognitive processes. Knowledge consisted of ideas so "clear and distinct" that they were beyond any possibility of doubt.

Descartes subsequently established his Rationalist method of inquiry, based on the notion of doubt and a process of reason, as a means to develop knowledge, particularly to distinguish knowledge from belief and opinion. Although this method had little direct bearing on concept development techniques as they are currently utilized, Descartes' emphasis on "clear and distinct" may have provided some incentive for later philosophers who also emphasized rigid clarity in regard to individual concepts. Most significant, however, was his dualism of the mind and body, which led later philosophers to focus their own arguments concerning concepts on one of the two identified aspects of human existence—on either the inner, mental realm (the world of ideas) or the outer, physical world.

John Locke

Locke (1690/1975) focused on "inner" reality (ideas and the mind) in his discussion of concepts in *An Essay Concerning Human Understanding*. Locke defined an "idea" as "the object of understanding when a man (sic) thinks . . . whatever it is, which the mind can be employed about in thinking" (p. 47). In contrast to Descartes' position that ideas could be innate, acquired prior to any experience, Locke argued that ideas were derived exclusively from experience. Experience, for Locke, consisted of observation either of the external world (which he called "sensation") or of the internal operations of the mind (referred to as "reflection").

According to Locke, experience involves a passive mind presented with "simple ideas." A "simple idea" represents "nothing but one *uniform appearance*" (p. 119), one particular or individual aspect of reality. The mind then creates generalizations from these simple ideas. Through a process referred to as *abstraction*, "ideas taken from particular beings become general representatives of all of the same kind" (p. 159). In other words, Locke argued that the mind discerned among ideas and categorized similar things. This process ultimately resulted in the formation of "complex ideas." These categories of complex ideas were developed through abstraction based on the particulars (the individual objects) encountered in reality. As a result, they had a relatively universal character and formed the basis for human knowledge. Actual knowledge, according to Locke, was "nothing but the perception of the connexion and agreement or disagreement and repugnancy of any of our ideas" (p. 525), a process that ultimately included the comparison and sorting of ideas to establish a consistent and coherent body of knowledge.

The active role taken by the mind in the formation of complex ideas led to the possibility that concepts could vary from one mind to the next, or become unclear or confused. Locke related such occurrences, however, to problems in individual thought processes (pp. 161-163), indicating that obscure or confused ideas resulted from either dull sensory organs or the inappropriate combination of simple ideas to form the more complex ones (concepts). Similarly, Locke argued that in some instances there may be a confused connection of a name or word symbol with an idea. This language problem led to difficulties in attempts to communicate or share concepts. Locke generally emphasized, however, that the ideas and the associated cognitive processes were at fault when problems existed with ambiguous or unclear concepts.

Locke and Descartes both present concepts as "ideas" in some form that serve as the objects of human thought. According to these philosophers, concepts are inherently private entities in that they reside exclusively in the individual mind. Locke did address the possibility that concepts could be communicated with other persons, but this could be accomplished only through a complex system of signs or symbols. Analysis, clarification, and development of concepts, as mental entities, could be accomplished only by gaining direct access to an individual's mind. Consequently, in these views, concepts were not amenable to any techniques currently employed for purposes of concept development. The only improvement or clarification of concepts that could be accomplished had to be focused on individual processes of thought and idea formation.

Locke's argument that all ideas were derived from experience presented another complication for concept development. This position suggested that a direct relationship exists between an idea and a sensory or reflective experience. Therefore, an understanding of a concept would require not only insight into actual thought processes (since concepts are "ideas") but examination of correspondence between the concept and the experience that produced it.

Immanuel Kant

Kant (1781/1965) also focused on concepts as ideas but, unlike Locke, did not view them as the result of experience. Instead, Kant argued that concepts existed in the mind even prior to any experience and, in fact, actually made experience possible. Knowledge, according to Kant, resulted in part from the combination of experience with the pre-existing content and capabilities (concepts) in the human mind. Concepts provided the *rules* necessary for this essential process of combination to occur.

In contrast to the views of many earlier philosophers, Kant denied that concepts had any direct relationship with objective reality. He also rejected the position that the definition of a concept revealed the essence of any associated object. In spite of these differences, Kant did discuss the possibility of defining concepts as a means to provide clarification, although he identified limitations as to the types of concepts that could be defined. A priori concepts, those that existed in the mind prior to experience, could not be defined since, according to Kant, gaining a complete definition of such a concept simply could not be accomplished; definition on this level "really only means to present the complete, original concept of a thing" (p. 586). Empirical concepts, similarly, "could not be defined at all but only made explicit" (p. 586). Only concepts that had been "arbitrarily invented" were amenable to any attempt at definition or clarification.

Conclusion

These prominent philosophers—Descartes, Locke, and Kant—made a tremendous contribution to current discussions of concepts. They postulated various ways in which concepts were acquired, the possibility that vague or ambiguous concepts impeded the development of knowledge, and the variety of types or levels of concepts that existed. Most significant for concept development purposes, however, was that they drew considerable attention to the importance of concepts in discussions about knowledge in general, even though there was tremendous diversity in their individual approaches to concepts and related epistemological questions. It is clear in the writings of these three philosophers that concepts are very important in developing knowledge.

In spite of the differences in their views, all three philosophers relied heavily on the notion of *ideas* and an emphasis on the inner workings of the human mind. This focus presented problems in regard to means by which concepts could be clarified or further developed. As noted previously, the emphasis on concepts as exclusively mental entities placed concepts in a realm where they were not accessible as a focus for inquiry. Locke did argue that concepts might be symbolized through words for purposes of communication, possibly providing some means for analysis or development. However, this position served only to raise questions about the connection among concepts, specific words, and other acts used to express individual thoughts. Some philosophers, most notably Frege (1952a, 1952b), reacted very negatively to such discussions of concepts and referred to them as "psychologism" in reference to the belief that the meaning of words was attributed only to specific mental processes. These concerns prompted a subsequent shift in the focus of discussions of concepts from the inner workings of the mind to an emphasis on external reality. This development undoubtedly was fueled even further by the advances that had been demonstrated in the natural sciences and the acceptance of positivism in discussions of scientific knowledge early in the twentieth century (Ayer, 1959; Silva & Rothbart, 1983; Webster et al., 1981), which placed an emphasis exclusively on empirical reality for the development of knowledge.

Concepts and Logic

Frege (1952a, 1952b) offered what can be considered a "realist" revolt against the mental or psychological focus of earlier discussions of concepts and knowledge. As with many of his predecessors, Frege (1952b) acknowledged the importance of concepts in the development of knowledge. He also recognized the existence of a great deal of confusion regarding the term, noting that "the word 'concept' is used in various ways; its sense is sometimes psychological, sometimes logical, and sometimes perhaps a confused mixture of both" (p. 42). In his own writings, Frege adopted principles of logic as they applied to language, and focused specifically on the distinction between concepts and objects as these elements were related to specific parts of language.

Earlier writers seemed to have confused the connection between concepts and objects. Previous philosophers had argued that concepts arose directly from experience with specific objects (Locke, 1690/1975) or that they made experience possible (Kant, 1781/1965). Although both positions treat concepts as "mental entities," things that exist solely in the mind, there is a difference in these views regarding whether they resulted from experience (Locke) or existed prior to experience (Descartes, Kant), and were necessary for a person even to have experience (Kant). Both views imply some relationship between concepts and objects and create significant problems in efforts to distinguish a concept from its corresponding object. This confused relationship between concepts and objects appears in the nursing literature as well when authors such as Jacox (1974) describe concepts as "words that describe objects . . ." (p. 5), or Keck (1986) indicates that "concepts represent some aspect of reality that can be quantified" (p. 16).

One solution to the problems raised by the connection between concepts and objects was proposed by the German philosopher Gottlob Frege. Frege attempted to resolve the confusion about concepts and objects by looking at the terms or denotative expressions that corresponded with concepts. He identified two primary categories of words: proper names and predicates. In this argument, proper names were said to represent specific objects and included terms such as *blue* and *two*, to use Frege's examples. Concepts, in contrast, were viewed as predicates; "[a concept] is, in fact, the reference of a grammatical predicate" according to Frege (1952b, p. 43). Concepts, therefore, represent the "existence of a property" (p. 48). As such, concepts are entities that may be true, or correctly applied, for some objects and false for others.

At first glance, the term "two" seems an unlikely example of a proper name to designate an object. However, a close examination of Frege's view of language helps to clarify his point. According to Frege, a concept, expressed by a grammatical predicate, constitutes an incomplete statement in the structure of language—for example, "is a prime number." This becomes a complete statement with the addition of a proper name, as in the resulting statement, "two is a prime number." In this example, the characteristic or concept ("prime number") is applied to the object named "two." The application of a concept to an object may be true or false; two *is*, or *is not*, a prime number.

For a concept to be predicated of an object appropriately, in other words, to present a characteristic of the object accurately, Frege (1952a) argued that the concept had to be absolutely clear. As he pointed out:

> A definition of a concept (of a possible predicate) must be complete; it must unambiguously determine, as regards any object, whether or not it falls under the concept . . . the concept must have a sharp boundary . . . a concept that is not sharply defined is wrongly termed a concept. (p. 159)

Without an exceptionally clear concept of prime number it would be impossible to determine whether or not the concept was appropriately predicated of the object known as "two." Similarly, according to this view, a person can be characterized accurately as "healthy" only if there is an absolutely clear definition of the concept of *healthy*.

Frege's emphasis on language and characterization of concepts as grammatical predicates made a unique contribution to discussions of concepts. One positive outcome of this view is that it avoids problems with concepts existing solely in the mind. Instead, the association of concepts with language indicates how concepts might be accessible for inquiry and development of effective concepts.

Frege's idea of what constitutes an adequate definition of a concept has had a lasting influence on discussions of concepts as well. According to Frege, the definition of a concept must be expressed as a set of necessary and sufficient conditions—the critical conditions or attributes necessary to define the concept and which, by themselves, were sufficient to distinguish it clearly from all other concepts. Frege's position regarding the boundaries and clarity of concepts indicated that concepts have an essence that is unchanging over time and across contexts. The requirement that the boundaries of each concept be clearly delineated emphasized that concepts are static in nature and the belief that any single concept could be viewed in isolation, not only apart from its context, but without regard to its relationship with other concepts. The ultimate goal for Frege was to ensure that concepts were so clearly delineated that the concepts could, indeed, be determined true or false in reference to any situation or object that was confronted.

The Search for an Ideal Language

The impact of Frege's realist approach to concepts was evident throughout the early twentieth century. The emphasis on language, a particularly significant aspect of Frege's works, provided a considerable basis for the writings of Wittgenstein, another prominent German philosopher. Wittgenstein's works can be divided into two periods, with radically different views expressed during each stage in the development of his thought. During his early period, Wittgenstein (1921/1981) produced his famous text, the *Tractatus Logico-philosophicus*. In discussing the importance of this work, Hartnack (1965) indicated that "The *Tractatus* is a book of just over eighty pages, but it has exercised a greater influence on twentieth-century philosophy than almost any other single work" (p. 45). This work provided a particularly great stimulus for members of the Vienna Circle, a group generally synonymous with the Logical Positivism movement in philosophy and which has influenced much of extant ideas about science and knowledge in general (Ayer, 1959; Carnap, 1956; Russell, 1914; Schlick, 1959; Webster et al., 1981).

The influence of Frege was evident in the *Tractatus* and in the notebooks Wittgenstein (1979) maintained, which showed the painstaking development of his ideas. However, Wittgenstein differed from Frege somewhat in his views of language and concepts. Frege regarded language as a system of symbols that clearly represented concepts; Wittgenstein, in contrast, discussed language in general as a system that directly corresponded to physical reality. According to Wittgenstein (1921/1981), words symbolized actual objects, not mental images or thoughts. The challenge, for Wittgenstein, was to develop and clarify language so that it could be used effectively to represent physical reality.

Wittgenstein agreed that there was a close relationship between concepts and language, but devoted very little attention to a specific discussion of concepts. Instead, he considered language itself to be the primary concern, and focused on language as a "picture" of reality, complete with rules for determining correspondence between language and reality (Wittgenstein, 1921/1981). In fact, Wittgenstein and the members of the Vienna Circle devoted considerable attention to the challenge of constructing an "ideal language" that would mirror precisely the structure of the external world. Such a language presumably would eliminate all ambiguity and enable the construction of statements that provided a picture of how reality really is. It was an ambitious goal, to say the least, and, by virtue of the many problems raised by such a language, not a very realistic or even appropriate focus.

Contributions and Problems with Entity Theories

All of the views previously addressed are representative of the entity theory of concepts, which has dominated much of philosophical thought on the subject of concepts. The contributions of philosophers associated with this general approach to concepts cannot be underestimated. There is little disagreement, for example, that concepts are mental or cognitive in nature. In addition, entity views provide an impetus and rationale for the clarification of concepts, establishing such work as a legitimate form of inquiry and providing numerous insights into methodologies for concept clarification and development.

However, as with any philosophical position, there are numerous problems associated with such views. One particularly glaring difficulty is related to Descartes' dualism, which contributed to philosophers emphasizing either internal thought processes or external reality in their discussions of concepts. Toulmin (1972) poignantly noted that this background contributed to "intractable conundrums about the relations between the 'inner' and 'outer,' or private and public, aspects of mental life" (p. 197). Language provided one means to establish a connection between the public and private realms of existence; through language, inner thoughts could be exposed to public scrutiny. However, the particular way in which philosophers such as Locke, Frege, and Wittgenstein discussed language only served to generate confusion about the precise connection between concepts and words. In fact, according to such views (especially those of Frege and Wittgenstein), the development of a concept was easily viewed as the clarification of a specific word, its reference, and the further development of language in general. Individual thoughts or "ideas" had little role in this process of knowledge development.

The emphasis on correspondence, whether between words and concepts, words and objects, or concepts and objects (or experience) is undoubtedly one of the most troublesome aspects of entity views and one of the "intractable conundrums." The term *health*, as just one example, is easily used to point out some of the difficulties with these views. The word *health* conjures considerably different images or concepts for different people. The specific idea or image (the concept) of *health* that a person possesses is based on that person's culture, socioeconomic status, and personal experience, along with a variety of other factors that contribute to formation of the concept. Health may be conceptualized as the absence of disease (another troublesome concept), in reference to individual functioning and independence, or in any number of diverse ways. It is clear that the concept typically expressed using the term *health* is not the same for all people.

None of the possible conceptualizations of health necessarily corresponds with any real object; there is no "fact" or "thing" called *health*, and it is difficult, perhaps even inappropriate, to say that someone's specific concept of health is false or in error. On a highly abstract level, there may be some object to which health (or hope, pain, or grief, as a few other examples) corresponds. There also may be certain empirical correlates that can be evaluated using accepted measurement tools, that help to determine the presence or absence of health. However, conceptualization of human experiences, such as health, cannot be accomplished definitively on the basis of measurement devices alone because these devices are not infallible. Consequently, the requirement that a concept correspond with some object on any level, and the attempt to determine the truth or falsity of a concept, are both philosophically troublesome and inconsistent with everyday existence.

In support of this criticism are studies conducted in the field of psychology that have shown a severe discrepancy between the positions advocated by entity views and actual human processes of conceptualization (Armstrong et al., 1983; Fehr, 1988; McCloskey & Glucksberg, 1978; Medin & Schaffer, 1978). First, studies have shown that, for many concepts, even experts in a field may be unable to specify the conditions that are essential (in other words, necessary and sufficient) to constitute a particular concept (Medin, 1989). Second, the "classical theory" of thinking, as such entity views often are called, implies that no one example of a concept is any better than another; all examples must possess the same core of essential attributes. Undoubtedly, however, it is possible to assemble a diverse group of people, all of whom might possess whatever are considered to be the essential attributes of health; yet some of these individuals certainly would be judged as more typical of the concept than others. The judgments of the "best" examples of the concept of health most likely vary with the personal characteristics of the judge. It is possible to argue that some of the judges would be false in their conceptualizations based on a strict interpretation of the notion of necessary and sufficient conditions. However, this view would require that individual perceptions be ignored. Equally significant, it would be incompatible with actual human practices and how people use the concepts they possess.

Finally, the classical view suggests that it is possible to determine definitively whether or not a particular instance does, indeed, exemplify a specific concept. However, there are numerous examples of situations that are vague in regard to conceptual category membership, such as the determination of whether or not addictive disorders are "diseases," a development that has challenged adherents to the popular "germ" interpretation of the concept of *disease*. Such challenges are not answered by an appeal to the necessary and sufficient conditions of the concept of disease, for these have changed over time and across cultural and even disciplinary contexts.

Entity views, therefore, have presented some philosophical difficulties in discussions of concepts, particularly in regard to the connection among concepts, language, and objects, and reliance on correspondence as the test for the "truth" of a concept. The requirement, imposed by Frege (1952a), that concepts have sharply defined boundaries and the lack of attention to context in discussions of concepts, raised additional questions. It is debatable whether or not reality can be so easily partitioned as to make an expectation of infallible distinctions and strict correspondence reasonable (Fehr, 1988). Similarly, the idea that concepts may change over time or across contexts raises concerns about how determinate and clearly delineated concepts can be, as more recent views demonstrate (Rodgers, 1989a, 1989b; Rorty, 1979; Toulmin, 1972; Wittgenstein, 1953/1968). The notion of conceptual change presents a strong case against the call for clear and rigid boundaries that cannot vary over time or across contexts.

Dispositional Theories of Concepts

Dispositional theories emerged partially in response to these problems with entity views. Interestingly, although it was the interpretation of Wittgenstein's early works (1921/1981, 1979) by Logical Positivists that provided much of the foundation for the views of concepts that dominated contemporary discussions noted previously, it also was Wittgenstein who later provided major criticisms of this approach and contributed to the transition toward dispositional views of concepts. In *Philosophical Investigations* (1953/1968), Wittgenstein denounced the "grave mistakes" (p. vi) contained in his earlier work and drew attention to the *use* of words, rather than the objects to which they refer, as the primary consideration in determining meaning. The rationale for an emphasis on use is presented clearly by Hallett (1967) in his discussion of Wittgenstein's writings:

> They, objects and shadows [facts that are absent but can still be held in thought], are unnecessary for speech. Use is obviously necessary. A word

must be used in a certain way if it is to have meaning, if it is to count as
speech rather than mere sounds.
They are sometimes missing; use never is.
Mental pictures are themselves signs; use is not.
Mental events are private; use is not . . . whatever the reason for
dissatisfaction with object or idea, use always gave satisfaction. (p. 76)

Consequently, Wittgenstein introduced the idea of language as a "game"
to emphasize the aspect of "use" and to replace the earlier "picture"
theory, which relied on correspondence for the determination of meaning.

Wittgenstein's (1953/1968) discussion of "language games" called
attention to the interactive nature of language, where "one party calls
out the words, the other acts on them" (1953/1968, p. 5). A language
game, therefore, is comprised of language and the actions associated
with its use. Unlike the picture theory, which advocated strict correspondence between words and objects, language games act as "objects
of comparison"; clarity is provided through identification of similar and
dissimilar features of various language acts. A language game serves as
a "measuring-rod; not as a preconceived idea to which reality *must*
correspond" (pp. 50–51). It provides a standard or a guide, not an
absolute determinant of truth or falsehood.

Wittgenstein (1953/1968) described his new position as based on a
principle of "family resemblances." According to this principle, it is
possible and reasonable to use "health" to describe diverse individuals
provided each person sufficiently *resembled* the concept of health and
displayed characteristics that resembled *health*. Application of the term
would not have to be based on whether each individual possessed a
finite core of essential attributes. This admits that concepts may have
rather blurred boundaries, far from the absolute clarity that Frege required. According to Wittgenstein, it was not reasonable to expect
perfectly clear "pictures" of all concepts. In a direct refutation of Frege's
earlier position that a concept with a blurred edge is not really a
concept, Wittgenstein presented the following questions for consideration:

Is an indistinct photograph a picture of a person at all?
Is it even always an advantage to replace an indistinct picture by a sharp
one? Isn't the indistinct one often exactly what we need? (p. 34)

Wittgenstein thus rejected the requirements that concepts have rigid
and distinct boundaries, that definitions be stated in terms of necessary
and sufficient conditions, and that there be strict correspondence between concepts and empirical reality.

Instead of correspondence, Wittgenstein (1953/1968) offered that
conceptualizations were based upon resemblances or commonalities in
the use of a word or concept. Conceptual clarity is based on the ability

to formulate comparisons, and efforts to clarify concepts were to be directed toward "seeing what is common" (p. 34) in the use of a word, not toward uncovering any "essence." Psychologists often refer to such a position appropriately as the "fuzzy set" theory, where "category membership [the applicability of a concept] is a matter of degree rather than all or none" (McCloskey & Glucksberg, 1978, p. 462).

The emphasis on the *use* of concepts was a prominent feature of Wittgenstein's *Philosophical Investigations* and set this work apart from many of the earlier contributions to discussions of concepts. However, in this text, as in some of his earlier related work (1921/1981, 1979), Wittgenstein was concerned primarily with language. The *Philosophical Investigations* text is devoted to the development of a complex thesis about language, its structure, and its relationship to reality rather than to a direct exposition of concepts. The views presented in this work are not totally exemplary of dispositional approaches in general because they lacked sufficient attention to individual capacities or abilities associated with concepts, the distinguishing feature of dispositional theories. However, the *Philosophical Investigations* was an important work in that it provided a transition in discussions of language and concepts and the foundation for dispositional views that subsequently were developed.

The "Use" of Concepts

The writings of the British philosopher Ryle (1949, 1971a, 1971b, 1971c) are more characteristic of a dispositional theory than those of Wittgenstein. Like Wittgenstein, Ryle (1971b) rejected the idea that reference to an object is the way to determine the meaning of a concept and adopted the idea of "use" as a central focus in his work. According to Ryle, "the use of an expression, or the concept it expresses, is the role it is employed to perform, not any thing or person or event for which it might be supposed to stand" (1971c, p. 364). Ryle charged philosophy with the task of identifying the criteria governing the logical application of an expression or concept, a task that was to be accomplished through analytic techniques (1949, p. 329). In other words, Ryle expected that philosophical analysis could produce the standards or guides needed to enable the appropriate use of a concept.

Ryle also considered concepts to be cognitive in nature, some form of mental entity. Yet, he attempted to overcome the difficulties presented by earlier philosophers who specifically emphasized mental processes in discussions of concepts. Refuting the dogma of the mind-body dualism, Ryle argued that there was, indeed, a strong connection between the two aspects of being. References to and, consequently, examination of mental processes could be made in terms of activities that could be witnessed by others:

. . . when we describe people as exercising qualities of mind, we are not referring to occult episodes of which their overt acts and utterances are effects; we are referring to those overt acts and utterances themselves. (Ryle, 1949, p. 25)

Discussions of cognition (thinking or conceptualizing) did not necessarily require an exploration of the actual processes of thought as they occurred inside the human mind. Rather, cognition could be discussed and even observed through its outward, public manifestations. Language provided a particularly important medium for such observations. For Ryle, a concept was not the same as a mere word; instead, a word or statement served as a means to express individual concepts and, therefore, was a source of observable evidence of the concepts.

Ryle also suggested that fundamental questions that served as the basis for discussions of concepts be reframed as well. Earlier philosophers asked primarily how concepts (or ideas) were acquired; Ryle (1971c) pointed out that the more appropriate question actually was "what were we unable to do until we had acquired it?" (p. 448). Ryle responded by indicating that the acquisition of a concept enables the management of a range of intellectual and conversational tasks that share features common to the concept. In other words, when a person has grasped a concept, the individual is able to think, converse, and categorize phenomena or situations. Without the possession or the grasp of a concept, an individual is unable to accomplish or even become involved in such activities.

In summary, a concept for Ryle is an abstracted feature of the world and is directly related to the ability to perform certain tasks. One of these tasks, and a critical one, is the effective use of language. In his view, concepts are neither objects nor the names of objects; they are not inherently true or false, nor are they the components of creating truths or falsehoods. Instead, they constitute the ability to move effectively through the world. As a result, concept development, the clarification and elaboration of concepts, can be viewed as the creation of improved abilities and new ways to function effectively.

Ryle formulated a number of theories of concepts through his writings. Consequently, to say that Ryle strictly equated a concept with a capacity would render an unusually narrow interpretation of this philosopher's contribution to discussions of concepts. What is most significant for a discussion of concept development is Ryle's idea that the use of a word may be an outward manifestation of an individual's grasp of a concept. By providing this insight, Ryle presented a way in which private, mental processes might be accessed and concepts, as mental abstractions, could be analyzed effectively. Individuals move through the world of everyday existence, and Ryle pointed out the role of concepts in that existence. With the influence of Ryle, concepts took on a more pragmatic role, and it was clear how practical gains could be made through efforts to clarify and develop concepts.

Both Ryle and the later Wittgenstein represented significant departures from previous ideas concerning the nature of concepts. Of particular importance, they offered a stark contrast to earlier views concerning correspondence between concepts and objects and a subsequent emphasis on a public or social aspect of concepts. In psychology the influence of these ideas, particularly Wittgenstein's emphasis on family resemblance, appears in an approach referred to as the "probabilistic" view (Medin, 1989; Smith & Medin, 1981), the "cluster concept" or "prototypical" view, or, as noted previously, the "fuzzy set" theory of concepts (Armstrong et al., 1983; Fodor & Lepore, 1996; McCloskey & Glucksberg, 1978).

These more recent psychological positions represent a substantial improvement over a typical dispositional theory such that the heading *dispositional* is inadequate to capture their uniqueness. Particularly, unlike the positions of Ryle and Wittgenstein, the emphasis in such views goes well beyond the mere use of concepts to their actual nature and how they are developed in the human mind. However, similar to a dispositional theory, the primary feature of all of these views is that the defining characteristics that comprise a concept are not "essential" or "necessary and sufficient." Instead, they are regarded only as demonstrating some degree of association with the concept. In a "probabilistic" view, there is additional concern for the probability with which a characteristic or attribute is associated with a concept. Such views allow for what is called the "typicality" effect, whereby some instances will be judged more typical of the concept than others, even though less typical instances still can be characterized using the same concept.

The concept of grief offers a practical example of the probabilistic view. Based on the idea of *family resemblances*, it is possible to describe an individual who has recently experienced the death of a loved one as demonstrating grief and as "typical" of grief. Yet, the concept of grief still may be used in reference to individuals who have experienced other types of loss, such as displacement from a job or home. In these latter instances, there is a sufficient *resemblance* or a reasonable probability concerning the defining characteristics of grief and the individual situations, even though they may be viewed as less typical of grief than the response to a death.

Peacocke (1992) has adopted dispositional principles to some extent in his elaborate theory of concepts. Throughout his discussion he adheres to what he calls the "principle of dependence" (p. 5), derived to some extent from Dummett's (1975) work. This principle indicates:

> There can be nothing more to the nature of a concept than is determined by a correct account of the capacity of a thinker who has mastered the concept . . . (a correct account of "grasping the concept"). (p. 5)

Peacocke blends this focus on capacity, however, with a somewhat essentialist view that also allows for identification of clear distinctions among concepts. This blending "opens up the possibility that we can simultaneously say in a single account what individuates a particular concept and also what it is to possess that concept" (p. 6).

In spite of the contributions of dispositional views, several other important concerns about concepts have continued to trouble philosophers and other interested scholars. Some problems have centered around the idea of *use*; Ryle (1971d) devoted an entire paper to a discussion of "use," yet failed to provide any clear explanation of what "use" really is. In addition, although dispositional approaches helped to dissolve the Cartesian dualism that has plagued discussions of concepts for some time by showing a relationship between private concepts and public activities such as language, the relationship between concepts and *knowledge* seemed to be of little interest to such authors. Along this line, it is worth pointing out that neither Ryle nor Wittgenstein was a methodologist. Consequently, their writings have not provided sufficient direction for procedures that might be employed for the clarification or development of concepts. As a result, there have been lingering concerns about how their philosophical positions might be translated into methods to enhance the growth of knowledge.

Other concerns about concepts in general warranted attention as well, yet were inadequately addressed by these more recent philosophers. For example, the argument that concepts are at least somewhat public or social in nature raised questions about the role of social and other contextual factors in the use or development of concepts. As Wittgenstein (1953/1968) pointed out, universal categories and concepts intelligible within all cultures can be found only to the extent that there are universal patterns of life and behavior. Because life patterns and behaviors do vary across contexts in many respects, so the associated concepts are likely to vary as well. This observation has significant implications for methodology in regard to the clarification or development of concepts in nursing. Relevant contexts may include cultural and ethnic backgrounds, other social groups, and even factors specific to different disciplines.

Time is another element of context that can have an effect on concepts. The problem of time can be viewed as a problem of *conceptual change* or variation. The predominant thought concerning concepts throughout much of history has focused on concepts as *universals*, unaffected by change and other forces in the world. This view, which lasted at least through the time of Frege, implored philosophers to "concern themselves with 'concepts' only as timeless, intellectual ideals, towards which the human mind struggles, at best, painfully and little by little" (Toulmin, 1972, p. 56). Such an absolutist tradition disregarded the possibility of historical and social influences having an effect on concepts and the existence of conceptual variation over time.

There can be little doubt, however, that concepts do change. In nursing, a vivid example concerns the concept of disease, which has varied widely over time and across a number of distinct cultural and disciplinary contexts. These dilemmas concerning conceptual variation were addressed rather extensively by Toulmin (1972). Examination of his views provides additional insights in an attempt to understand the diversity of approaches to the discussion of concepts.

The Evolution of Concepts

Toulmin (1972) failed to define the term *concept*, but his discussion still added a new dimension to an understanding of this topic. Particularly significant about Toulmin's contribution was his emphasis on the process of conceptual change and the relationship between concepts and scientific progress and development. Following the line of thought that concepts are social in nature, Toulmin based his argument on this critical assumption:

> We acquire our grasp of language and conceptual thought . . . in the course of education and development; and the particular sets of concepts we pick up reflect forms of life and thought, understanding and expression current in our society. (p. 38)

Toulmin thus considered concepts to be developed through social interaction and a process referred to as "enculturation," which may be accomplished through simple interaction, imitation, or formal education.

Toulmin's work is distinct particularly for this emphasis on the social aspect of concepts. In fact, Toulmin discussed concepts explicitly as the collective possession of a community of concept users, emphasizing the importance of context and socialization in his discussions. Focused specifically on scientific disciplines as the community and context of interest, he also provided an interesting description of the relationship between concepts and the advancement of knowledge in various fields of study.

According to Toulmin, intellectual disciplines are characterized by specific sets of "explanatory ideals"; the "professionals," the human individuals associated with a particular discipline or knowledge base, are driven by certain phenomena that the group desires to explain. Problems result when existing capabilities fall short of reaching these ideals (p. 152). Conceptual problems often accounted for the gap between current understanding and intellectual goals. The development or clarification of concepts, therefore, was viewed as an important component of overall scientific progress.

According to Toulmin, concepts possess "explanatory power" demonstrated by their utility in characterizing phenomena or situations of interest in the discipline. Through a process that entails continuing application of the concept and critical analysis of its contribution to problem solving, the concepts of the science can be altered, refined, or changed altogether, yielding a concept with continually improved content and "explanatory power." Toulmin argued that in any "rational enterprise" concepts survive "because they are still serving their original intellectual functions, or else because they have since acquired other, different functions . . ." (p. 130). Concepts, therefore, are continually changed or refined, or new concepts are introduced to enhance the problem solving abilities of the discipline. Consequently, the process of concept development occupies a critical role in solving the problems relevant to a science.

By pointing out the social nature of concepts and the factors and processes associated with concept development and change, Toulmin provided several new possibilities for the conduct of inquiry. First, his arguments about the social nature and disciplinary context of concepts demonstrated the need for researchers to consider these aspects in inquiry oriented toward concept development. The likelihood of conceptual change raises similar concerns and challenges earlier assumptions that a concept may be defined in only one way. Similarly, the notion of essences and rigid and unwavering boundaries for concepts must be reevaluated in light of Toulmin's position and actual examples that demonstrate the existence of conceptual variation and change (Rodgers, 1989a, 1989b).

Toulmin did not specifically address the implications of his views for methods of concept development. However, it is clear in his work that concept development can be of vital importance in the growth of knowledge in a discipline. He pointed out the role of concepts in ensuring continuity and, hence, the identity of a discipline over time and in solving relevant problems within the discipline. The development of concepts, therefore, can be seen as a significant research and intellectual activity in the scientific enterprise of nursing. In addition, because concepts have a particular function in a discipline and are viewed as changing and developing over time, it is reasonable and, in fact, desirable, to work toward concepts that are increasingly clear, useful, and effective in problem solving. Rodgers (1989) elaborated on and adapted, in part, Toulmin's views to develop an interpretation of concept analysis that shows the implications of conceptual change and the context-dependent nature of concepts for nursing inquiry (see Chapter 6).

Toulmin's point that concepts exist in the context of scientific disciplines is expanded somewhat in the views of cognitive psychologists who argue that different perspectives can influence the formation of concepts. As Medin (1989) pointed out, "something is needed to give concepts life, coherence, and meaning" (p. 1474). This ingredient may be the context or "theory" in which specific exemplars are viewed. In other words, perspectives provided by theories or other contextual bases affect what features are viewed as similar in order to determine the relationship (or resemblance) between certain situations and specific concepts (Medin & Schaffer, 1978; Spalding & Murphy, 1996; Wisniewski & Medin, 1994). Concepts, therefore, may be not only context-dependent in regard to specific scientific disciplines, as Toulmin (1972) argued, but may show even greater variation through the influence of diverse theories.

Psychologists conducting research in regard to concepts provide other clues as to how they are formed or learned. For psychologists, discussion of "concept development" typically concerns how an individual person develops a particular concept. This focus is quite different from a methodological or philosophical interest in the development of concepts to enhance the knowledge base of a discipline such as nursing. Still, philosophical views can gain a great deal from work done in psychology and a coherent philosophical position on concepts should account for the evidence provided through research.

Research provides overwhelming evidence that concepts are not absolute and that individual development of concepts is based on "similarity" or "family resemblance" rather than on a finite set of criteria that define the concept (McCloskey & Glucksberg, 1978; Rosch & Mervis, 1975; Spalding & Murphy, 1996). Research demonstrates that "concept learning" and the ability to apply concepts effectively are influenced by existing knowledge (Spalding & Murphy, 1996), theory (Wisniewski & Medin, 1994), memory (Barsalou & Medin, 1986), general perspectives (Oden & Lopes, 1982), and other cues or stimuli (Gelman & Medin, 1993; Goodman, 1972; Medin & Bettger, 1994; Medin & Schaffer, 1978). All of these factors need to be considered in efforts to devise methods to deal with conceptual problems within the discipline and to develop concepts that will be useful and applicable in nursing (Rodgers, 1989a, 1989b).

IMPLICATIONS FOR CONCEPT DEVELOPMENT IN NURSING

The views presented in this discussion of the philosophical foundations of concept development reveal the tremendous diversity in attempts to answer questions concerning the nature and role(s) of concepts and the relationship between concepts and the development of knowledge. These views undoubtedly raise numerous questions about methodological issues concerning concept development in nursing. Unfortunately, in spite of the tremendous volume of literature on the subject of concepts, there is little specific information available to assist researchers in identifying appropriate designs and procedures for concept development. Even the literature that does include a discussion of methods still leaves the investigator to make many decisions independently.

There are many approaches that researchers can use to develop concepts. The choice of approach may be varied according to the concept of interest and the purpose of the inquiry. Quite a few authors of written reports of concept analyses or other concept development activities have indicated that they selected their methods based primarily, if not solely, on ease of use or what has been used most often. Such an approach to method selection in any research runs a great risk of compromising the rigor of the inquiry and the usefulness of the results. The selection of methods must be based on sound philosophical rationale and appropriateness for the purpose of the study. Because of the variety of conceptual problems that can be addressed in nursing, the researcher may have to make independent methodological decisions in many instances to ensure a worthwhile study and the production of meaningful results. These decisions should not be made arbitrarily. Overall, productive use of concept development techniques is dependent upon the investigator recognizing the assumptions that underlie the approach employed and the philosophical basis of all methodological decisions.

A reasonable approach to concept development is contingent upon a variety of factors. First, since the purpose of concept development is to resolve some type of conceptual problem, the researcher should begin by identifying clearly the nature of the problem to be addressed by the research. There is little discussion of conceptual problems in the majority of the literature of philosophy of science. Laudan (1977) described two major classifications of conceptual problems: "internal" conceptual problems, or problems related to the lack of clarity of basic concepts, and "external" conceptual problems, in which there is a conceptual conflict between competing theories (pp. 49-54). In his 1996 work, Laudan expanded this classification to include four types of conceptual problems (Laudan, 1996, p. 79). However, all of these problems concerned conceptual weaknesses in the context of existing or developing theories. For the nurse researcher, conceptual problems may appear in numerous different forms, many of which have little to do with an examination of theory.

On a practical level, conceptual problems can be confronted in a variety of ways: confusing terminology or ambivalent word use in attempts to characterize certain situations or phenomena; difficulty synthesizing existing knowledge on a topic, particularly because key concepts have been defined in diverse ways and, often, arbitrarily;

problems defining important concepts for research or theory development; problems or questions concerning the origin of a particular concept and potential change in definition over time; concerns about differences in existing concepts across disciplines that hinder knowledge synthesis, growth, and communication; potential conflicts between concepts and actual situations encountered in nursing; the need for new or more effective concepts to characterize experiences encountered in nursing; and the appropriateness of combining two or more concepts to generate a useful construct. These problems clearly indicate that concept development methods may be appropriate and beneficial in further knowledge development. A single concept may be associated with many of these problems. As with any inquiry, the nurse researcher should identify the primary problems that are of interest prior to beginning a study for purposes of concept development. A clear problem is important to ensure that the study is designed appropriately and results will be useful to alleviate the problem. The researcher may find that different techniques may be appropriate for confronting different types of conceptual problems.

A second concern that needs to be addressed in selecting an approach to concept development involves the nature of the concept of interest. Concepts that are "scientific" or "natural" may be amenable to more precise definition, particularly when the concept is relatively new and, thus, less likely to have been redefined numerous times. Similarly, such concepts may be evaluated more easily than others in reference to some tangible or measurable aspect of reality. Physiological concepts are likely to fall into this category. Psychosocial concepts and other "artifact" concepts (Bloom, 1996; Malt, 1994; Malt & Johnson, 1992), on the other hand, are likely to evidence greater ambiguity, variation, and overlap, and more difficulty in linking them to objective empirical situations.

Concepts that are related to a "process" (Kim, 1983) present a unique situation as well. Part of the act of defining, clarifying, or otherwise developing concepts often concerns the connection between the concept and specific events or occurrences. Process concepts, however, may not have a clearly identifiable beginning or end point and may be more difficult to clarify in general because of variations that occur at specific points in the process. Clarification of concepts such as grief (Cowles & Rodgers, see Chapter 7) or other concepts that pertain to a process (Westra & Rodgers, 1991) may require special consideration because of the internal variations inherent in the concept.

Another consideration in selecting an approach to concept development concerns the history of the concept. History, in this sense, pertains to the general length of time the concept has been in existence, its estimated time and context of origin, and the translations and adaptations that have occurred over time. Concepts that have been in existence for multiple decades are likely to have undergone change and to be applied differently than when initially developed. Although the passing of time theoretically provides the opportunity for further development of a concept, in reality concepts often become more vague and ambiguous over time. In some situations the concept may have been retained in its original form, without attempts to bring about the changes that may have been appropriate as life situations in general changed. The result may be a gross lack of conceptual clarity or a concept that is no longer relevant or effective in application to the situations that are confronted in nursing. Concepts that are fairly well developed with some consensus about definition may warrant a different slant in inquiry. In such cases, research may be needed to evaluate the applicability of the concept in different settings. A "social" or critical approach might be useful as well to identify individual and cultural influences on the concept. Often an initial analysis based on review of existing literature can serve as an important heuristic to clarify the nature of the conceptual problem and to help the researcher determine a productive approach for inquiry.

Methods for concept development offer a significant contribution to expanding the knowledge base of nursing. For these methods to be useful, it is important that the researcher be attentive to the variety of philosophical issues associated with concepts. Particularly, the current status of the concept of interest and the nature of associated conceptual problems need to be considered in selecting appropriate techniques for further development. In addition, the basic assumptions adopted by the investigator have a profound effect on the specific approach to concept development and the interpretation and application of the findings.

In spite of the long history of discussions of concepts and the tremendous diversity of opinion, at present there is only a beginning answer to the question "What is a concept?" There is a consensus that concepts are cognitive in nature and that they are comprised of attributes abstracted from reality, expressed in some form and utilized for some common purpose (Rodgers, 1989b). Consequently, concepts are more than words or mental images alone. In addition, an emphasis on "use" alone is not sufficient to capture the complex nature of concepts.

There also are substantial empirical data, along with philosophical rationale, to support a "family resemblance" (cluster concept or fuzzy set) approach to conceptualization. It may be practical, and even desirable, to aim for a high level of clarity and precision in the definition or development of certain concepts. However, this aim does not support an emphasis on entity views with their focus on reduction, necessary and sufficient conditions, rigid boundaries, and context-free interpretations. Instead, in such cases, clarity still must include recognition of the possibility of temporal and contextual change and an appreciation for connections, rather than reduction, to be consistent with current philosophical thought.

Further work is needed to determine whether or not any position can be universally applicable to all types of concepts (natural, artifact, and process concepts, for example). As philosophers, psychologists, nurses, and other scholars continue to explore the fundamental questions concerning concepts, new answers will emerge and, undoubtedly, new questions as well. At this time it is most important for nurse researchers to recognize the importance of resolving conceptual problems in nursing and to be aware of the philosophical foundations of concept development and their implications for expanding the knowledge base of nursing. A strong and defensible philosophical rationale for decisions made by researchers ultimately is the primary ingredient in efforts to promote conceptual progress in nursing.

REFERENCES

Aristotle. (1947). Posterior analytics (G. R. G. Mure, Trans.). In R. McKeon (Ed.), *Introduction to Aristotle* (pp. 9-109). New York: Random House.

Aristotle. (1984). Categories (J. L. Ackrill, Trans.). In J. Barnes (Ed.), The complete works of Aristotle (pp. 3-24). Princeton, NJ: Princeton University Press.

Armstrong, S. L., Gleitman, L. R., & Gleitman, H. (1983). What some concepts might not be. *Cognition, 13,* 263-308.

Ayer, A. J. (Ed.). (1959). *Logical positivism.* Glencoe, IL: Free Press.

Barsalou, L. W., & Medin, D. L. (1986). Concepts: Static definitions or context-dependent representations? *Cahiers de Psychologie Cognitive,* 6, 187-202.

Beck, C. T. (1996). A concept analysis of panic. *Archives of Psychiatric Nursing, 10,* 265-275.

Becker, C. H. (1983). A conceptualization of concept. *Nursing Papers, 15,* 51-58.

Bloom, P. (1996). Intention, history, and artifact concepts. *Cognition, 60,* 1-29.

Bohlander, J. R. (1995). Differentiation of self: An examination of the concept. *Issues in Mental Health Nursing, 16*(2), 165-184.

Boyd, C. (1985). Toward an understanding of mother-daughter identification using concept analysis. *Advances in Nursing Science, 7*(3), 78-86.

Carnap, R. (1956). *Meaning and necessity.* Chicago: University of Chicago Press.

Chinn, P. L., & Jacobs, M. K. (1987). *Theory and nursing: A systematic approach* (2nd ed.). St. Louis: C. V. Mosby.

Chinn, P. L., & Kramer, M. (1991). *Theory and nursing: A systematic approach* (3rd ed.). St. Louis: C. V. Mosby.

Coyne, I. T. (1996). Parent participation: A concept analysis. *Journal of Advanced Nursing, 23,* 733-740.

Descartes, R. (1960). Meditations on first philosophy. In M. C. Beardsley (Ed.), *The European philosophers from Descartes to Nietzsche* (pp. 25-96). New York: Random House. (Original work published 1644)

Diers, D. (1979). *Research in nursing practice.* Philadelphia: J. B. Lippincott.

Duffy, M. E. (1987). The concept of adaptation: Examining alternatives for the study of nursing phenomena. *Scholarly Inquiry for Nursing Practice, 1,* 179-192.

Duldt, B. W., & Giffin, K. (1985). *Theoretical perspectives for nursing.* Boston: Little, Brown.

Dummett, M. (1975). What is a theory of meaning? In S. Guttenplan (Ed.), *Mind and language* (pp. 97-138). Oxford: Oxford University Press.

Fehr, B. (1988). Prototype analysis of the concepts of love and commitment. *Journal of Personality and Social Psychology, 55,* 557-579.

Fodor, J., & Lepore, E. (1996). The red herring and the pet fish: Why concepts still can't be prototypes. *Cognition, 58,* 253-270.

Forsyth, G. L. (1980). Analysis of the concept of empathy: Illustration of one approach. *Advances in Nursing Science, 2*(2), 33-42.

Frege, G. (1952a). *Grundgesetze der Arithmetic* (P. T. Geach, Trans.). In P. Geach & M. Black (Eds.), *Translations from the philosophical writings of Gottlob Frege* (pp. 159-181). Oxford: Basil Blackwell.

Frege, G. (1952b). On concept and object (P. T. Geach, Trans.). In P. Geach & M. Black (Eds.), *Translations from the philosophical writings of Gottlob Frege* (pp. 42-55). Oxford: Basil Blackwell.

Gelman, S. A., & Medin, D. L. (1993). What's so essential about essentialism? A different perspective on the interaction of perception, language, and conceptual knowledge. *Cognitive Development, 8,* 157-167.

Gibson, C. H. (1991). A concept analysis of empowerment. *Journal of Advanced Nursing, 16,* 354-361.

Goodman, N. (1972). Seven strictures on similarity. In N. Goodman (Ed.), *Problems and projects* (pp. 437-447). New York: Bobbs-Merrill.

Haddock, J. (1996). Towards further clarification of the concept 'dignity.' *Journal of Advanced Nursing, 24,* 924-31.

Hadzikadic, M., Hakenwerth, A., Bohren, B., Norton, J., Mehta, B., & Andrews, C. (1996). Concept formation vs. logistic regression: Predicting death in trauma patients. *Artificial Intelligence in Medicine, 8,* 493-504.

Hallett, G. (1967). *Wittgenstein's definition of meaning as use.* New York: Fordham University Press.

Hardy, M. K. (1974). Theories: Components, development, evaluation. *Nursing Research, 23,* 100-107.

Hartnack, J. (1965). *Wittgenstein and modern philosophy* (M. Cranston, Trans.). New York: New York University Press.

Jacox, A. (1974). Theory construction in nursing: An overview. *Nursing Research, 23,* 4-13.

Johns, J. L. (1996). A concept analysis of trust. *Journal of Advanced Nursing, 24,* 76-83.

Kant, I. (1965). *Critique of pure reason* (N. K. Smith, Trans.). New York: St. Martin's Press. (Original work published 1781)

Keck, J. F. (1986). Terminology of theory development. In A. Marriner (Ed.), *Nursing theorists and their work* (pp. 15-23). St. Louis: C. V. Mosby.

Kim, H. S. (1983). *The nature of theoretical thinking in nursing.* Norwalk, CT: Appleton-Century-Crofts.

King, I. M. (1988). Concepts: Essential elements of theories. *Nursing Science Quarterly, 1,* 22-25.

Knafl, K. A., & Deatrick, J. A. (1986). How families manage chronic conditions:

An analysis of the concept of normalization. *Research in Nursing & Health, 9*, 215-222.

Laudan, L. (1977). *Progress and its problems.* Berkeley, CA: University of California Press.

Laudan, L. (1996). *Beyond positivism and relativism.* Boulder, CO: Westview Press.

Lebowitz, M. (1987). Experiments with incremental concept formation: UNIMEM. *Machine learning, 2*, 103-138.

Locke, J. (1975). *An essay concerning human understanding.* Oxford: Oxford University Press. (Original work published 1690)

Malt, B. C. (1994). Water is not H_2O. *Cognitive Psychology, 27*, 41-70.

Malt, B. C., & Johnson, E. C. (1992). Do artifact concepts have cores? *Journal of Memory and Language, 31*, 195-217.

Matteson, P., & Hawkins, J. W. (1990). Concept analysis of decision making. *Nursing Forum, 25*(2), 4-10.

McCloskey, M.E., & Glucksberg, S. (1978). Natural categories: Well defined or fuzzy sets? *Memory & Cognition, 6*, 462-472.

Medin, D. L. (1989). Concepts and conceptual structure. *American Psychologist, 44*, 1469-1481.

Medin, D. L., & Bettger, J. G. (1994). Presentation order and recognition of categorically related examples. *Psychonomic Bulletin & Review, 1*, 250-254.

Medin, D. L., Goldstone, R. L., & Gentner, D. (1993). Respects for similarity. *Psychological Review, 100*, 254-278.

Medin, D. L., & Schaffer, M. M. (1978). Context theory of classification learning. *Psychological Review, 85*, 207-238.

Meize-Grochowski, R. (1984). An analysis of the concept of trust. *Journal of Advanced Nursing, 9*, 563-572.

Meleis, A. I. (1985). *Theoretical nursing.* Philadelphia: J. B. Lippincott.

Meleis, A. I. (1991). *Theoretical nursing* (2nd ed.). Philadelphia: J. B. Lippincott

Meleis, A. I. (1997). *Theoretical nursing* (3rd ed.). Philadelphia: J. B. Lippincott

Oden, G. C., & Lopes, L. (1982). On the internal structure of fuzzy subjective categories. In R. R. Yager (Ed.), *Recent developments in fuzzy set and possibility theory* (pp. 75-89). Elmsford, NY: Pergamon.

Peacocke, C. (1992). *A study of concepts.* Cambridge, MA: The MIT Press.

Rawnsley, M. M. (1980). The concept of privacy. *Advances in Nursing Science, 2*(2), 25-31.

Rew, L. (1986). Intuition: Concept analysis of a group phenomenon. *Advances in Nursing Science, 8*(2), 21-28.

Rodgers, B. L. (1989a). Concepts, analysis, and the development of nursing knowledge: The evolutionary cycle. *Journal of Advanced Nursing, 14*, 330-335.

Rodgers, B. L. (1989b). The use and application of concepts in nursing: The case of health policy (Doctoral dissertation, University of Virginia, 1987). Dissertation Abstracts International, 49-11B, 4756.

Rorty, R. (1979). *Philosophy and the mirror of nature.* Princeton, NJ: Princeton University Press.

Rosch, E., & Mervis, C. B. (1975). Family resemblances: Studies in the internal structure of categories. *Cognitive Psychology, 7*, 573-605.

Russell, B. (1914). *Our knowledge of the external world.* Chicago: Open Court.

Ryle, G. (1949). *The concept of mind.* Chicago: University of Chicago Press.

Ryle, G. (1971a). Systematically misleading expressions. In *Collected papers* (Vol. 2, pp. 39-62). London: Hutchinson.

Ryle, G. (1971b). The theory of meaning. In *Collected papers* (Vol. 2, pp. 350-372). London: Hutchinson.

Ryle, G. (1971c). Thinking thoughts and having concepts. In *Collected papers* (Vol. 2, pp. 446-450). London: Hutchinson.

Ryle, G. (1971d). Use, usage and meaning. In *Collected papers* (Vol. 2, pp. 407-414). London: Hutchinson.

Schlick, M. (1959). The turning point in philosophy (D. Rynin, Trans.). In A. J. Ayer (Ed.), *Logical positivism* (pp. 53-59). Glencoe, IL: Free Press.

Silva, M. C., & Rothbart, D. R. (1983). An analysis of changing trends in philosophies of science on nursing theory development and testing. *Advances in Nursing Science, 6*, 1-13.

Simmons, S. J. (1989). Health: A concept analysis. *International Journal of Nursing Studies, 26*, 155-161.

Smith, E. E., & Medin, D. L. (1981). *Categories and concepts.* Cambridge, MA: Harvard University Press.

Spalding, T. L., & Murphy, G. L. (1996). Effects of background knowledge on category construction. *Journal of Experimental Psychology: Learning, Memory & Cognition, 22*, 525-538.

Tadd, W., & Chadwick, R. (1989). Philosophical analysis and its value to the nurse teacher. *Nurse Education Today, 9*, 155-160.

Toulmin, S. (1972). *Human understanding.* Princeton: Princeton University Press.

Walker, L. O., & Avant, K. C. (1988). *Strategies for theory construction in nursing* (2nd ed.). Norwalk, CT: Appleton & Lange.

Walker, L. O., & Avant, K. C. (1995). *Strategies for theory construction in nursing* (3rd ed.). Norwalk, CT: Appleton & Lange.

Watson, J. (1979). *Nursing: The philosophy and science of caring.* Boston: Little, Brown.

Webster, G., Jacox, A., & Baldwin, B. (1981). Nursing theory and the ghost of the received view. In J. C. McCloskey & H. K. Grace (Eds.), *Current issues in nursing* (pp. 26-35). Boston: Blackwell Scientific.

Westra, B. L., & Rodgers, B. L. (1991). The concept of integration: Á foundation for evaluating outcomes of nursing care. *Journal of Professional Nursing, 7*, 277-282.

Wilson, J. (1963). *Thinking with concepts.* London: Cambridge University Press.

Wisniewski, E. J., & Medin, D. L. (1994). On the interaction of theory and data in concept learning. *Cognitive Science, 18*, 221-281.

Wittgenstein, L. (1968). *Philosophical investigations* (3rd ed.) (G. E. M. Anscombe, Trans.). New York: Macmillan. (Original work published 1953)

Wittgenstein, L. (1979). *Notebooks: 1914-1916* (2nd ed.) (G. E. M. Anscombe, Trans.). Chicago: University of Chicago Press.

Wittgenstein, L. (1981). *Tractatus logico-philosophicus* (D. F. Pears & B. F. McGuinness, Trans.). London: Routledge & Kegan Paul. (Original work published 1921)

Knowledge Synthesis and Concept Development in Nursing

Kathleen A. Knafl and Janet A. Deatrick

In an editorial in *Nursing Research,* Florence Downs (1989) criticized the noncumulative nature of nursing research, stating, "We all need to become much more sensitive to the fact that 'stop and go' activity ends in proliferation of isolated findings. Classification and synthesis remain essential to furthering realistic theory development and an understanding of how conditions are related within a nursing context" (p. 323). Although not disputing the validity of Downs' critique, it also is true that there has been a growing interest in knowledge synthesis in nursing. Nurse scholars have both utilized and developed a variety of approaches to knowledge synthesis. To date, much of the work in this area has been directed to concept analysis.

Nursing has evinced a long-standing recognition of the importance of concept development for the advancement of nursing theory and practice (Hardy, 1974; Jacox, 1974; Norris, 1982). Concept analysis was given a major impetus in the early 1980s when both Chinn and Jacobs (1983) and Walker and Avant (1983) published books on nursing theory that offered guidelines for conducting concept analysis. Since then, authors have continued to publish both guidelines for concept analysis and results of analyses (Chinn & Jacobs, 1987; Knafl & Deatrick, 1986, 1990; Rew, 1986; Rodgers, 1989a, 1989b; Schwartz-Barcott & Kim, 1986; Tilden, 1985; Walker & Avant, 1988). Concept analysis typically entails synthesizing existing views of a concept and distinguishing it from other concepts. There are also other approaches to knowledge synthesis including a variety of approaches for reviewing the literature

(Artinian, 1982; Cooper, 1982, 1984, 1989; Ganong, 1987; Noblit & Hare, 1988).

Little attention has been given to comparing the relative merits of these different approaches to knowledge synthesis. As a result, readers may not understand why a particular approach was selected, and authors may not consider the full range of approaches when undertaking a knowledge synthesis project. The aim of this chapter is to present an overview of several broad approaches to knowledge synthesis and a more detailed comparison of approaches to concept analysis and development.

APPROACHES TO KNOWLEDGE SYNTHESIS

The strategies summarized in Table 3-1 are directed toward evaluating knowledge development in a particular domain. Using each, the analyst critically reviews literature, occasionally gathers data, and draws conclusions regarding what is known and what further work needs to be done in a particular area of interest. If successful, the synthesis conveys to the reader the "state of the art" in a given area.

Literature Reviews

Guidelines for conducting integrative reviews and critiques of existing reviews can be found in the literature. Both Jackson (1980) and Cooper (1982, 1984, 1989) distinguished various types of integrative reviews and conceptualized integrative reviews as a research process. Jackson (1980) maintained that such reviews could serve a variety of substantive, methodological, and theoretical purposes. Similarly, Cooper (1989) noted that "reviews can focus on research outcomes, research methods,

Table 3-1   Strategies for Synthesizing Knowledge

Strategy	Purpose	Data Source	Proponents

Literature review
  Integrative
  Meta-analysis
  Meta-ethnography
  Conceptual mapping
	Knowledge synthesis/ aggregation	Literature	Artinian (1982); Cooper (1982, 1984, 1989); Devine & Cook (1983); Ganong (1987); Glass (1976); Jackson (1980); Noblit & Hare (1988)

Concept analysis	Identification, clarification, or refinement of a concept	Literature; empirical data; constructed cases	Chinn & Jacobs, (1983, 1987); Chinn & Kramer (1991); Rodgers (1989a); Sartori (1984); Schwartz-Barcott & Kim (1986); Walker & Avant (1983, 1988, 1994); Wilson (1969)

theories, and/or applications" (p. 13). Ganong (1987) provided guidelines for conducting integrative reviews and critiqued 17 published reviews of nursing research. He emphasized the importance of being explicit in the review as to one's purpose, sampling design, and data collection methods.

Other authors (Abraham & Schultz, 1983; Devine & Cook, 1983; Glass, 1976; Smith & Naftel, 1984) addressed how statistical techniques can be used in integrative literature reviews. Glass (1976) described this approach, known as *meta-analysis:*

> Meta-analysis refers to the analysis of analyses. I use it to refer to the statistical analysis of a large collection of analysis results from individual studies for the purpose of integrating the findings. (p. 3)

These publications cite the results of specific meta-analyses: Beck, 1996; Kinney et al., 1996; Krywanio, 1994. Smith and Naftel (1984) listed existing analyses. In the past several years, the emphasis has shifted in meta-analysis from the single purpose of measuring effect size to a more encompassing goal of concept clarification (Booth-Kewley & Friedman, 1987; Broome, 1993).

Noblit and Hare (1988) outlined a framework for synthesizing the results of qualitative studies, a technique they termed *meta-ethnography.* Meta-ethnography is an inductive approach that Noblit and Hare describe as a series of overlapping phases relying on the technique of metaphoric reduction to translate the interpretations of one qualitative study into the interpretations of another. As in meta-analysis, the reviewer synthesizes the results of existing research. However, meta-ethnography is viewed by its developers as unique from other approaches to knowledge synthesis. Noblit and Hare (1988) maintained:

> We use the term meta-ethnography to highlight our proposal as an interpretive alternative to research synthesis. For us, the meta in meta-ethnography means something different than it does in meta-analysis. It refers not to developing overarching generalizations but, rather, translations of qualitative studies into one another. (p. 25)

Noblit and Hare highlight their description with examples throughout the text. Certainly, meta-ethnography offers a promising approach for integrating the results of the numerous ethnographic, grounded theory, and phenomenological studies published in nursing. Although not explicitly following Noblit and Hare's approach, Dixon's (1996) analysis of 16 articles reporting qualitative studies of parents' experiences with health care providers identified common underlying concepts that characterized the interactions between parents and professionals. As such it points to the usefulness of these kinds of integrative reviews for advancing concept development in nursing.

In an effort to understand the comparative merits of quantitative and qualitative approaches to conducting integrative reviews, Brown and Hellings (1988) compared the results of their meta-analysis of studies of maternal-infant attachment with Lamb and Hwang's (1982) qualitative review of the same topic. They found that important advantages of meta-analysis are avoidance of type 11 errors and investigator bias. On the other hand, qualitative reviews give the reader a better sense of individual studies, combine results from methodologically diverse studies, allow for the investigation of the influence of multiple variables, and are not limited by the author's failure to report certain statistics. Given the distinct advantages of the approaches, Brown and Hellings (1988) concluded that both types of reviews are useful.

In contrast to the analytic techniques associated with integrative reviews and the specific statistical techniques of meta-analysis, Artinian (1982) developed conceptual mapping for depicting "the relationships among variables linking the independent variables to the dependent variable" (p. 379). As described by Artinian, the purpose of conceptual mapping is to clarify the research problem in the context of proposal development. Conceptual mapping requires the explicit identification of concepts of interest and facilitates identification of how these concepts have been related to one another in previous research. Artinian described conceptual mapping as an especially useful educational technique for graduate students embarking on their first research project, and provided detailed examples of conceptual maps completed by former students. Unlike other synthesizing approaches, conceptual mapping was not presented as resulting in a "stand alone" scholarly outcome.

Although the aforementioned techniques offer general and specialized approaches for knowledge synthesis, they do not explicitly address concept clarification and development as a primary goal. Methods for concept analysis fill that gap.

APPROACHES TO CONCEPT ANALYSIS

As shown in Table 3–2, scholars have developed several approaches to concept analysis. While all approaches share a common focus on concept clarification, authors linked their approaches to distinct intellectual underpinnings and identified somewhat different analytic goals. Moreover, they specified varying steps or phases as comprising the work of concept analysis. Table 3–2 summarizes these differences across the approaches with regard to the following: intellectual underpinnings, analytic purposes, and analytic steps or phases. Exemplar references for each approach are also included in the table.

Chinn and Jacobs

Chinn and Jacobs (1983, 1987) described their approach to concept analysis as an adaptation of Wilson's (1969) method. Like Wilson's, their approach relies heavily on the development of exemplary cases (model, contrary, related, borderline) that are used to identify the defining criteria of the concept. Criteria, which are described as always tentative, reflect what is learned about the concept from developing cases and from selectively reviewing the literature.

In one of the earliest publications of a concept analysis, Forsyth (1980) used Chinn and Jacob's approach in analyzing the concept of empathy. She presented a model case of empathy followed by a discussion of defining criteria for the concept as reflected in the model case. Her discussion incorporated validating evidence from the literature. The concept and the provisional criteria were further refined and expanded through the presentation and analysis of contrary, related, and borderline cases and through further review of the literature. Forsyth described her review of the literature as selective and not exhaustive.

Throughout her presentation, Forsyth (1980) emphasized the simultaneous nature of the activities of concept analysis and stated, "The techniques are not necessarily used in step-by-step fashion; rather they tend to emerge simultaneously once the initial steps of analysis have been undertaken" (p. 34). She noted that concept analysis is best done as a collaborative endeavor.

More recently, Warren (1993) used this approach as a vehicle for explaining the concept of social isolation. Although not explicitly stating her sampling criteria, Warren reviewed numerous nursing and nonnursing sources and followed her identification of defining criteria with an insightful discussion of their implications for nursing assessment and intervention.

In the 1991 edition of *Theory and Nursing: A Systematic Approach,* Chinn and Jacobs (now Kramer) introduced several refinements to their approach to concept analysis, which is presented as a strategy for creating meaning. They stated that "conceptual meaning is something that is created. It does not 'exist' as an 'out there' reality, but it is deliberately formed from empiric experience" (p. 80).

As shown in Table 3-2, Chinn and Kramer credited both Wilson (1969) and Walker and Avant (1983, 1988) as influencing their approach to what they termed *concept clarification.* Although the underlying purpose and steps of the clarification process remained similar to those in the first two editions, the authors expanded the data sources they recommended considering as part of the analysis. Under data sources they discussed definitions, cases (model, contrary, related, and borderline), visual images, popular and classical literature, music, professional literature, and people. The presentation of data sources was couched

TABLE 3-2 Approaches to Concept Analysis/Development

Approach	Underpinnings	Purpose	Phases/Steps	Example
Chinn & Jacobs (1983, 1987)	Wilson (1969)	"To arrive at a tentative definition of the concept and a set of criteria by which one can judge whether or not the empirical phenomena associated with the concept exist in a particular situation" (Chinn & Jacobs, 1983, p. 90).	1. Identify concept 2. Specify aims 3. Examine definitions 4. Construct cases 5. Test cases 6. Formulate criteria	Forsyth (1980)/empathy; Warren (1993)/social isolation
Chinn & Kramer (1991)	Wilson (1969); Walker & Avant (1988)	"Produce tentative definition of the concept and a set of tentative criteria for determining if the concept 'exists' in a particular situation" (Chinn & Kramer, 1991, p. 88).	1. Select concept 2. Clarify purpose 3. Identify data sources 4. Explore context and values 5. Formulate criteria	None
Walker & Avant (1983, 1988)	Wilson (1969)	"To distinguish between the defining attributes of a concept and its irrelevant attributes" (Walker & Avant, 1988, p. 35).	1. Select concept 2. Determine aim of analysis 3. Identify all uses of concept 4. Determine defining attributes 5. Construct a model case 6. Construct additional cases 7. Identify antecedents and consequences 8. Define empirical referents	Boyd (1985)/mother-daughter identification; Henson (1997)/mutuality; Rew (1986)/intuition

Author	Theoretical sources	Purpose	Steps	Applications
Rodgers (1989a)	Price (1953); Rorty (1979); Toulmin (1972); Wittgenstein (1968)	To clarify the current use of a concept with attention to contextual and temporal aspects; to provide a clear conceptual foundation as a heuristic for further inquiry (Rodgers, 1989a; see chapter 6)	1. Identify the concept of interest 2. Identify surrogate terms 3. Identify sample for data collection 4. Identify attributes of the concept 5. Identify references, antecedents, and consequences of concept 6. Identify related concepts 7. Identify a model case 8. Conduct interdisciplinary and temporal comparisons	Rodgers (1989a, 1989b)/ health policy; Cowles & Rodgers (see Chapter 7)/grief; Westra & Rodgers (1991)/ integration
Sartori (1984)	Ogden & Richards (1946)	"To arrive at a definition of the concept that is both adequate and harmonious" (Sartori, 1984, p. 56).	1. Reconstruct concept 2. Select designating term 3. Reconceptualize the concept	Knafl & Deatrick (1990)/ family management style
Schwartz-Barcott & Kim (1986)	Reynolds (1971); Schatzman & Strauss (1973); Wilson (1969)	"To identify, analyze, and refine concepts in the initial stage of theory development" (Schwartz-Barcott & Kim, 1986, p. 91).	1. Theoretical phase 2. Fieldwork phase 3. Analytical phase	Madden (1990)/ therapeutic alliance; Phillips (1991)/chronic sorrow

in an explicit recognition of empirics, ethics, aesthetics, and personal knowing as distinct ways of knowing. In their discussion of the use of multiple data sources, Chinn and Kramer argue that "although case techniques that are associated with creating conceptual meaning are very useful, when they are supplemented with other data sources, a richer meaning for concepts evolves" (p. 93). Also new in this edition was their consideration of how the meaning of a concept varies across contexts and their recommendation that clarification strategies be adapted to the specific purpose of the analysis.

Walker and Avant

Walker and Avant (1983, 1988, 1994) identified concept analysis as one of three approaches to concept development. Other strategies included concept synthesis for the development of new concepts and concept derivation for the translation of concepts across disciplines.

Like Chinn and Jacobs (1983, 1987) and Chinn and Kramer (1991), this approach to concept analysis builds on Wilson's (1969) seminal work. As noted in Table 3-2, the approaches differ somewhat in the steps and ordering of the analytic process. Although the authors of these approaches pointed out that concept analysis usually does not proceed in a strictly linear fashion, their differential ordering of steps leads to a somewhat different emphasis in the analytic process. For Walker and Avant (1988), case construction followed identification of defining criteria and served to illustrate the presence or absence of the criteria across the concept of interest and related concepts; for Chinn and Jacobs (1987), case construction preceded formulation of defining criteria and played a key role in the defining process. Chinn and Kramer (1991) incorporated case construction as one of many possible data sources that contributed to the formulation of defining criteria. Walker and Avant included the specification of antecedents, consequences, and empirical referents as components of the analysis, whereas Chinn and Kramer encouraged the exploration of various contexts and values associated with the concept.

Henson (1997) used Walker and Avant's approach to analyze the concept of mutuality. Although using a somewhat different ordering of the analytic steps, Henson demonstrated the usefulness of the approach for distinguishing across concepts (e.g., mutuality, autonomy, reciprocity, collaboration, paternalism) and identifying antecedents and consequences of a concept. Like earlier, more traditional applications of the approach by Boyd (1985) and Rew (1986), Henson's review of the literature was highly selective with minimal specification of sampling strategy.

Rodgers

Rodgers (1989a) offered an approach to concept analysis that "overcomes difficulties with a positivistic or reductionistic view and that addresses contemporary concerns valuing dynamism and interrelationships within reality" (p. 332). Rodgers integrated the views of several prominent philosophers (Price, 1953; Rorty, 1979; Toulmin, 1972; Wittgenstein, 1953/1968) in developing her evolutionary view of concepts as continually subject to change, and as developing through significance, use, and application. *Significance* is "the concept's ability to assist in the resolution of problems, its ability to characterize phenomena adequately, thus furthering efforts toward the achievement of intellectual ideals" (Rodgers, 1989a, p. 332). Use of the concept refers to the manner in which it is employed and its application refers to actual instances of use. According to Rodgers, it is through the process of application that concepts are further refined and developed.

Rodgers maintained that her approach differed from traditional approaches to concept analysis in several important ways. She emphasized that the analytic process was nonlinear and involved a series of overlapping phases rather than sequential steps. Rodgers also maintained that the singular, fundamental purpose of concept analysis was to clarify the concept of interest. At the same time, she pointed out that such clarification was an essential dimension of nursing diagnosis development and clinical problem solving (1993). Moreover, she stated that only a model case should be presented, since the use of other types of cases such as contrary and borderline reflected a view of concepts as unchanging. She stated, "Such cases are not consistent with the view of concepts that underlies this revised method. Instead, their functions are addressed in the form of related concepts, a change that recognizes the interconnectedness of the world and the likelihood of change" (p. 333). Rodgers also favored identifying real-life model cases rather than constructing such cases solely for the purpose of the analysis. She contended, "A model case of a concept enhances the degree of clarification offered as a result of analysis by providing an everyday example that includes the attributes of the concept" (p. 334).

In a separate publication of the results of an analysis of the concept of health policy, Rodgers (1989b) employed her approach in order to clarify the current use of the concept. The analysis proceeded through a series of flexible phases rather than invariate steps and included a detailed account of procedures for sampling the literature. Based on her evolutionary view of concepts, she presented only an empirically based model case of the concept.

Sartori

Sartori's approach to concept analysis builds on Ogden and Richards's (1946) work and focuses on words, meanings, and referents and the relationships among the three. Sartori's (1984) book, *Social Science Concepts: A Systematic Analysis,* included a description of his method of concept analysis as well as concept analyses by different authors on a variety of topics such as consensus, development, ethnicity, and power. Sartori described a three-step process in which the concept was reconstructed, named, and reconceptualized. Concept reconstruction entailed reviewing and synthesizing existing knowledge about the concept. Concept formation and reconceptualization encompassed selecting a term to name the concept, and then refining the concept. Sartori's approach does not use case presentations.

Although basing their analyses on Sartori's framework, authors who contributed concept analyses to his book employed somewhat different applications of his three-step process, adapting it to their purposes and to the body of literature related to the concept. In general, each author's analysis was based on a selective review of research literature. In their applications of Sartori's approach, authors typically used descriptive grids to summarize characteristics of the concept reflected in the literature. Figures were used to show the relationship between the concept of interest and related concepts.

For example, Jackson (1984) used Sartori's framework to analyze the concept of ethnicity. His analysis focused on existing definitions of the concept and the identification of empirical referents. Jackson (1984) noted that he selected definitions because they were "prominent in the literature on ethnicity and rather typical" (p. 219). As a result of this reconstruction phase of the analysis, he identified "core characteristics" of the concept. Based on these core characteristics, he named the concept *ethnic collectivities* and concluded his presentation with a series of summary definitions of the concept and related concepts such as ethnic category and ethnic group. Taken as a whole, Sartori's book provides a detailed elaboration of one approach to concept analysis and a series of diverse analyses exemplifying the wide-ranging applicability of the approach. In one of the few applications of this approach in nursing, Knafl and Deatrick (1990) used Sartori's method to analyze the concept of family management style. They noted that the approach was especially appropriate for the analysis of concepts in the beginning stages of development since it encompassed (re)naming and refining the concept of interest.

Schwartz-Barcott and Kim

Schwartz-Barcott and Kim (1986) presented a "hybrid model" for concept development that explicitly incorporated both theoretical and empirical activities. The hybrid approach consists of three sequential phases: theoretical, fieldwork, and final analytical. It builds on Reynolds's (1971) composite approach to the development of scientific knowledge, Wilson's (1969) approach to concept analysis, and Schatzman and Strauss's (1973) book *Field Research: Strategies for a Natural Sociology.*

During the theoretical phase, the literature is reviewed with an eye to selecting a working definition of the concept of interest. This working definition then serves to focus the fieldwork phase of concept development, which is "aimed at refining a concept that has been analyzed in the theoretical phase" (Schwartz-Barcott & Kim, 1986, p. 96). Refinement serves to validate and elaborate the concept through qualitative research. During the final analytical phase, the results from the two previous phases are integrated in order to define the concept and identify measurement issues and strategies. At this point, the concept's applicability and importance to nursing is evaluated.

The authors provided a detailed example of how the hybrid model was used by a graduate student to develop the concept of withdrawal. To date, the hybrid model has been used primarily as an educational device for students working on their master's research projects and doctoral dissertations (D. Schwartz-Barcott, personal communication, March 3, 1989). Madden (1990) and Phillips (1991) used the hybrid model to analyze and develop further the concepts of therapeutic alliance and chronic sorrow. Based on a review of the literature, Madden formulated a working definition of the concept that she subsequently used to direct her observations of interactions between community health nurses and their clients. Observational data were analyzed systematically and used to expand the initial working definition of the concept. During the final analysis phase, the revised definition of therapeutic alliance was discussed in terms of existing nursing theories. In both the theoretical and fieldwork phases of the analysis, Phillips emphasized measurement as well as definition of the concept. Chronic sorrow originally had been used to describe the experiences of parents with a child with mental retardation, and Phillips was interested in exploring its applicability to other groups. Her analysis demonstrated how the hybrid approach could be used to identify the linkages between concepts and explore the varying contexts in which the concept is useful.

DISCUSSION

Scholars engaged in knowledge synthesis have a wide range of approaches at their disposal. These approaches address a variety of purposes. Whereas some are geared to knowledge aggregation in a substantive area, others focus on refining and clarifying a single concept. Some, such as conceptual mapping and hybrid concept development, have been initiated and applied primarily as educational techniques for beginning researchers in graduate programs. Other approaches, such as integrative reviews and concept analysis, have a long history of mainstream scientific endeavors. Two of the techniques, meta-analysis and meta-ethnography, are relatively new. Given the variety of approaches, it is best to look at the strategies presented in Tables 3-1 and 3-2 as a menu of possibilities that should be tailored to one's purposes and desired outcome at the outset. The rationale for using a particular strategy should be justified because it will help to clarify the approach and the nature of the phenomenon being explored in the synthesis activity.

Although current information is available on each approach, the extent to which they have been applied by nurse scholars varies considerably. There are numerous published examples in nursing of integrative reviews, meta-analyses, and concept analyses. In contrast, few authors have reported meta-ethnographies, hybrid-model concept development, or conceptual mapping. It is hoped that an awareness of such alternative strategies will result in their use and further development.

Regarding concept analysis, explicit comparison of the approaches revealed important differences among them. As different methods of concept analysis were explored, it became apparent that the nature of the literature review and the use of illustrative cases varied considerably.

Chinn and Jacobs (1983, 1987) said little about the literature review stage of the analysis, and the applications of their approach by others tended to rely heavily on the presentation of cases. Typically, the cases were constructed early in the analysis to help identify defining criteria, which were tested and refined throughout the course of analysis. Chinn and Jacobs recommended the development of multiple types of cases (e.g., model, contrary, related) and did not distinguish between empirically based cases and those created for the purpose of the analysis.

Chinn and Kramer (1991) identified cases (model, contrary, related, and borderline) as one of several data sources to be used in generating and refining defining criteria. Like the other sources of data, cases were used to stimulate thinking about the concept. While they emphasized using many diverse sources of data, Chinn and Kramer (1991) gave few guidelines for reviewing or synthesizing such data. They maintained that concept clarification should be a thoughtful, systematic process.

Walker and Avant (1983, 1988) stressed the centrality of the literature review to concept analysis. Although they did not provide explicit guidelines for carrying out such a review, they encouraged the analyst to do extensive reading in widely varying sources and to maintain a systematic record of the various ways in which the concept was used in the literature. They maintained that cases usually were used to illustrate the defining criteria of a concept. They acknowledged, however, that with a new concept, cases may be used to help identify defining criteria. Like Chinn and Jacobs, they recommended the development of multiple types of cases.

Rodgers (1989a) also emphasized the importance of the literature review. Moreover, unlike other authors, she specified guidelines for sampling the literature and suggested that a model case be identified at the end of the analysis to clarify and illustrate the concept. She advised that the model case be based on an everyday example of the concept, a position she maintained was consistent with her evolutionary view of concepts. Cases are not used to identify defining attributes in this approach.

The literature review was also a major aspect of Sartori's approach and comprised the initial phase of the analysis, concept reconstruction. Although he did not specify guidelines for sampling the literature, he did suggest that the analyst note differences in usage across disciplinary boundaries. He did not discuss the use of case development in his approach.

Like Sartori, Schwartz-Barcott and Kim recommended initiating their hybrid approach to concept analysis with a review of the literature. Although they did not address the topic of case development, their empirical phase entailed data collection for the purpose of both developing the concept and illustrating its *real world* existence. Their approach speaks to the importance of balancing reliance on existing literature and new data when the intent is the further refinement of a relatively new or undeveloped concept.

The strategies described in this paper provide an overview of selected approaches to knowledge synthesis and concept development. They accommodate a wide variety of purposes and knowledge bases. Most can be used either to prepare for further research or as free-standing scholarly endeavors. We recommend that the strategies described be viewed as a "menu of possibilities." Selection of a specific item from the menu might reasonably begin by considering the scope of your interests. If the focus of interest is a particular concept rather than a broader substantive or theoretical area, you can consider menu items specific to concept analysis. Within this narrower range of choices, it is important to keep in mind that different approaches to concept analysis are geared to somewhat different purposes. Rodgers (1989a, 1989b) and Sartori (1984) focus their attention solely on concept clarification; Chinn and Jacobs (1983, 1987), Chinn and Kramer (1991), and Walker and Avant (1983, 1988) cite a wider range of purposes including such aims as developing an operational definition or refining a nursing diagnosis. Chinn and Kramer (1991) point out that concept analysis is a way to create conceptual meaning and that different purposes can advance that more general goal. Schwartz-Barcott and Kim's (1986) approach is specifically geared to using formal concept analysis as a starting point for further empirical work geared to elaborating the concept.

Persons interested in synthesizing knowledge in a more encompassing substantive or theoretical domain can choose from a variety of approaches for conducting reviews of the literature. If the field of interest is characterized primarily by experimental studies, meta-analysis may be an ideal way to synthesize knowledge. In contrast, meta-ethnography is especially tailored to fields of study dominated by qualitative work. The conventional integrative review provides a useful alternative for scholars who do not choose to limit their review to studies using a particular type of methodology. Whatever approach to knowledge synthesis is finally chosen, scholars embarking on such a project are encouraged to consider the full array of possibilities and to select the one most suited to their purposes.

REFERENCES

Abraham, I. L., & Schultz, S. (1983). Univariate statistical models for meta-analysis. *Nursing Research, 32,* 312–315.

Artinian, B. (1982). Conceptual mapping: Development of the strategy. *Western Journal of Nursing Research, 4,* 379–393.

Beck, C. T. (1996). A meta-analysis of predictors of postpartum depression. *Nursing Research, 45*(5), 297–303.

Booth-Kewley, S., & Friedman, H. S. (1987). Psychological predictors of heart disease: A quantitative review. *Psychological Bulletin, 101,* 343–362.

Boyd, C. (1985). Toward an understanding of mother-daughter identification using concept analysis. *Advances in Nursing Science, 7*(3), 78–86.

Broome, M. E. (1993). Integrative literature reviews in the development of concepts. In B. L. Rodgers & K. A. Knafl (Eds.), *Concept Development in Nursing* (pp. 193–215). Philadelphia: W. B. Saunders.

Brown, M., & Heffings, P. (1988). A case study of qualitative versus quantitative reviews: The maternal-infant bonding controversy. *Journal of Pediatric Nursing, 4,* 104–111.

Chinn, P., & Jacobs, M. (1983). *Theory and nursing: A systematic approach.* St. Louis: C. V. Mosby.

Chinn, P., & Jacobs, M. (1987). *Theory and nursing. A systematic approach* (2nd ed.). St. Louis: C. V. Mosby.

Chinn, P., & Kramer, M. (1991). *Theory and nursing. A systematic approach* (3rd ed.). St. Louis: C. V. Mosby.

Cooper, H. M. (1982). Scientific guidelines for conducting integrative research reviews. *Review of Educational Research, 52,* 291–302.

Cooper, H. M. (1984). *The integrative research review. A systematic approach.* Beverly Hills: Sage.

Cooper, H. M. (1989). *Integrating research. A guide for literature reviews* (2nd ed.). Beverly Hills: Sage.

Devine, E. C., & Cook, T. D. (1983). A meta-analytic analysis of psychoeducational interventions on length of postsurgical hospital stay. *Nursing Research, 32,* 267–274.

Dixon, D. M. (1996). Unifying concepts in parents' experiences with health care providers. *Journal of Family Nursing, 2*(2), 111–132.

Downs, F. (1989). New questions and new answers. *Nursing Research, 38,* 323.

Forsyth, G. L (1980). Analysis of the concept of empathy: Illustration of one approach. *Advances in Nursing Science, 2*(2), 33–42.

Ganong, L. H. (1987). Integrative reviews of nursing research. *Research in Nursing and Health, 10,* 1-11.

Glass, G. (1976). Primary, secondary, and meta analysis of research. *Educational Researcher, 5,* 3-8.

Hardy, M. K. (1974). Theories: Components, development, evaluation. *Nursing Research, 23,* 100-107.

Henson, R. H. (1997). Analysis of the concept of mutuality. *Image: Journal of Nursing Scholarship, 29*(1), 77-81.

Jackson, G. B. (1980). Methods for integrative reviews. *Reviews of Educational Research, 50,* 438-460.

Jackson, R. (1984). Ethnicity. In G. Sartori (Ed.), *Social science concepts: A systematic approach* (pp. 205-233). Beverly Hills: Sage.

Jacox, A. (1974). Theory construction in nursing: An overview. *Nursing Research, 23,* 4-13.

Kinney, M. R., Burfitt, S. N., Stullenbarger, E., Rees, B., & DeBolt, M. R. (1996). Quality of life in cardiac patient research: A meta-analysis. *Nursing Research, 45*(3), 173-180.

Knafl, K. A., & Deatrick, J. A. (1986). How families manage chronic conditions: An analysis of the concept of normalization. *Research in Nursing and Health, 9,* 215-222.

Knafl, K. A., & Deatrick, J. A. (1990). Family management style: Concept analysis and development. *Journal of Pediatric Nursing, 5,* 4-14.

Krywanio M. L. (1994). Meta-analysis of physiological outcomes of hospital-based infant intervention programs. *Nursing Research, 43,* 133-137.

Lamb, M., & Hwang, C. (1982). Maternal attachment and mother-neonate bonding: A critical review. In M. Lamb & A. Brown (Eds.), *Advances in developmental psychology* (Vol. 2, pp. 1-39). Hillsdale, NJ: Eribaum.

Madden, B. (1990). The hybrid model for concept development: Its value for the study of therapeutic alliance. *Advances in Nursing Science, 12*(3), 75-87.

Noblit, G., & Hare, R. (1988). *Meta-ethnography: Synthesizing qualitative studies.* Beverly Hills: Sage.

Norris, C. M. (Ed.). (1982). *Concept clarification in nursing.* Germantown, MD: Aspen Systems.

Ogden, C.Y., & Richards, I. A. (1946). *The meaning of meaning.* New York: Harcourt Brace Jovanovich.

Phillips, M. (1991). Chronic sorrow in mothers of chronically ill and disabled children. *Issues in Comprehensive Pediatric Nursing, 14,* 111-120.

Price, H. H. (1953). *Thinking and experience.* London: Hutchinson House.

Rew, L. (1986). Intuition: Concept analysis of a group phenomenon. *Advances in Nursing Science, 8*(2), 21-28.

Reynolds, P. (1971). *A primer in theory construction.* Indianapolis: Bobbs-Merrill.

Rodgers, B. L. (1989a). Concepts, analysis, and the development of nursing knowledge: The evolutionary cycle. *Journal of Advanced Nursing, 14,* 330-335.

Rodgers, B. L. (1989b). Exploring health policy as a concept. *Western Journal of Nursing Research, 11,* 694-702.

Rodgers, B. L. (1993). Concept analysis: An evolutionary view. In B. L. Rodgers & K. A. Knafl (Eds.), *Concept development in nursing* (pp. 73-92). Philadelphia: W. B. Saunders.

Rorty, R. (1979). *Philosophy and the mirror of nature.* Princeton, NJ: Princeton University Press.

Sartori, G. (1984). *Social science concepts: A systematic analysis.* Beverly Hills: Sage.

Schatzman, L., & Strauss, A. (1973). *Field research. Strategies for a natural sociology.* Englewood Cliffs, NJ: Prentice Hall.

Schwartz-Barcott, D., & Kim, H. (1986). A hybrid model for concept development. In P. L Chinn (Ed.), *Nursing research methodology: Issues and implementation* (pp. 91–101). Rockville, MD: Aspen.

Smith, C., & Naftel, D. (1984). Meta-analysis: A perspective for research synthesis. *Image, 16,* 9–13.

Tilden, V. (1985). Issues of conceptualization and measurement of social support in the construction of nursing theory. *Research in Nursing and Health, 8,* 199–206.

Toulmin, S. (1972). *Human understanding.* Princeton, NJ: Princeton University Press.

Walker, L. O., & Avant, K. C. (1983). *Strategies for theory construction in nursing.* Norwalk, CT: Appleton-Century-Crofts.

Walker, L. O., & Avant, K. C. (1988). *Strategies for theory construction in nursing* (2nd ed.). Norwalk, CT: Appleton and Lange.

Walker, L. O., & Avant, K. C. (1994). *Strategies for theory construction in nursing* (3rd ed.). Norwalk, CT: Appleton and Lange.

Warren, B. J. (1993). Explaining social isolation through concept analysis. *Archives of Psychiatric Nursing, 7*(5), 270–276.

Westra, B. L., & Rodgers, B. L. (1991). The concept of integration: A foundation for evaluating outcomes of nursing care. *Journal of Professional Nursing, 7,* 277–282.

Wilson, J. (1969). *Thinking with concepts.* New York: Cambridge University Press.

Wittgenstein, L. (1968). *Philosophical investigations* (3rd ed.). (G. E. M. Anscombe, Trans.). New York: MacMillan. (Original work published 1953)

The Wilson Method of Concept Analysis

Kay C. Avant

In the preface to his book *Thinking with Concepts* (1963), Wilson explained that the text was written expressly to be "worked through" by students (in particular, his sixth form—or high school—students) in an effort to gain skill in answering questions of a conceptual nature. He proposed that analysis of concepts "gives framework and purposiveness to thinking that might otherwise meander indefinitely and purposelessly among the vast marshes of intellect and culture" (p. ix). Throughout the book, Wilson continued to emphasize that concept analysis is a technique that aids the user in clear thinking and communication.

Wilson spent the first part of his book discussing the methods and techniques of concept analysis. Parts 2 and 4 are extensive examples of the use of the techniques and some practice exercises for the reader or student. Part 3 is a brief discussion of the links between philosophy and concept analysis. For further explanations of Parts 2, 3, and 4, the reader is referred to the original source. For the purposes of this chapter, Part 1 of Wilson's book will be the primary source of information.

In this chapter, the techniques Wilson advocated will be explained and then will be used in examining a concept of interest to nursing. The concept to be examined will be *science.*

Wilson listed 11 steps in concept analysis:

1. Isolating questions of concept
2. Finding right answers
3. Model cases
4. Contrary cases
5. Related cases
6. Borderline cases
7. Invented cases
8. Social context
9. Underlying anxiety
10. Practical results
11. Results in language

Each of these 11 steps will be considered separately with a nursing example used to illustrate each step.

ISOLATING QUESTIONS OF CONCEPT

Wilson distinguished among three types of questions: questions of fact, questions of values, and questions of concept. Questions of fact can be answered with knowledge that is already available in some form. Questions of value are answered based on moral principles present within an individual or a society. Questions of concept, however, are about meaning; the way questions of concept are answered depends entirely on the angle from which the analyst is looking at them. Wilson uses the example of the question "Is a whale a fish?" (1963, p. 4). The answer to this question, according to Wilson, might vary depending on whether the one posing the question was a marine biologist or working in the Ministry of Agriculture and Fisheries. To the marine biologist, because a whale is a mammal, it may not "count" as a fish. On the other hand, to someone from the Ministry of Agriculture and Fisheries, a whale probably would be considered a fish since it swims in the sea with the other fish.

Wilson (1963) made it clear that questions are rarely in their pure form. Many questions are mixed; that is, they require more than one type of analysis in order to answer them. He gave the example of the question "Should people in mental asylums [sic] ever be punished?" (p. 23). To answer this question clearly, the analyst must know some facts about the kinds of people usually found in psychiatric hospitals, know what is meant by the concept of punishment, and make a value or moral judgment about whether punishment is appropriate for such people. Therefore, before embarking on a concept analysis, the analyst should be sure that the question being answered is one of concept and not one of fact or value.

What is of concern in questions of concept are the actual and possible uses of words. When asking a question of concept, one is asking "what counts" as the concept or "what criteria" are being used to determine the meaning of the concept. Wilson suggests that one should take concepts seriously by becoming self-conscious about how words are used.

Concepts, and the words used to express them, are meant to serve human purposes and to do so efficiently. The way a person decides to use a word is of considerable importance. Words often do not have a single meaning. Individuals in various geographical regions may use the same word, but the meaning may be entirely different. Meanings for words change over time and over generations. For instance, in the West and Southwest, a *dude* meant someone who was unfamiliar with a working farm or ranch and who often wore inappropriate clothing for such work. A *dude* was an object of derision. Now, a *dude* is "cool" to youngsters, thanks to a popular movie concerning mutant turtles and Bart Simpson.

Two disciplines may use the same label for a concept that may have different meanings in those two disciplines. For instance, the concept of *support* is somewhat different in architecture and in nursing. In architecture, the concept of support is used to express the idea of a physical structure underlying and upholding an edifice. In nursing, however, the concept of support is more often used to mean emotional or social assistance.

A question often asked in nursing is "Is nursing a science or an art?" A corollary to this question is "Should nursing be a science?" These two questions demonstrate Wilson's ideas about questions of fact, values, and concept. The first question is a question of concept. The second one is a question of value. The issue of whether nursing *should* be a science is not one that can be answered by either facts or analysis of the concept. It can only be answered by examining values. However, the question about whether nursing is an art or a science *is* a question of concept. It requires an understanding of what nursing is and also what science is. What counts as nursing? What counts as science? These questions can be answered by determining what nursing is and what science is and then comparing the essential elements of nursing to the essential elements of science to determine the fit. For the purposes of this chapter, we will assume that the reader already knows the essential elements of nursing and thus will focus only on the concept of science.

"RIGHT" ANSWERS

Often questions about concepts do not have a single "right" answer. It may be inappropriate to speak of *the* meaning of a word. It is also unwise, however, to assume that concepts are completely limitless and may be defined any way one pleases. Some ways in which a concept is used are closer to the heart or core of the concept than others. The uses that are somehow farther from the core are frequently metaphors, extensions, derivations, or borderline uses of the concept. The analyst needs to determine which elements are essential to the core of the concept and which are not.

A concept may be used in two contexts, each of which implies a different meaning. For example, a period in history is a particular and circumscribed length of time in which certain significant events occurred; but a *period* in grammar is a mark of punctuation. The two contexts lend different shades of meaning to the same concept. By looking closely at the various uses of *period,* however, you can determine that there are some essential elements that remain constant over all contexts, such as the element of an end point. Wilson points out that it is the sensitivity of the analyst to these *essential* and *nonessential* elements that makes for a successful analysis. In all concept analyses, the goal is clarity of language and cogency of communication. Therefore, determining the really essential or typical features of a concept is a priority.

In the case of *science,* many definitions have been formulated over time. In the interests of brevity, only the most common ones will be used here.

Webster's New Universal Unabridged Dictionary (1983) defines science as

> a) state or fact of knowing; knowledge; b) systematized knowledge derived from observation, study, and experimentation carried on in order to determine the nature or principles of what is being studied; c) a branch of knowledge or study, especially one concerned with establishing and systematizing facts, principles, and methods, as by experiments and hypotheses; d) the systematized knowledge of nature and the physical world; e) skill, technique, or ability based upon training, discipline, and experience.

Shapere (1984), a sociologist of science, defined science as the "process by which areas or fields of scientific investigation are formed" (p. xxii). Woolgar (1988), also a sociologist of science, stated that "what counts as science varies according to the particular textual purposes for which this is an issue" (p. 21). In effect, he argues that science is basically a social activity engaged in by participants who define science within the context of their interactions. Griffin (1988), a philosopher of science, defined science as "the attempt to establish truth through demonstrations open to experiential replication" (p. 26).

MODEL CASES

One of the best ways to begin a good analysis is to find an instance that the investigator is absolutely sure is an example of the concept under study. The instance should be so obvious that you could say, "Well if *that* isn't an example of so-and-so, then nothing is" (Wilson, 1963, p. 28). The model case is used to help the analyst see what the essential features are that allow a person to use the word correctly. Model cases are the paradigm, or exemplary, cases of the concept under study. Therefore they are critical to a good analysis. Most model cases are chosen based on the analyst's working definition of the concept. Moreover, the development of the model case is iterative; that is, the analyst works back and forth between the various cases and the working definition until the essential features of the concept become clear.

Wilson also suggested using more than one model case and comparing them. In this way, he said, the analyst can compare the essential features of each to see which ones are present in all cases. These would then be the essential features of the concept. Wilson warned, though, that some concepts do not have critical or essential features but do have typical features. That is, there may be concepts that have no single feature in common but that are linked by a group of characteristics. He gave the example of the concept of *games,* in which a typical feature is that two or more people can play. Yet it is not an essential feature because there are games like solitaire that do not require two people and that still clearly count as games.

In the example of science, a model case might be one such as this: A chemist is running a series of experiments in the laboratory. Based on previous work in the field, the chemist hypothesizes that a particular combination of chemicals will produce a drug that will reduce blood pressure in experimental rats. Over time, the chemist tries many combinations and amounts of the chemicals until a set is found that does reduce blood pressure in the rats. After many trials with that combination of chemicals, the chemist publishes an article in a refereed journal reporting the findings of the studies, linking them to other studies that have been done previously, proposing some changes in the underlying theory, and suggesting areas for further study.

Another case might be that of a nurse, who in the course of practice, observes certain recurring behaviors in a particular set of patients with a particular nursing diagnosis. On the basis of both literature review and clinical judgment, the nurse sets up a series of experimental therapies using volunteers from among the patients with the relevant diagnosis. Analysis of the data leads the nurse to believe that one treatment is substantially better than the others in outcome. After publishing the initial results, the nurse conducts several more studies to confirm the findings. Finally, the nurse writes a theoretical paper synthesizing the results of all the studies and proposes a therapeutic model for the treatment of the particular diagnosis.

These are cases easily recognized by people as examples of *science.* What are the distinguishing characteristics as seen in these two cases? The elements common to both cases are knowledge generation, knowledge testing, knowledge organization, and knowledge accumulation. There is also an element of experience involved, as both scientists are skilled practitioners. In addition, both scientists communicated their work to others in their respective disciplines, and both were concerned with real world problems. That is, each scientist expects his or her work to have some practical significance in the future. There is a sense of ongoing activity as well.

CONTRARY CASES

The opposite method can also be helpful. That is, one can find an instance in which one could say "Well, whatever so-and-so is, *that* certainly isn't an instance of it" (Wilson, 1963, p. 29). Again, Wilson suggested using more than one contrary case, if necessary, and comparing across cases to discover what it is about them that makes them cases of *not*-the-concept. The features of the cases that make them contrary furnish clues to what features might be essential to the concept under study.

In the case of science, a contrary case is the following: A mother is watching her twins play in the back yard with a friend. She observes that the twins behave differently with one another than with their friend. She does not understand why this is so. After watching for a few moments, she turns away and begins washing the dishes.

This is clearly not an instance of science. The mother makes observations, but there is no effort to interpret them, to study the phenomenon systematically, or to accumulate or communicate the knowledge in any way.

RELATED CASES

Most concepts are not studied in isolation. As a rule, the concept under study is connected to other concepts that are similar or that occur in similar contexts. One must examine the network of concepts of which the concept under study is a part in order to truly understand how the study concept is the same and how it is different from those in the same network with it. It is through the critical examination of the network of related concepts that the analyst can gain insight into which features of the study concept are essential and which are not.

For the concept of science, *philosophy* is a related concept, as is *scholarship*. In *philosophy* the case might be that of a professor writing a series of treatises on the origins of ethical reasoning in the Celtic culture. For *scholarship* the case might be that of a student carefully examining all the literature on a given topic and writing a paper synthesizing the knowledge.

Neither of these cases is an example of science, although they are closer to it than the contrary case. Both are cases of scholarly endeavor, but they do not encompass all the essential elements of science. In the case of philosophy, there is no knowledge testing and no evidence in the case that the professor has plans to share the treatises with his professional colleagues. Nor is there evidence that the activity will be ongoing. In the scholarship case the student is synthesizing accumulated knowledge but is not generating it, testing it, or sharing it. Nor is the student likely to continue with the activity once the paper is turned in.

BORDERLINE CASES

Borderline cases are those in which the analyst is not sure whether a case fits as an example of the concept or not. The analyst deliberately uses instances that are difficult to classify. By understanding what makes them difficult to classify, the analyst can often determine which elements are essential to the concept and which are not. This activity helps the analyst clarify what counts as the concept and what does not.

In the case of science, one borderline case might be a single study and another might be, for example, a car mechanic searching for the solution to a problem until it is found. In a study, hypotheses are generated and tested and results are obtained. The difference between science and a single study is that a single study can either generate knowledge or test knowledge, but unless that knowledge is published it does not add to a body of knowledge. The researcher may or may not be skilled and the research may or may not be concerned with a real world problem. A single research study does not imply any ongoing work. Research is only a method of science; it is not science itself. The case of the car mechanic is also a borderline case because hypotheses are tested until a solution is found. Moreover, no knowledge may be generated, no additions are made to the body of knowledge of the field, and the mechanic may or may not be skilled in his or her practice.

INVENTED CASES

Sometimes, the concept under study is such that the scientist cannot discover a sufficient number of different instances to clarify the concept. In this case, it is often helpful to take the concept outside of one's own experience. Wilson (1963) used the concept of "man" to illustrate his point (p. 32). Finding the essential criteria for a man is particularly difficult when in our world men are so easily classified as *men*. This may seem confusing since it suggests that one might need to invent cases when concepts are rare and also when concepts are very familiar. This is, however, exactly what Wilson meant. It is not the rarity of the concept or its frequency but the generalized agreement across cultures about what counts as the concept that is problematic.

To determine what the essential elements of *man* are, since there is such universal agreement across cultures about what a *man* is, one cannot find enough different instances of it to clarify the concept. Wilson suggested that taking a concept out of its context and using our imagination to understand our actual experience is often a fruitful way to grasp the essential elements of the concept under study. For instance, Wilson asked whether a creature who lives on the earth, has intelligence, and looks like a man but has no emotions, no art, and no sense of humor would count as a man. Since we identified relatively clear cases for the concept of science, no invented case was developed.

SOCIAL CONTEXT

Language only occurs within a social context. Thus, concepts take on meaning within that social context. But, social contexts differ across cultures, across regions, and even across disciplines. Therefore, the sensitive analyst must take into account the social milieu in which the concept under study is used. The analyst might ask who might use the concept, when it might be used, why it might be used, and so forth as a way of determining the context in which it is likely to be used.

There seems to be more controversy over how *science* is defined than over the context in which it occurs. Most discussions of the term seem to hold to the view that science occurs in laboratories, in academic sites, in industry and commerce, and in clinical settings. Nevertheless, there may be subtle variations in the conceptual context even when there is general agreement about where it occurs. For instance, a chemist in an industrial setting might see science somewhat differently from a social worker in a family abuse shelter. Although the essential elements of science remain the same, the foci of the two disciplines may be such that what is seen as "good" science may be somewhat different. The choices of research methods may be different, or the emphasis on the individual essential elements may have different weights.

UNDERLYING ANXIETY

Associated with the idea of a social context for concepts is the idea that most persons use concepts for a purpose. That is, there is an underlying feeling or tone with all use of language. If the analyst can determine what feelings might be associated with the concept under study, some important insights about the concept may emerge. For instance, the analyst might ask, Has the concept generated strong feelings or controversy? Is there debate about the issue? Is it generally positive, or is it negative?

In nursing, the underlying anxiety about *science* seems to be a need to justify the discipline's existence and make it a legitimate academic enterprise. Interestingly, this is true not only of nursing but of other young sciences such as sociology and social work as well. There seems to be a feeling in the young disciplines that until the discipline achieves *science,* it is not valid. Moreover, in many of the young sciences the methods of the more established natural sciences are not always useful. The newer disciplines are working, along with nursing, to find better ways to acquire and accumulate knowledge; the analysts in these fields are thereby shaping and refining their understanding of the concept of science.

PRACTICAL RESULTS

Wilson said that understanding a concept ought to make some difference in our lives. In other words, there ought to be some practical result from understanding the essential elements of a concept. If there is no practical result from analysis of a concept, then something is seriously amiss with the language in which the question of concept was put. He suggests that if we understand the concept, we are more likely to understand the underlying worries of the person who is using it. And by understanding the underlying worries, we are more likely to respond to those worries appropriately.

In terms of the example concept with which we have been working, there seem to be four essential elements of the term *science*. The first is that science is concerned with knowledge—its generation, testing, organization, and accumulation. The second is that science is an experiential process that involves highly developed skills. The third is that science is a social activity within a group of like-minded scholars. The fourth is that there is some concern for truth in science; that is, the scientist is interested in at least some relationship between the knowledge developed and the world as it is experienced day by day.

RESULTS IN LANGUAGE

The final step in Wilson's procedure for concept analysis is obtaining results in language. Since words often have ambiguous meanings, it is not always possible to be decisive about *the* single or central meaning of a word. It is, however, still sensible to adopt one meaning over another. The purpose in doing so is to find the one meaning that works most efficiently, but that is not so restricted that it ceases to have any function at all. In other words, Wilson suggested that when one is choosing the essential features of a concept, one should choose those that are most useful. Wilson (1963) said that after careful concept analysis, one should be able to say, "Amid all these possible meanings of the word so-and-so, it seems most sensible and useful to make it mean such-and-such: for in this way we shall be able to use the word to its fullest advantage" (p. 37).

For the concept of *science,* the following is the most useful definition: the knowledge seeking, knowledge acquiring, knowledge accumulating, knowledge organizing, and knowledge disseminating activities of scholars in a particular field. These activities require a significant degree of skill, are experientially based, and are expected to produce knowledge that relates in some way to the world as it is experienced.

CONCLUSION

The Wilson (1963) method of concept analysis is an effective, easy-to-use method for discovering the essential features of a concept. Although it often seems a lengthy process to novices, it can be a helpful strategy, particularly in cases in which the concept is vague or has more than one meaning. His method is not complex and can be accomplished by persons as young as teenagers. It is an extremely useful strategy for classroom use in small groups and as a way of stimulating lively discussions. It is also very helpful for novice researchers as they attempt to arrive at operational definitions for their variables of interest.

Wilson suggested that the best way to conduct a good concept analysis is to follow all the steps in order. Yet he admitted that in some cases one or more of the last four steps may be either too obvious or irrelevant. In analyses in which that is so, the irrelevant steps may be omitted. The sensitivity of the analyst will enable her or him to make good use of the appropriate steps of the strategy.

In nursing, one of the most important tasks facing us as we develop our own science is the naming and development of our concepts. Until we have identified our concepts of concern, our science will not grow very rapidly. Concept analysis is extremely useful as a tool for clarifying potential concepts of interest.

Concept analysis is also valuable prior to tool development. Nursing lacks appropriate tools to measure many important concepts. A good concept analysis yields essential elements of the concept that can then be incorporated into tools for measuring the concept. And when a tool is developed using concept analysis as a base, the researcher already has a head start on construct validity.

There are limits to what concept analysis can do, however. It cannot generate new concepts. It cannot give answers to all our questions about which concepts should have the most emphasis in the discipline, nor can it tell us which concepts are the best for nursing.

A single concept, by itself, is only useful for naming a phenomenon. But when it is related to other concepts, it becomes more useful to the discipline. Concepts in relationships or patterns are what drive nurse scholars to ask questions, to try to answer those questions, and to contribute to the development of nursing *science.*

REFERENCES

Griffin, D. R. (1988). *The reenchantment of science.* New York: State University of New York Press.

Shapere, D. (1984). *Reason and the search for knowledge.* Boston: D. Reidel.

Webster, N. (1983). *Webster's new universal unabridged dictionary* (2nd ed.). New York: Dorset & Baber.

Wilson, J. (1963). *Thinking with concepts.* Cambridge: Cambridge University Press.

Woolgar, S. (1988). *Science: The very idea.* New York: Tavistock.

5

Wilsonian Concept Analysis: Applying the Technique

Kay C. Avant and Cynthia Allen Abbott

In this chapter the technique suggested by Wilson (1963) will be used to examine a concept relevant to nursing practice. We have chosen the concept of delegation for analysis. It is abstract enough to lend itself to analysis; it is relevant to nursing practice; and it may have several different meanings. Because nurses are involved in delegation in all aspects of their work, a clear understanding of the essential elements of delegation is appropriate. This chapter is organized around Wilson's (1963) 11 steps in concept analysis. The reader is referred to Chapter 4 for a full explanation of each of the steps.

ISOLATING QUESTIONS OF CONCEPT

Questions are often raised about the nature of delegation and nursing care. Certain questions may be at issue, such as, Should nursing care ever be delegated? If a situation calls for delegation, is there ever one in which the authority is delegated but the responsibility is not? and To whom is it appropriate to delegate certain nursing care? However, these are not pure questions of concept. The first question is a question of value. It calls for both an analysis of the concept of delegation and a value judgment about its use. The second question is also a mixed question. It calls for a concept analysis for three different concepts (delegation, authority, and responsibility) and also for a policy analysis of the appropriate use of the concepts analyzed. The third question calls for a concept analysis and also is a question requiring the use of facts about the nature and qualifications of those to whom the delegated

---

These are the views of the author (Cynthia Abbott) and do not represent the views of the
U.S. Army, Department of Defense.

action might be given. A true question of concept would be, What is the logical nature of the concept of delegation? Therefore, this concept analysis will attempt to provide the answer to this last question.

RIGHT ANSWERS

Wilson (1963) pointed out that there are no final right answers in a concept analysis. However, he did emphasize that there are primary and central uses for *concepts* that can be distinguished by a thoughtful analysis. The effort is to determine which elements of the concept of delegation are the important or essential ones and which ones are extensions, derivations, or metaphors of the concept.

The concept of delegation has two principal uses. The first has to do with the act of assigning. The second use refers to a group with a mission.

In the first case the process of delegation includes ideas such as supervision and assignment of duties, the transfer of authority to subordinates to complete work (Johnson, 1996), as well as using time and expertise effectively (Conger, 1994; Rees, 1988). Delegation also includes the ideas of communication, responsibility, monitoring, supervision, and work (Johnson, 1996). To maximize the outcome of successful delegation, the superior must assess the subordinate (Johnson, 1996; Keenan et al., 1990; McAlvanah, 1989; McConkey, 1986; Poteet, 1984; Rees, 1988), the complexity of the work or task to be done (American Association of Critical Care Nurses [AACN], 1990; Bentley, 1985; Conger, 1994; Ericksen et al., 1992; Harbin, 1990; Keenan et al., 1990; McAlvanah, 1989; McConkey, 1986; Murphy, 1984; Olivant, 1984; Poteet, 1984, 1986), and the context or situation in which the work is to be done (AACN, 1990; Bass et al., 1975; Blau & Scott, 1962; Conger, 1994; Hoy & Bousa, 1984; Johnson, 1996; Leana, 1986, 1987; Runnie, 1985; Vinton, 1987) before making the assignment.

The superior assigns the subordinate to complete a specific task (AACN, 1990; Anders, 1988; Anderson, 1984, Haynes, 1974; Hoy & Bousa, 1984; Johnson, 1996; Leana, 1986; Poteet, 1984, 1986; Rees, 1988; Vinton, 1987). The superior communicates to the subordinate (Bass et al., 1975; Harbin, 1990; Johnson, 1996; McAlvanah, 1989; Olivant, 1984; Poteet, 1984; Runnie, 1985; Shapira, 1976; Vinton, 1987; Watson, 1983) the needed performance criteria (Harbin, 1990; McConkey, 1986; Poteet, 1984; Rees, 1988; Watson, 1983), time allowed (Poteet, 1986), and plans for providing feedback (AACN, 1990; Bentley, 1985; Keenan et al., 1990; Rees, 1988). The superior transfers to the subordinate the authority (AACN, 1990; Anderson, 1984; Hoy & Bousa, 1984; Leana, 1986, 1987; Murphy, 1984; Rees, 1988; Runnie, 1985; Shapira, 1976; Vinton, 1987), resources (Bentley, 1985; Conger, 1994;

Haynes, 1974; Rees, 1988; Vinton, 1987), and responsibility necessary to complete the task or work (Anders, 1988; Anderson, 1984; Bentley, 1985; Haynes, 1974; Keenan et al., 1990; McAlvanah, 1989; McConkey, 1986; Murphy, 1984; Poteet, 1986; Rees, 1988; Simpson & Sears, 1985). The superior does not interfere with task completion unless assistance is sought by the subordinate (Hay & Bousa, 1984; Keenan et al., 1990; Leana, 1986, 1987; Rees, 1988; Simpson & Sears, 1985; Vinton, 1987). The superior completes the work through the subordinate (Conger, 1994; Drucker, 1963).

In the second case the person (delegate) is selected, elected, or appointed by another person, a group of persons, or an organization to represent their interests, usually to an even larger body of persons or organizations. A set of such selected persons is referred to as a *delegation*. The delegation here is a body of people and is not the activity itself. This second use of the concept *delegation* appears to be an extension of the primary concept in that the delegates are the ones who receive the assignment. The real delegation occurs from the group or organization that selects or appoints the delegates. Therefore, it is the first use of the concept that will be considered here because it is the primary concept, or the activity of delegation, that is of interest to us.

MODEL CASES

Case 1

A working mother is feeling overwhelmed with all the tasks she must accomplish in two hours to prepare for a dinner party for six close friends. She considers ways to decrease the number of things she must do. She reviews which tasks are most complicated and decides that only she can plan the menu and prepare the meal for the dinner party. Two other tasks are vacuuming the carpets and dusting the furniture. She believes her 10-year-old daughter can vacuum and dust reliably because the daughter has done these chores several times before under the mother's supervision.

The mother directs the daughter to vacuum the carpets and dust before 6 PM. She needs to vacuum the hall, living room, and dining room to remove the visible dirt and lint on the floors. She should dust the furniture in those same three rooms. The mother tells the daughter she is to ask her if more information or assistance is needed in doing the task.

As the daughter vacuums, the father comes down the hall in muddy shoes. The daughter cries out, "Stop, you have to take your shoes off! I'm cleaning the floor for mom and I don't want to vacuum the hall again!" The father follows his daughter's direction and takes off his shoes before continuing down the hall. The mother occasionally checks the progress and quality of vacuuming and dusting completed. Finally, the mother examines the completed job, provides approval of the work, and rewards the daughter by allowing her to have a friend over the next night to play.

Case 2

A second model case, taken from nursing, is the case of the nursing team leader making assignments for the upcoming shift. She reviews the case load, the patient acuity status, and the number and type of staff she will have on duty. She knows that several of the patients are very sick and will need her best staff nurses. A number of patients are not so sick and will need less skilled care. When her staff arrives, she discusses the case load with them and assigns the care of specific patients according to her knowledge of the competency levels of her staff and the predictability, severity, and needs of the patients. She tells staff members what her expectations are and tells them to ask for help if they need it.

Later in the morning, as she makes rounds to check on the patients and the staff, the new staff nurse asks for help calibrating an infusion pump. The team leader shows the nurse how to calibrate the pump, then watches as the nurse calibrates the infusion properly. She commends the new nurse on his skill and on his willingness to ask for help.

Conclusions. In both of these cases, there are common elements. In each case there is work to be done, a person who is responsible for the work to be done (superior or delegator), and another person to whom the work is assigned (subordinate or delegate). In each case the delegator communicates what work is to be done and her expectations for the completion of the work. Access to needed resources is provided to the delegate. The delegator monitors the progress of the work and rewards the delegate at the successful completion of the work. The delegate in each case assumes the responsibility, demonstrates the competency, and takes the authority to complete the work.

CONTRARY CASES

Contrary cases are those cases that clearly do not apply to the concept under study. Contrary cases help to clarify the essential elements of the concept by focusing on the opposite of it. Sometimes it is easier to say what a thing is not than to say what it is. The contrary cases give a different view of the concept and allow the analyst to compare one case against its opposite.

Case 1

A contrary case from the model case might be that of a working mother who is feeling overwhelmed with all the tasks she must accomplish in two hours to prepare for a dinner party for six close friends. She goes over the tasks and prioritizes them. She decides to dust the furniture but not to vacuum, to clean the bathroom but not the bedrooms, and to simplify the menu by purchasing dessert instead of making it herself. She picks up the dessert on the way home from work. When she gets home, she hastily completes all the tasks she has listed and with dinner in the oven, finds she has just enough time to change her clothes before the guests arrive.

Case 2

A contrary case in nursing might be that of Mr. Smith, one of two team leaders on his unit. Mr. Smith walks through a bad snowstorm to get to work one morning only to discover that he is the only one on his team who has managed to get to work so far. There are messages from three others on the team that they are on their way but that they are delayed because of unplowed streets. He calls the nursing supervisor to report his plight, but she tells him he is not alone. The same situation has happened all over the hospital. She tells him that she has asked some night staff to stay on for at least another hour or so and that she has called an agency for help. In the meantime, he must just do the best he can until she can send him some help. Sighing, Mr. Smith reviews the patient load, prioritizes the tasks to he done, and taking the highest priorities first, begins to work. He continues to complete the high-priority tasks as best he can and hopes fervently for more help to arrive soon.

Conclusions. These cases are not cases of delegation. Although the woman has a lot of work to do, she never seeks to assign any of it to anyone else. She does review the tasks and determines priorities, but she never communicates them to anyone and does not ask for help. Mr. Smith also does not delegate. He does review the tasks and assigns priorities. If more of his team arrives later, he will delegate some of the work at that point. However, since he is alone, he cannot delegate.

RELATED CASES

Related cases are cases that somehow are similar to or connected with the concept under analysis. In the case of the concept of delegation, the concepts of trust and of referring and transferring seemed to be the most germane because delegation is often difficult when trust has not been established between the delegator and the delegate and because referring and transferring are often used as synonyms for delegation. Distinguishing among these concepts should aid the analysis of delegation.

Case 1

Jonathan is the commander of a garrison on the frontier. His scout, David, tells him there are enemy troops just over the hill from the garrison headquarters. Although Jonathan does not see the enemy soldiers, he calls his officers together and tells them to prepare for a possible enemy attack. His officers question why he is preparing for attack when no enemy is in sight. He replies, "I trust David's report."

Conclusion. The concept of trust is defined in *Webster's Ninth New Collegiate Dictionary* as "assured reliance on the character, ability, strength, or *truth* of someone or something" (1983). It involves a relationship between two persons in which one can be confident of the other's abilities and values and can depend on the other to behave in certain ways under certain conditions. Trust between a superior and a subordinate is antecedent to delegation because the delegator must be confident of the delegate before giving him or her the assignment.

Case 2

Mrs. Loners, the high school counselor, is called to the teacher's lounge by Mr. Clark, the math teacher. When she arrives, she finds Mr. Clark and Dorothy, a junior student. Dorothy is crying, wringing her hands, and looking fearfully toward the corner of the room. Mr. Clark tells Mrs. Loners that Dorothy began acting strangely in class, mumbling at first and then yelling "Get away from me! Get away!" even though no one was near her at the time. Mr. Clark says, "I am not equipped to handle this one. I will leave her in your capable hands." He leaves the room and returns to class.

Conclusion. The concept of referring is sometimes used as a synonym for delegation. To refer is to "think of; regard, or classify within a general category or group; to send or direct for treatment, aid, information or decision" (*Webster's,* 1983). From the case and from the definition it can be seen that to refer something involves giving up the decision-making task altogether. The person making the referral may not retain any of the responsibility for further decision making once the referral is made. The referring individual does not communicate how the job is to be done, does not provide resources to do the job, and does not monitor the results.

Case 3

Mrs. Loners attempts to talk to Dorothy but is unable to get her to respond. After several attempts she takes Dorothy to her office and calls Dorothy's parents. She explains the situation to the parents and tells them that they must come and pick Dorothy up. She explains that the school system is not prepared to deal with such a situation. When the parents arrive, Mrs. Loners urges them to seek immediate treatment for Dorothy and provides the names of several psychologists who treat teenagers. She hands Dorothy over to them and sadly watches as the family leaves the school.

Conclusion. The concept of transferring is also related to delegation. It is defined as "to convey from one person, place, or situation to another; to cause to pass from one to another" (*Webster's,* 1983). In the case of transfer, the person transferring again retains no authority or responsibility for the item or work that is passed to the other. Little or no communication about the item or work may take place between the transferring person and the person to whom the item or work is transferred.

BORDERLINE CASES

Borderline cases are those in which one is not sure whether the case is one of delegation. The borderline cases are particularly useful because by trying to see what makes them borderline, it is possible to determine what there is in the model case that is essential. Two borderline cases are used in this analysis to point out essential features of delegation.

Case 1

The high school needed a significant curriculum change. The principal was asked by a group of faculty to consider a revised curriculum. The principal formed a task force of teachers to consider all areas of possible change such as content areas, recommended textbooks, teaching styles, and ancillary support required to implement a new curriculum. She gave the task force access to all needed resources and gave the members authority to ask other faculty for additional information. The principal gave the task force performance criteria, time expectations, and planned weekly meetings to guide job completion. She stated that if the aforementioned criteria were met and if the faculty reached 100 percent agreement on all aspects of the proposed curriculum, the group would be able to implement the proposed curriculum as a pilot program. During weekly meetings the principal insisted that the task force make significant changes in their ideas and plans. Within the allotted time the task force completed the formal proposal with required criteria and support of all faculty. The principal did allow the faculty to implement the proposed curriculum as a pilot program.

Conclusion. The critical attributes of assignment, communication, and reward are present, but the attribute of transfer of authority is altered. Although access to needed resources was given, the principal did not allow the task force to complete the assignment without interference in their decision making. Her need to direct the task force when not asked interfered with the transference of authority to subordinates.

Case 2

Julia is a new head nurse who is trying to introduce a more participatory management style on her unit. Therefore, upon reviewing the case load and acuity level of patients and finding that most of the patients were no longer critical, she decides to let her staff make the assignments as a group after shift report. When the shift report is finished, she asks the staff, "Now, how are we going to arrange it so all these patients get the best care we can give them?" The staff decides to discuss the needs of each patient, and decide as a group who will take care of each one. The head nurse is pleased with the resulting decisions and smiles to herself as the staff leaves discussing how pleased they are with their work assignments.

Conclusion. This case is also a borderline case. Some of the essential elements of the model case are present, but some are not. There is work to be done. There is a superior and a group of subordinates, but they are not treated strictly as subordinates by the superior. Assignments are made but not by the superior. There is communication about the work to be done and expectations about how it should be done, but both are defined by the group and not by the superior. The superior does monitor the proceedings but does not interfere. The staff assumes responsibility for the work and carries it out.

INVENTED CASES

Invented cases are used when the concept under study does not provide a sufficient number of instances of the concept to clarify it (Wilson, 1963). In the case of delegation there are numerous instances, and an invented case is not strictly necessary. However, for the purposes of demonstrating the application of all of the steps in Wilson's (1963) method, an invented case has been included here.

Case Study

The king rat on planet Noah was a biblical historian and an astrologer. Wise men of his planet had predicted since his birth that his reign as king would end in the destruction of the planet. The king rat realized the predictions would soon be true, for in two months the planet Noah would collide with the sun. However, he had a plan to save the various species on the planet, based on knowledge of biblical literature.

The king rat devised a master plan and called his most trusted experts to meet. He charged the experts, such as anthropologists, sociologists, biologists, and nurse scientists, to choose one male and one female of fertile age from each species on the planet to represent inhabitants of the planet. He set the day the selection was to be complete and told the experts to use his name if anyone obstructed their mission. He proclaimed all of the experts to have supreme access to needed transportation, food, housing, staff, and any additional support requested. Additionally, he commissioned the air force high command to ready a spaceship with sufficient supplies and adequate environmental conditions to sustain all life for three years or until a safe haven was identified. The planet Earth was deemed a possible haven since it had reportedly undergone a similar crisis with flood millennia ago.

The king rat made it clear that he was available for counsel. He stated that he would oversee the results of the plan as experts progressed in their mission. Each expert was expected to contact him if problems that interfered with progress were encountered. Additionally, he reminded each member of the seriousness of the mission and of the potential consequences for the future life on planet Noah if even one individual did not succeed in effectively completing the collection of the species. At the completion of the mission and departure of the space ship from the planet Noah, the king rat praised the experts in public and knighted them for their success in completing the mission.

Conclusion. A superior-subordinate relationship involving trust and subordinate expertise is seen between the king and his subordinates. Additionally, this case illustrates the planning the king rat completed before assigning missions and charging the experts. Once assignments were made, the king transferred the authority to the experts by allowing them to use his name if they encountered resistance. Monitoring was addressed by supervising the progress of results as they occurred incrementally. Expecting the subordinate to tell the king if problems interfered with progress implies a transfer of responsibility for progress of the mission. Additionally, reviewing the consequences for the entire project should a mission fail transferred a piece of responsibility for the mission success to each subordinate. Access to all resources to include additional staff was transferred. And finally, the subordinates were rewarded for their work.

SOCIAL CONTEXT

The social context in which a concept is used can provide the analyst with insight into the essential nature of the concept. For instance, the concept of delegation is most often used in the context of business and management. Persons in positions of authority, and often those in subordinate positions as well, may be concerned about the proper use of delegation. When it is appropriate and when it is not, to whom tasks can or should be delegated, and how much monitoring and supervision are sufficient for delegated tasks are recurrent issues. Nurses are concerned with delegation at all levels. Nurse managers delegate to staff; staff delegate to assistive personnel; and, of course, physicians delegate to nurses as well. The complexity of the social contexts of health care agencies and systems, when considered alongside the social mandate for nurses to provide the best quality care in the most cost-effective manner, makes delegation a critical issue. To understand the concept of delegation, one must understand the complex nature of the health care system in which it occurs and the moral, legal, and technical issues surrounding delegation in that context.

The aspects of delegation most reflected in the social context have to do with the superior's assessment of the tasks to be done, the prioritizing of those tasks, the abilities of the subordinates, and the trust she or he has in those subordinates. In a system as complex as a health care agency, the superior manages tremendous responsibility for decisions involved in tasks delegated. If the superior is new to the system, for instance, or is inexperienced as a supervisor, the quality of this assessment may suffer. As a consequence of an inadequate assessment, tasks may be delegated inappropriately, leading to ineffective or perhaps unsafe patient care. On the whole, inappropriate delegation in nursing care may result in harm to patients or clients when delivered by those with inadequate skill, knowledge, or insufficient supervision by a nurse (Johnson, 1996).

UNDERLYING ANXIETY

Closely associated with considering the social context of a concept is examining the underlying anxiety associated with it. It seems to us that there are at least two underlying anxieties associated with the concept of delegation. First is the issue of whether any nursing task ought to be delegated at all. If a task is a nursing task, should it not be performed by a nurse? And yet, there are too many tasks and not enough nurses to carry out them all. Management decisions regarding hospital staffing levels may require that nurses delegate many tasks to non-nurses in order that patients receive adequate care.

A second underlying source of anxiety is which nursing tasks are safe to delegate and to whom? Does the context in which the tasks are to take place make a difference in whether they can be delegated? For instance, delegating the bath and linen change for a patient who is recovering from elective surgery and ready for discharge on the following day is potentially different from delegating the bath and linen change for a newly admitted, critically ill patient in medical intensive care. The issue of trust in the superior-subordinate relationship is important in resolving the underlying anxieties associated with delegation.

Both the social context and the underlying anxiety of the concept of delegation demonstrate that the issue of complexity of task, superior-subordinate trust, and ability of the delegate are important aspects of delegation. It must be the responsibility of the delegate or supervisor to clearly understand the task and the person delegated to perform the task.

PRACTICAL RESULTS

Wilson (1963) pointed out quite accurately that analyzing a concept should have some practical results. That is, one should consider what the purpose is in analyzing a concept. If the results are not useful, analyzing the concept is a waste of time. In the case of the concept of delegation, we feel that understanding the logical structure of the concept will help us to teach nurses what delegation entails (Conger, 1994; Johnson, 1996), to evaluate nurses' skill in delegating, to direct and coordinate patient care through others (Parsons, 1998), and to help us measure the concept in research. An understanding of the logical structure of the concept will provide a frame of reference for our work.

RESULTS IN LANGUAGE

Wilson (1963) suggested that in defining a logical structure for a concept, one should take care to choose the most useful criteria for the concept of interest. That is, care must be taken not to delimit the concept so much that it is essentially banned from one's working vocabulary. On the other hand, the concept should not be so loosely limited that it can be used in almost any situation and thus, in effect, become meaningless. Therefore, the priority of the analyst of any concept should be to choose the critical elements in such a way as to allow the use of the concept to its fullest advantage.

CONCLUSIONS

Having progressed through Wilson's 11 steps, we can now examine the results of our analysis to determine the logical structure of the concept of delegation. The premier consideration of an analysis, for Wilson, is the identification of the essential elements of the concept under analysis. Therefore, as a result of our analysis, the essential elements of the concept of delegation are as follows:

1. There must be a superior-subordinate relationship in which the superior has both responsibility and authority.
2. There must be a level of trust between the superior (the delegator) and the subordinate (the delegate).
3. There must be a task or set of tasks to be accomplished.
4. The delegator must assess the situation in terms of the complexity, priority, and potential risks of the task as well as the abilities of the delegate.
5. The delegator must assign the task to the delegate.
6. The delegator must communicate to the delegate any expectations about the way the task is to be completed.
7. The delegator must provide the delegate with access to resources needed to complete the task.
8. The delegate must assume responsibility for the task.
9. The delegator must monitor the completion of the task and provide feedback to the delegate about the effectiveness of task completion.
10. Both delegator and delegate benefit from the experience.

From this list of essential elements or characteristics, a clear picture of the process of delegation appears. It would be possible, using this list of essential elements, to prepare a lesson plan to teach the process of delegation to beginners in management and to determine the effectiveness and safety in delegating certain nursing tasks to assistive personnel. To Wilson, the process of concept analysis is undertaken to clarify one's thinking and to make communication easier. This concept analysis of delegation has served that purpose for us. We hope it will serve the same purpose for our readers.

REFERENCES

American Association of Critical Care Nurses (AACN). (1990). *Delegation of nursing and non-nursing activities in critical care.* Laguna Niguel, CA: AACN.

Anders, G. T. (August 15, 1988). Duties you should—and shouldn't—delegate. *Medical Economics,* pp. 182-191.

Anderson, J. G. (1984). When leaders develop themselves. *Training and Development Journal, 38*(6), 1822.

Bass, B. M., Valenzi, E. R., Farrow, D. L., & Solomon, R. J. (1975). Management styles associated with organizational, task, personal, and interpersonal contingencies. *Journal of Applied Psychology, 60*(6), 720-729.

Bentley, C. (1985). MI through the night. *Australian Nurses Journal, 14*(10), 41-44.

Blau, P. M., & Scott, W. R. (1962). *Formal organizations.* New York: Chandler.

Conger, M. (1994). The nursing assessment decision grid: Tool for delegation decision. *Journal of Continuing Education in Nursing, 25*(1), 21-27.

Drucker, P. (1963). Managing for business effectiveness. *Harvard Business Review, 41*(3), 18-26.

Ericksen, L., Quandt, B., Teinert, D., Look, D. L., Loosie, R., Mackey, G., & Strout, B. (1992). A registered nurse-licensed vocational nurse partnership model for critical care nursing. *Journal of Nursing Administration, 22*(12), 28–38.

Harbin, R. E. (1990). Practicing effective delegation. *Pediatric Nursing, 16*(1), 91–92.

Haynes, M. E. (1974). Delegation: Key to involvement. *Personnel Journal, 53,* 454–456.

Hoy, W. K., & Bousa, I. D. A. (1984). Delegation: The neglected aspect of participation in decision making. *Alberta Journal of Educational Research, 30,* 320–331.

Johnson, S. H. (1996). Teaching nursing delegation: Analyzing nurse practice acts. *Journal of Continuing Education in Nursing, 27*(2), 52–58.

Keenan, M. J., Hurst, J. B., Dennis, R. S., & Frey, O. (1990). Situational leadership for collaboration in health care settings. *Health Care Supervisor, 8*(3), 19–25.

Leana, C. R. (1986). Predictors and consequences of delegation. *Academy of Management Journal, 29,* 754–774.

Leana, C. R. (1987). Power relinquishment versus power sharing: Theoretical clarification and empirical comparison of delegation and participation. *Journal of Applied Psychology, 72,* 228–233.

McAlvanah, M. E. (1989). A guide to delegation. *Pediatric Nursing, 16,* 379.

McConkey, D. D. (1986). *No-nonsense delegation* (rev. ed.). New York: American Management Association.

Murphy, E. C. (1984). Delegation—from denial to acceptance. *Nursing Management, 15*(1), 54–56.

Olivant, M. (1984). Delegation problems. *Nursing Times, 80*(31), 43–44.

Parsons, L. C. (1998). Delegation skills and nurse job satisfaction. *Nursing Economics, 16*(1), 18–26.

Poteet, G. W. (1984). Delegation strategies a must for the nurse. *Executive Journal of Nursing Administration, 14*(9), 18–21.

Poteet, G. W. (1986). Delegation strategies for the pediatric nurse. *Journal of Pediatric Nursing, 1,* 271–273.

Rees, R. (1988). Delegation: A fundamental management process. *Education Canada, 28*(2), 26–32.

Runnie, R. J. (1985). School centered management: A matter of style. *School Business Affairs 51*(4), 64–67.

Shapira, Z. (1976). A facet analysis of leadership styles. *Journal of Applied Psychology, 61*(2), 136–139.

Simpson, K., & Sears, R. (1985). Authority and responsibility delegation predicts quality of care. *Journal of Advanced Nursing, 10,* 345–348.

Vinton, D. (1987). Delegation for employee development. *Training and Development Journal, 4*(1), 65–67.

Watson, C. (1983). Third-stage limits and delegation. *Nursing Mirror, 156*(18), 35.

Webster's ninth new collegiate dictionary. (1983). Frederick C. Mish (editor-in-chief). Springfield, MA: Merriam-Webster.

Wilson, J. (1963). *Thinking with concepts.* Cambridge: Cambridge University Press.

6

Concept Analysis: An Evolutionary View

Beth L. Rodgers

Historically, popular views of concepts and concept analysis have been based on a philosophical position known as essentialism. The purpose of analysis has been to define the concept of interest in terms of its critical attributes or "essence." This essence typically is presented as a set of conditions that are both necessary and sufficient to delineate the domain and boundaries of the concept. Consistent with an essentialist viewpoint, in such analyses the concept is examined apart from its context or any relationship with other concepts. Reports of this type of inquiry give the impression that the concept is both universal (that is, without contextual variation) and unchanging. In other words, the results are presumed to reveal precisely what the concept *is*.

Recently, philosophical discussions of concepts have presented views in opposition to the essentialist position and that show the flaws in this approach. The current tendency has been to consider concepts as dynamic, rather than static; "fuzzy," rather than finite, absolute, and "crystal clear"; context dependent, rather than universal; and to possess some pragmatic utility or purpose, rather than an inherent "truth" (Ryle, 1971; Toulmin, 1972; Wittgenstein, 1953/1968; see also Rodgers, Chapter 2 of this text). This contemporary view of concepts has gained considerable support from empirical research in the field of psychology (Barsalou & Medin, 1986; Fehr, 1988; McCloskey & Glucksberg, 1978; Medin & Bettger, 1994, Smith & Medin, 1981). It is worth noting as well that this position is compatible with the perspective generally accepted in nursing, which espouses a view of reality, and of human beings and related nursing phenomena, as constantly changing, comprised of numerous interrelated and overlapping elements, and interpretable only in regard to a multitude of contextual factors.

Unfortunately, researchers have not operationalized fully the implications of contemporary philosophical positions in actual methods of concept analysis. Adherence to essentialism has compromised the significance and utility of attempts to clarify and develop concepts in nursing. One alternative approach to concept analysis, which has been referred to as the "evolutionary" view (Rodgers, 1989a, 1989c, 1993), is derived from contemporary philosophical thought and was designed to overcome some of the difficulties associated with traditional positions.

THE PHILOSOPHICAL BASIS OF THE EVOLUTIONARY VIEW

The evolutionary approach to concepts represents the integration of views expressed primarily by Toulmin (1972) and Wittgenstein (1953/ 1968), although Price (1953) and Ryle (1971) also were influential. According to this approach, a concept is considered to be an "abstraction that is expressed in some form" (Rodgers, 1989a, p. 3). In other words, concepts are formed by the identification of characteristics common to a class of objects or phenomena and the abstraction and clustering of these characteristics, along with some means of expression (most often a word). Although concepts are individual and private in nature, the process of abstraction, clustering, and association of the concept with a word (or other means of expression) is influenced heavily by socialization and public interaction. The development of a concept for a person takes place with guidance from the social context in which the person interacts and develops concepts. As contextual factors vary, there will be variations in concepts over time or across situations.

Toulmin (1972) discussed this process in relation to socialization within a discipline, yet his term *enculturation* is appropriate to describe this process regardless of the specific context in which it occurs. An example of this process of enculturation is apparent in examination of the concept of health. In nursing, formal education and professional socialization both support the conceptualization of health as "more than the absence of disease," as expressed in this common axiom. This conceptualization is quite distinct from that of persons in other disciplines, and may be different from the concept held by a student upon entering a program of nursing education. The social interaction, education, and other aspects of professional development constitute a context of "enculturation" that supports a variation of the concept of health for nurses.

The forms of expression that are acquired along with a concept enable an individual to share his or her concepts publicly with others.

These forms of expression typically are discursive or linguistic, such as the use of the word "health" to express the concept of well-being noted above. It is important to recognize, however, that there may be nondiscursive forms of expression as well—for example, through various means of artistic expression, such as music, dance, or the visual arts. The work (1994) of noted choreographer Bill T. Jones provides an excellent example of how artistic forms can serve this purpose of expression as well. Jones worked with a multitude of individuals, people from all sorts of backgrounds who were diagnosed with terminal illness, and helped them to express their experience of terminal illness through dance. This work, created with members of the general population, led to the development of a multimedia dance performance (entitled *Still/Here*) to capture the expressions of these unique individuals. It is easy to imagine how difficult it might be to express through words what it is like to be terminally ill. However, the people involved in this project were quite capable of expressing their experiences through movements and dance. Similarly, the visual arts, such as paintings and sculpture, are widely recognized as significant media for expression. The power of such forms of expression has yet to be utilized as a focus of inquiry, yet may have tremendous potential for clarification of significant concepts in a discipline such as nursing.

These expressions, regardless of form, provide access to an individual's concepts and reflect the individual's use of the concept. Consequently they provide the basis for concept analysis. Words, as noted previously, are the most common focus of inquiry, and a ubiquitous form for expression of concepts. It is important to note, however, that a concept is not merely the word or expression but the mental cluster that lies behind the word. Words are manifestations of concepts (Price, 1953), not the concepts themselves.

Examination of the common use of a concept, through these expressions, provides a means to explore the underlying concept and to identify its attributes (definition). In other words, a concept can be defined by analyzing the ways in which it is used, and this use is apparent in the ways the associated term is used. It is important to remember that it is not the word (expression) that is of primary interest, but the idea (concept) that is expressed using the identified word.

Although many scholars view the process of defining concepts as important, in existing discussions relatively little attention has been given to the relationship between concepts and knowledge. In other words, what purpose(s) do concepts serve in the general enterprise of knowledge development? According to Toulmin (1972), concepts, especially what he termed "scientific" concepts, contribute to knowledge because of their inherent "explanatory" powers. (A thorough reading of Toulmin's work reveals that he used the terms *scientific* and *explanatory* quite loosely. Nonetheless, it is probably more appropriate to refer to concepts as having explanatory or descriptive power.) One of the primary functions of concepts is to facilitate categorizations. In other words, concepts are important in determining how to refer to or discuss certain situations, events, or phenomena, and how various conceptual categories may be related to each other. When concepts are clear, which means that their definitions are articulated and understood, it is possible to "explain" phenomena as belonging to or indicative of a particular concept and, consequently, as possessing certain attributes. Clear concepts are necessary to characterize phenomena of interest, to describe situations appropriately, and to communicate effectively.

When the attributes (definition) that comprise the concept are not clear, the ability to communicate and categorize phenomena is severely limited. For example, several nurses engaged in a discussion of "professionalism" may have a great deal of difficulty understanding each other if each nurse possesses a different concept of *professionalism*. Similarly, each might give different example of professionalism or, if asked to identify an incident as indicative of professionalism, may disagree on their assessments. It is easy to see how such a situation can contribute to confusion and miscommunication. One alternative, of course, is to always ask the individual with whom we are communicating "What do you mean by that?" However, this would be quite a hindrance to communication and is not an option in situations other than verbal discourse. Nursing inquiry certainly would be hampered by the need to communicate in such a way, and the need to define important concepts in a study on an individual basis raises problems with integration of results. Indeed, this is not unlike the current situation with much research because different definitions used across multiple studies contribute to difficulty synthesizing results of inquiry to identify a cohesive and consistent body of knowledge.

Clarification of concepts is an important step in the process of developing concepts that are useful and meaningful in the discipline. It is not an end point, but a critical step in the process of developing knowledge related to concepts of interest in nursing. The task of clarification can be accomplished by analyzing the common use of the concept through the ways in which the concept is expressed. Analyzing the concept in this way makes it possible for the researcher to identify the cluster of attributes that constitute the concept and, hence, to define the concept. As a result, the concept may be used more effectively. With a clearly defined concept, it is possible to classify or characterize phenomena and, in turn, to evaluate the strengths and limitations of the concept. Variations subsequently can be introduced and tested, moving toward the development of a concept that is even more useful and that reflects a contemporary context for its use.

This process of definition, evaluation, and refinement is important in the development of knowledge. The goal is to clarify and develop concepts that are clear and useful. Most important, however, is the generation of concepts that resolve existing conceptual problems. This notion of development and refinement reveals the emphasis placed on conceptual change or "evolution" within this view of concepts. The attributes of a concept do not constitute a fixed set of necessary and sufficient conditions, or the *essence* of the concept. Instead, according to this view, the cluster of attributes that constitutes the definition of the concept may change over time, by convention or by purposeful redefinition, to maintain a useful, applicable, and effective concept.

The Concept Development Cycle

The process of concept development can be described and illustrated as a cycle that continues through time and within a particular context (Figure 6-1). The context may be that of a particular discipline, cultural group or, on some occasions, the context provided by a particular theory. Three distinct aspects of concept development are apparent, and include the significance, use, and application of the concept. The significance of the concept reflects Toulmin's (1972) observation that "concepts acquire a meaning through serving the relevant human purpose in actual practical cases" (p. 168). This "relevant purpose" is the concept's ability to resolve problems and to characterize phenomena adequately, thus furthering progress in the development of knowledge.

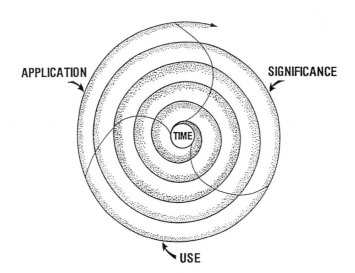

Figure 6–1 Cycle of concept development. (Reprinted with permission from B. L. Rodgers [1989]. Concepts, analysis, and the development of nursing knowledge: The evolutionary cycle. *Journal of Advanced Nursing, 14,* 330–335.)

As Toulmin indicated, the significance given to a particular concept at any point in time is related to a variety of factors. The importance attached to a particular concept or conceptual problem, for example, provides a strong incentive internal to a discipline to focus efforts on the development of the concept. Other factors, referred to as external because they lie beyond the boundaries of the particular discipline, include various rewards and incentives to develop particular concepts. Overall, a concept that is considered significant will be used often, emphasized, and studied, all of which enhance the development of concepts that are more clear and useful (Rodgers, 1989a, 1989c).

Significance thus has a profound effect on the use of the concept. Use, in this sense, refers to the common manner of employing the concept and the situations appropriate for its use. Consistent with the definition of *concept* provided previously, the use of a concept includes means of expression and carries with it the attributes of the concept. Consequently, *use* is a relevant and important focus in efforts to define the concept.

As the concept takes on a particular use, and understanding of this use is passed on through education and socialization, the concept is applied in a succession of new situations. Through application of the concept, its range or scope becomes clear, along with situations that are characterized effectively using the concept. Consequently, application reveals not only the strengths of the concept but its limitations. Based on this knowledge of the abilities provided by the concept, directions for further development are generated. Certain aspects of the concept undoubtedly gain significance because of needs that exist at the time, thus stimulating the work necessary to develop, use, apply, and continually reevaluate and refine the concept.

Implications for Concept Development

This philosophical foundation has several significant implications for methods of concept development. The emphasis on conceptual change points to the idea that concept development must be an ongoing process, with no realistic end point, except that work on a particular concept may decrease as the concept loses significance. As phenomena, needs, and goals change, concepts must be continually refined and variations introduced to achieve a clearer and more useful repertoire. Attempts to delineate precise or definitive boundaries, to distinguish a concept from its context, or to view it apart from a network of related concepts, as often done with concept analysis, are not consistent with this view.

The emphasis on context calls attention to an important concern in the selection of settings and samples for concept development. As noted previously, the relevant context may be disciplinary, social, cultural, or theoretical. For example, inquiry into the concept of health requires the researcher to acknowledge that health may be conceptualized quite differently relative to the group membership of the person who uses the concept. Similarly, time must be considered as a factor in sample selection because historical variations in concepts are common as well.

METHODS OF EVOLUTIONARY CONCEPT ANALYSIS

The methods of concept analysis play a particularly important role in this cycle of concept development. As a result of conventional use, over time a concept may become ambiguous or vague. In some situations, concepts may seem to be in conflict, and persons who use the concepts may not be able to describe the attributes of the concept or situations appropriate for their application. The thinking that lies behind many regularly performed activities often takes place without awareness of it, and so the use of concepts often occurs without knowledge or clarity concerning the definition of the concept. Concept analysis is focused on the *use* phase of development and is directed toward clarification of the concept and its current use, and uncovering the attributes of the concept as a basis for further development. Through analysis, the researcher can identify a current consensus or "state of the art" regarding the concept, which provides a foundation for further development. The focus here is on identification, an inductive approach to analysis, as the researcher seeks to identify what is common in the use of the concept, not to impose any strict criteria or expectations on the analysis.

The actual procedure of concept analysis consistent with this philosophical approach resembles the approach presented by Wilson (1963) and popularized in nursing by Walker and Avant (1983, 1988) and Chinn and Jacobs (1983; Chinn & Kramer, 1991). Different approaches to concept analysis are likely to share common features simply due to the nature of concepts and characteristics common to any analytic process. A *concept*, by definition, is a cluster of attributes. Analysis entails the breaking apart of a thing to identify its constituent components. Therefore, concept analysis in any form will involve the discovery of the attributes of the concept. As a form of inquiry, divergent approaches to concept analysis may have some procedural similarities as well. Inquiry involves the collection of data in some manner, and inquiry into concepts often is focused on analysis of written or spoken communication as a primary data source. Consequently, it is inevitable that divergent methods for concept analysis will show some similarities. However, classification of this evolutionary view as "Wilsonian," as a few writers have done due to the fact that it shares some features with approaches that were derived directly from the work of Wilson (1963), reflects both a superficial and erroneous interpretation of this methodology.

The differences between this evolutionary view and other extant approaches to concept analysis are subtle, especially as they concern the philosophical underpinnings of the method. Nonetheless, they are significant as the philosophical orientation has a profound effect on the focus of inquiry and on the ways in which results are interpreted and used. In this evolutionary approach the emphasis is on inductive inquiry and rigorous analysis, rather than beginning the investigation with the researcher's own preconceived ideas of the concept as the process appears in some investigations. The researcher also is encouraged to adhere to conventional standards for inquiry, rather than proceed with the investigation on an ad hoc basis. In regard to the nature of a concept, the emphasis on context, including sociocultural and disciplinary contexts as well as time, represents a radical departure from other approaches to analysis of concepts. In general, in this approach, concepts are not seen as static, timeless entities with identifiable boundaries, a perspective that is highly evident in Wilson's (1963) discussion of the analysis process. The results do not reveal precisely what the concept *is* or *is not*, or what is or is not an instance of the concept. Instead, consistent with the idea of a cycle of continuing development, results serve as a *heuristic* by providing the clarity necessary to create a foundation for further inquiry and development. In using this approach, the investigator should not intend, or expect, that the results will be adopted immediately for application in practice and research. Instead, the intent is to produce results that can be applied and tested as another phase in the continuing cycle of concept development as the range of the concept is evaluated and its contribution to the discipline assessed and expanded.

Concept analysis methods can be used with any form of communication. Possible data sources include printed media, such as newspapers or professional literature; interviews or other spoken language; and the performing arts. The most common use is with print media, especially the professional literature. The conduct of analysis using existing literature sources will be emphasized in this discussion for purposes of describing the method and because of the popularity of that approach.

The researcher who conducts inquiry using concept analysis should always begin with a clear understanding and documentation of a conceptual problem. Once the problem has been identified, and concept analysis has been determined as an appropriate form of investigation, the researcher can proceed with the processes of data collection, analysis, and interpretation. This evolutionary method of concept analysis involves the following primary *activities*:

1. Identify the concept of interest and associated expressions (including surrogate terms).
2. Identify and select an appropriate realm (setting and sample) for data collection.
3. Collect data relevant to identify:
   a. the attributes of the concept; and
   b. the contextual basis of the concept, including interdisciplinary, sociocultural, and temporal (antecedent and consequential occurrences) variations.
4. Analyze data regarding the above characteristics of the concept.
5. Identify an exemplar of the concept, if appropriate.
6. Identify implications, hypotheses, and implications for further development of the concept.

Many of these activities are carried out simultaneously throughout the investigation. Consequently, they represent tasks to be accomplished rather than specific steps in the process. To facilitate discussion, these activities will be described as if they are distinct.

Identifying the Concept of Interest

Although this process of concept analysis is iterative, in that the investigator works back and forth among the various activities involved in the inquiry, the first activity always is to identify the concept of interest and appropriate expressions. One of the most common ways of expressing a concept is through written or spoken language. Consequently, the major focus at the beginning of the study is to determine the concept of interest and appropriate terminology to guide the analysis. This is a crucial step in concept analysis, and not always as simple a task as it may seem. For example, a researcher interested in concepts applicable to a human response to a major life change may be confronted with an array of confusing concepts from which to choose, including depression, denial, sorrow, grief, and hopelessness. In a more positive view, concepts such as optimism, acceptance, coping, adaptation, accommodation, transition, or hope might be appropriate. The selection process often is complicated by the fact that the same concept may be expressed using different terminology. Terms such as *adaptation, accommodation,* and *coping,* for example, often are used interchangeably (hence, they are surrogate terms) to express the same or, at least, a highly similar idea. Familiarity with the literature at this phase of the analysis is essential as it enables the researcher to select the concept and terminology appropriate to focus the study. It is important to remember that a concept is not a word, but the idea or characteristics associated with the word. Words are used to express concepts; they are not the concepts themselves.

At this point in the process the researcher also must be clear about the particular direction to take with the analysis. Concept analysis always is oriented toward definition and subsequent clarification of the selected concept. Nevertheless, there are several secondary outcomes associated with clarification in general that may be of interest to the researcher and that can be accomplished through this analysis procedure. For example, the researcher may desire to explore changes that have occurred in the concept over time, or areas of agreement and disagreement across disciplines or other contexts. In an exploration of the concept of health policy (Rodgers, 1989b; 1989c), both of these interests were pursued by examining the literature from four disciplines within an extensive time frame. This procedure made it possible to identify the initial emergence of the concepts in an historical context as a specialized derivative of the superordinate concepts of social and public policy. It also revealed unique aspects of the concept of health policy as it was viewed within different fields of study. The results provided useful insight into the context for the origin of the concept (its emerging significance) and the particular perspective on the concept of health policy within each group. The results revealed substantially different perspectives on the concept across disciplines and over time that illuminated the values and orientations of the disciplines involved in discussions of health policy.

In some instances, the goal might be to expand the repertoire of concepts available to characterize situations encountered in nursing practice or research. Westra and Rodgers (1991) analyzed the concept of integration for its applicability in nursing situations. Through her professional contact with chronically ill older adults in their homes, Westra had become aware of the lack of concepts applicable to these individuals as they responded to the many changes in their lives. Concepts such as coping, accommodation, or adaptation, commonly applied in such situations, did not capture effectively the interactive nature of these older adults in their relationships with their personal, physical, and social environments. Rather than merely coping with or adjusting to changes, they were much more involved in actually shaping and directing their lives, taking into account the new situations, abilities, and limitations they encountered. Mutual change, on the part of both the person and other aspects of the environment, was a prominent feature of this process.

Westra had seen references to *integration* in some of the existing literature, although it was not found in regard to the types of situations with which she was concerned. Wondering if this might be a useful way to characterize the experiences of these older adults, she pursued an analysis of the concept. As a result, it was found that this concept could indeed be useful in nursing, providing an effective way of characterizing a particular human response and offering guidelines for evaluating the outcomes of nursing care (Westra & Rodgers, 1991).

Choosing the Setting and Sample

The specific goals of the researcher in using the evolutionary concept analysis procedure have a strong influence on selection of the setting and a sample for data collection. In a literature-based analysis, the setting refers to the time period to be examined and the disciplines or types of literature to be included. As with any research, decisions related to these aspects are made based on the initial questions asked by the researcher and the desired outcomes. The ultimate goal is to generate a rigorous design consistent with the purpose of the study.

Decisions regarding which disciplines to include can be made based on familiarity with the literature and awareness of which fields of study have an interest in, and frequently employ, the concept of interest. In the analysis of the concept of health policy (Rodgers, 1989b), this concept was found to be of great interest in the fields of nursing, medicine, health care administration, and the policy sciences. Consequently, the sample was selected from the population of literature published in these domains. Similarly, in exploring the concept of integration, Westra and Rodgers (1991) drew the sample from the disciplines of education, psychology, sociology, and allied health literature for the same reasons noted above. Nursing literature also was included in this study because of our interest in the concept as it appeared in our own discipline.

For many concepts, particularly those commonly used in nursing and health care, it may be important to include the popular literature as well. Many people gain a considerable amount of information regarding health and health care through the popular media. Undoubtedly, these sources shape their individual concepts. Analysis of a concept that includes this type of literature may be beneficial in bridging the gap between the perspectives of providers and those who are the recipients of care.

When the specific domains of literature to be included in the study have been identified, the next activity involves selection of the sample to be used in the research. In studies of concepts it is not uncommon for researchers to describe their samples (if any methodological description is provided) as comprised of the literature that either was "available," "relevant," or "pertinent" to the investigation or, in some cases, to describe the sample as consisting simply of "existing literature" concerning the concept (Boyd, 1985; Brubaker, 1983; Evans, 1979; Forsyth, 1980; Matteson & Hawkins, 1990; Meize-Grochowski, 1984; Rew, 1986; Simmons, 1989; Smith, 1981). Such samples raise questions about the rigor of the design and the credibility of the findings. The use of literature samples offers a strong advantage to the researcher, unavailable in many types of research, in that it is possible to identify the total (indexed) population of literature through both computerized and printed data bases. Literature can be identified by categorical listing (i.e., major headings), by title, abstract, or keyword searches, or by a combination of these search procedures. Consequently, a more stringent sampling design may be used in the study to increase the likelihood of a credible sample.

The investigator cannot identify the actual, entire population of relevant literature that exists using this procedure. It is possible, however, to identify the total population of indexed literature. Samples drawn from this population represent a significant improvement over completely accidental or convenience samples, which are common in many reports of completed analyses. Furthermore, these data sources are particularly relevant for sample selection in concept analysis because of their role in institutionalizing concepts within disciplines. For example, a person in the field of education who is interested in the concept of integration is likely to consult a literature index or data base in the discipline as an early step in acquiring knowledge related to this concept. Consequently, these data bases not only contain references to literature appropriate to the concept of interest but also may serve to institutionalize the use of a concept within a discipline.

Using the indexes and computer data bases to identify the total indexed population of literature, standard means of probability sampling can be used to select the sample for use in the investigation. In early studies (Rodgers, 1989b, 1989c), in which the ultimate goal was to combine data from multiple disciplines to arrive at a consensus on the concept of interest, the population lists (the citation list obtained from the indexes) first were stratified by discipline and then by year within each discipline stratum. Next, lists were combined to represent the total population of indexed literature. Stratified systematic sampling with a random starting point then was used to select the actual literature items to be used in the analysis. This procedure resulted in a comprehensive sample with proportionate representation of each discipline and of each year included in the design.

Although this procedure is effective, in many cases it often is appropriate to treat each discipline as a separate population to enable rigorous interdisciplinary comparisons for the concept of interest. A random number table or computer-generated random numbers can be used to select an appropriate sample from each discipline. Like systematic sampling, this procedure requires the researcher to number each item on the list of literature, and then to select the desired number of items to represent each discipline. As a general guide, at least 30 items from each discipline or stratum, or 20 percent of the total population, whichever is greater, should be selected for the sample. A sample size of 30 is quite small to identify a consensus in the literature or to achieve convergence in the data. Yet, in some investigations in which the concept is relatively new or has received little attention, it may be difficult assembling a larger sample. This volume of literature usually can provide an adequate basis for identifying consensus within the discipline and for substantiating the conclusions of the researcher. When there is substantial vagueness in authors' discussions and uses of the concept of interest, or there is great diversity in approaches, a larger sample may be needed before it is possible to identify a consensus in the use, and thus a definition, of the concept. The researcher always should be prepared to select additional sources according the decision criteria used in the study as needed to identify convergence in the literature or to explore further ideas that emerge during analysis.

Several concerns typically emerge using these sampling designs. First, there may be considerable overlap among disciplines in the literature indexed. The *Index Medicus*, for example, includes references to numerous publications that are considered representative of the nursing literature. Many computerized data bases provide the capacity to delete such listings from one data base when desired, while still enabling them to appear in the appropriate population. The researcher also can eliminate overlap by reviewing a printed list of citations and manually deleting or cross-referencing items that are commonly associated with another discipline (Rodgers, 1989c). Because health care is a highly interdisciplinary field, the researcher may need to make decisions regarding how to treat journals that reflect an interdisciplinary focus. There is no rule for handling such literature, other than the researcher must have a defensible rationale and be consistent in whatever decisions are made. As interdisciplinary journals proliferate, it may be meaningful to include articles from such sources in their own stratum. Another option would be to classify the article according to some logical criterion such as the discipline of the primary author or, perhaps, the theoretical foundation for the work that is reported in the article.

Another concern with this type of sampling procedure is related to the volume of literature that may be identified. In the study of the concept of health policy (Rodgers, 1989b, 1989c), one intent was to identify the emergence of the concept and to examine change over time. Consequently, the population included literature that spanned a 13-year period, which predated the origin of the concept. The population that was identified through these means consisted of 4,343 articles and 210 book reviews. This resulted in a very time-consuming, and rather costly, process and foundation for sample selection. However, even this number of items in the total population is manageable for use in sample selection.

This particular investigation (Rodgers, 1989b, 1989c) was conducted to a great extent to substantiate the view of concepts associated with this evolutionary approach; most researchers are not likely to find such a large-scale analysis necessary. However, large volumes of literature are identified in many analyses. In such situations, the researcher can reduce the population and subsequent sample to a manageable size by constricting the time frame, choice of disciplines, or choice of literature sources. Conversely, problems associated with an inadequate sample size for some concepts occasionally arise. These difficulties often can be overcome by expanding the scope of the study or by including other search procedures. For example, a search accomplished initially based on title alone can be expanded to include abstract and keyword searches to enlarge the population from which the sample will be selected.

The investigator also must be attentive to indexing procedures used by the developers of the various data bases. References sometimes are encountered that seem inappropriate to the guidelines used in the search, especially when the search is conducted using major headings. Selecting a sample of adequate size can compensate for such variances in indexing procedures. Similarly, there is the possibility that important works will be missed if the literature search is limited to computerized data bases or printed indexes alone. If the researcher feels it is appropriate, based on experience or knowledge concerning the concept of interest, works considered to be "landmark" or "classic" and special searches to identify books, book reviews, dissertations, or theses may be included (Rodgers, 1989b, 1989c). Publications that appear frequently as citations in other works may have been influential in the development of the concept and might be pursued as possible "classic" or "landmark" writings. A panel of experts may be solicited as well to provide their recommendations regarding essential works on a topic (Galante, 1990; Rodgers, 1989c). The most important consideration at this stage of the investigation is to ensure a sample that is rigorously selected, with a strong rationale for all decisions, as a means to obtain effective representation of the literature and to diminish researcher bias in the study.

Collecting and Managing the Data

In the evolutionary method of concept analysis, the emphasis is on an inductive, discovery approach focused on identification of the relevant aspects of the concept. Consequently, the actual analysis focuses on the collection and analysis of raw data and not on the construction of "cases," as is advocated in some approaches (Chinn & Jacobs, 1983; Walker & Avant, 1988; Wilson, 1963). The specific data collected, however, resemble that collected in other approaches to concept analysis, with minor variations. Specifically, the researcher reviews the literature to identify data relevant to the attributes of the concept, its contextual features (antecedents, consequences, and sociocultural and temporal variations), surrogate terms, and related concepts, along with data pertaining to applications of the concept (references). Additional data that portray changes in the concept over time also may be of interest, although researchers often will not have identification of this aspect of the concept as a goal. The fact that this approach is based on a philosophical position that concepts are dynamic and evolve over time should not be misconstrued as indicating that such analysis must be accomplished in every investigation. Identification of change over time can contribute significantly to understanding the origins, development, and functions of a concept. Yet this developmental perspective is not always necessary to clarify the current status and applications of a concept.

Identification of the attributes of the concept represents the primary accomplishment of concept analysis. The attributes of the concept constitute a *real* definition, as opposed to a *nominal* or dictionary definition that merely substitutes one synonymous expression for another (Rodgers, 1989c). It is this cluster of attributes that makes it possible to identify situations that fall under the concept, or, in other words, those that can be characterized appropriately using the concept of interest.

The researcher often has to work diligently to identify data relevant to the attributes of the concept. Actual definitions provide helpful, important data regarding the attributes, but authors rarely provide such definitions in their writing. Consequently, the researcher must look for all statements that provide a clue to how the author defines the concept. In the search for these data, it may be helpful for the researcher to keep in mind the question, "What are the characteristics of (the concept)?" In actual practice, the question often comes up in a more colloquial form, "What is this 'thing' the writer is discussing?" Any statements that provide insight into the answer to these questions constitute data relevant to the attributes.

Identifying the contextual basis of the concept refers to the situational, temporal, and sociocultural and disciplinary contexts for application of the concept. Relevant questions to ask in collecting data to identify these aspects of the concept include "What is happening when (an instance of the concept) occurs?" "What happens before . . ." and "What happens after . . ., or as a result of (the concept)?" "Is the concept used differently in different situations? By different people?" The focus in exploring the contextual aspects of the concept is to gain understanding of the situations in which the concept is used, the use of the concept in those varying situations, and its use by people with potentially diverse perspectives.

For further clarification, the investigator also collects data regarding the references of the concept. References indicate actual situations to which the concept is being applied. For example, the concept of grief (see Chapter 7) most often is used in *reference* to people who have experienced the death of a significant person in their lives, although it also is used in *reference* to other experiences of loss. All of these outcomes of the analysis help to identify the scope of the concept to enhance its clarity and effective application.

Surrogate terms and related concepts constitute the remaining data to be collected. Surrogate terms are means of expressing the concept other than the word or expression selected by the researcher to focus the study. Surrogate terms must be identified, to some extent, before beginning formal analysis. This is necessary because terms that are used interchangeably to express the same concept need to be used to identify an appropriate population for sampling. Additional surrogate terms may be identified readily during data collection through the interchange of terminology. The researcher must be careful to distinguish between surrogate terms and related concepts, which are concepts that bear some relationship to the concept of interest but do not seem to share the same set of attributes. In collecting these types of data, it is helpful for the researcher to keep in mind whether the author is merely using a different word for the same idea or is referring to something different altogether. The notion of surrogate terms is derived from the position that there may be multiple ways of expressing the same concept. The purpose of identification of related concepts is based on the philosophical assumption that every single concept exists as a part of a network of related concepts that provide a background and help to impart significance to the concept of interest. Identifying these related concepts adds to the contextual basis of the concept of interest by situating the concept in the context of a broader knowledge base.

In some approaches to concept analysis, there is an attempt to capture this idea of interconnection through the development of "related cases" (Walker & Avant, 1988; Wilson, 1963). Related cases pose some significant limitations, however. First, as described in the existing literature, they are constructed by the researcher, thereby providing considerable opportunity for the introduction of bias. Most important, however, related cases are limited to a focus on application of the specific concept of interest, or situations that demonstrate perhaps some, but not all, of the attributes of the concept being analyzed. Although this may be of some value in clarifying the use of the concept of interest, such cases do not provide any insight into what *other* concepts might be relevant in similar situations. For example, emphasis on only related cases in the analysis of the concept of hope (Zorn, 1988) would not have revealed that optimism and faith, as a few examples, actually are important *concepts* that should be considered in viewing this human response and its potential variations. Consistent with the philosophical basis for this evolutionary perspective, the identification of related concepts is an important contribution to concept clarification overall. Significantly, this outcome can provide a useful direction to clarify additional concepts, thus adding to knowledge relevant to a broad area of concern. The work of Haase and others (see Chapter 12) demonstrates further the value of identifying and clarifying related concepts.

As with any research, data management is an important concern in concept analysis, and one that is subject to numerous variations. Undoubtedly, every researcher will develop an individual style for collecting, organizing, and managing the data. In developing individual procedures, however, it is important to keep in mind both the purpose of the investigation and the analytical techniques that will be used in the study. Specifically, in recording relevant data, it is helpful to note verbatim passages in quotation marks and to note the source and page number for future reference.

One procedure consists first of gathering together items selected to be included in the sample. As the literature is obtained, each item is assigned an identification number to indicate the discipline and the number of the item. Disciplines can be distinguished using letters of the alphabet followed by the number of the item, which is the number assigned to the article on the population list. Using this identification system provides an easy means of noting a source when collecting data, helps to differentiate among the various disciplines addressed in the study, and also provides a simple cross-referencing system between each item and the original population list.

Data collection begins by reading each item at least one time to identify the general tone of the work and to gain a sense of the writer's use of the concept. This step also helps the researcher become immersed in the work, which facilitates identification of data relevant to the analysis. For actual data collection, separate sheets of paper can be used to record data relevant to each of the major categories: attributes, antecedents, consequences, references, surrogate terms, and related concepts. Each coding sheet is identified as to both category of data and the discipline from which the data were generated. At the conclusion of data collection, the data already will be organized by category to conduct analyses relevant to each significant aspect of the concept and to conduct separate analyses for each discipline to facilitate subsequent comparison.

One other type of data that is collected throughout the analysis consists of notes or records maintained by the investigator. As with any qualitative study, the researcher needs to keep track of all methodological decisions made throughout the investigation and to keep records of thoughts and perceptions as data collection and analysis proceed. Recording these impressions assists the researcher in grouping and labeling the major themes that emerge relative to each category of data and in keeping track of thoughts regarding other aspects of the analysis. Such records also provide a basis for an audit, enabling the researcher to retrace the steps of the inquiry as a means to substantiate neutrality and credibility in the investigation (Lincoln & Guba, 1985; Rodgers & Cowles, 1993).

Analyzing the Data

Although data collection and literature retrieval frequently occur simultaneously, investigators may find it most effective to delay the final, formal analysis until near the end of data collection. This procedure is contrary to that of most qualitative research. However, there are significant differences between field studies and the type of data collection and analysis conducted for purposes of concept development. In a typical field study, concurrent analysis is necessary to provide direction for the next step in the investigation, particularly in regard to the questions to ask and appropriate sources of data. Because there is not this same element of an emergent design in concept analysis as a result of the more focused inquiry and the rather circumscribed processes, formal analyses may be conducted at or near the conclusion of data collection.

Undoubtedly, the researcher will have numerous thoughts and insights regarding the concept as data collection progresses, and these may be recorded appropriately in the researcher's journal. Yet, delaying formal analysis is helpful for many investigators to avoid premature closure, or "jumping to conclusions," and the difficulty in seeing beyond the early impressions that may result. There are few occurrences more detrimental in concept analysis than the researcher getting stuck on a particular idea and, consequently, being unable to allow the characteristics of the concept to emerge from the data. Perhaps this avoidance of premature closure and preconceived notions—seeing what the researcher thinks the concept *should* be—presents the greatest challenge in concept analysis. It is not uncommon for investigators to select concepts that are of great interest to them, and that they would like to be able to present in a specific way after the analysis. In other words, the researcher wants the analysis to validate his or her pre-existing views on the concept. Because the researcher may not be totally aware of this tendency, additional measures are warranted to decrease the impact of personal bias.

Concurrent analysis also seems to lead to a premature belief that the data are "saturated" when considerable redundancy is discovered. Invariably, however, the next article or book examined provides a new insight or, at least, a suggestion of a better way to express ideas related to the concept of interest. Consequently, there are considerable benefits to delaying extensive analysis until near the conclusion of data collection. The investigator should remember, however, that it always is possible, perhaps even desirable, to return to the literature for clarification of ideas or to pursue new items for the sample as questions and insights are generated during analysis. In this sense, data collection and analysis may be concurrent. The researcher may, indeed, collect more sources and data before the analysis is complete. However, this process still varies appropriately from typical field studies.

Generally, analysis is carried out according to a standard procedure of thematic analysis. Each category of data (attributes, contextual information, and references) is examined separately to identify major themes presented in the literature. Essentially, this phase of analysis is a process of continually organizing and reorganizing similar points in the literature until a cohesive, comprehensive, and relevant system of descriptors is generated. Related concepts and surrogate terms generally are exempt from this specific analysis procedure. These typically need no further reduction, as they are recorded in simple one- or two-word units of data. Nevertheless, the researcher may find it interesting to note the frequency of their occurrence in the literature examined and to make cross-disciplinary comparisons if desired.

It is unlikely that every piece of data recorded by the investigator ultimately will be clustered under some heading in the analysis phase. In most studies the researcher will have recorded some data that seemed relevant at the time yet, on further analysis, are found to have little significance when the data are viewed collectively. Because the intent of the analysis is to identify a consensus, failure to incorporate occasional extraneous bits of information along with predominant themes is not a cause for great concern. It is inappropriate, however, to ignore data that seem to represent "outliers," as these do provide important insights into the concept. Instead, they may be addressed appropriately in a discussion of the findings or, in some cases, may indicate emerging trends or the need for additional research.

As the data are organized and appropriate "labels" are identified to describe the major aspects of the concept, analysis takes on a more theoretical focus. The researcher may examine the data for areas of agreement and disagreement across disciplines, change over time, or for insight into emerging trends concerning the concept. These findings are subtle at times, yet are worth pursuing because they provide important information regarding contextual aspects of the concept, its current status, emerging use, and directions for future development.

Identifying an Exemplar

The identification of exemplars in some form is a common and useful part of concept analysis. Because the evolutionary method is an inductive technique, exemplars should be *identified* rather than constructed by the investigator. The purpose of an exemplar is to provide a practical demonstration of the concept in a relevant context. The researcher may need to review additional literature beyond the actual sample included in the study to locate a quality exemplar. As an alternative, the researcher may pursue field observations or interviews to identify a clear example of the concept.

The ultimate goal with this activity is to illustrate the characteristics of the concept in relevant contexts and, as a result, enhance the clarity and effective application of the concept of interest. The researcher must be cautious, however, to avoid certain pitfalls that can be associated with the identification of exemplars. Most important, as in all research, is the investigator maintaining neutrality as much as possible. Bias can be introduced easily at this stage by the researcher's selecting exemplars that represent personal interests. For example, the choice of an exemplar related to critical care may limit the utility of the case for audiences from other settings when the results of the analysis are disseminated. Similarly, extraneous or excessive detail in the description of an exemplar may distract the reader from the concept itself. The *ideal* exemplar, if only one will be provided, is generic or universal enough to illustrate the concept clearly as it might appear in a variety of instances. The researcher may find it appropriate to present multiple exemplars to ensure clarity. Further, in some analyses the researcher may discover that there is considerable variation in the use of the concept. Typically this variation will be associated with the context for its use or it will vary across the range of application. In such situations, the presentation of multiple exemplars may be appropriate. This exemplar does not constitute a model case or prototype of the concept. Instead, it serves to provide a practical example of how the concept might appear in "real life" for purposes of clarity. As noted above, multiple exemplars may be preferred or needed to accomplish this purpose.

A common difficulty encountered in this phase of the inquiry is the inability to locate an appropriate exemplar. There may be a strong desire at this point to terminate the search and simply construct a case. Nevertheless, the researcher cannot consider the inability to identify an appropriate exemplar as a limitation of the study. Instead, it reveals important information about the developmental status of the concept. The researcher should be cautious in presenting an exemplar in these situations to avoid premature closure, giving the impression that the concept is more clear, better developed, or more useful than it really is in its current state. An exemplar still may be used to illustrate the current status of the concept, although the researcher should explain the limitations or "fuzzy" areas of the concept that are vague and in need of further development.

Interpreting the Results

The philosophical basis for this approach to analysis has a strong influence on the interpretation of the results. As noted previously, concept analysis is viewed here as an inductive procedure, as a means of identifying a consensus or the "state of the art" of the concept, and thus provides an important foundation for further research. The results of analysis, therefore, do not provide *the* definitive answer to questions concerning what the concept is. Instead, they may be viewed as a powerful heuristic, promoting and giving direction to additional inquiry. Criticisms that concept analysis has failed to resolve conceptual problems in nursing may be grounded in failure to recognize the importance of the heuristic function of the inquiry and, perhaps, an essentialist ideology. The purpose is not to provide a final solution, a "crystal clear" notion of what the concept is, as would be expected with an essentialist orientation. Instead, the aim is to provide the foundation and clarity necessary to enhance the continuing cycle of concept development. The results are, in that sense, a starting point, rather than an end.

Interpretation thus proceeds along two lines: shedding insight on the current status of the concept and generating implications for inquiry based on this status and identified gaps in knowledge. Interpretation of data regarding the current status of the concept can be pursued in many ways dependent upon the interests of the researcher. Cross-disciplinary comparisons can be particularly useful and enlightening in many concept analyses. In the study of the concept of health policy (Rodgers, 1989b, 1989c), a comparison of the concept across the four disciplines revealed beneficial information about the perspectives of the individual disciplines. Nurse authors, for example, frequently addressed health policy in reference to health care personnel, a focus that was conspicuously absent in the literature of medicine. Identifying these differences may lead to a greater understanding of the perspectives of nurses and other professionals, recognition that not only enhances understanding across disciplines but may contribute to improved collaboration as well.

Interdisciplinary comparisons also may be useful in situations in which a concept in nursing is considered to have been "borrowed" from another discipline. (The reader is referred to the large volume of nursing theory literature beginning in the late 1960s that dealt with the notion of "borrowed" versus "unique" knowledge in nursing. For example, see Johnson [1968] for historical background on this topic.) Although I do not subscribe to arguments regarding "borrowed" versus "unique" knowledge in nursing, in some situations there may be legitimate concerns about changes in perspective or the translation of the concept across contexts.

Comparisons can be conducted with regard to time as well as disciplinary contexts. Again, using health policy as an example, considerable change was noted over the 13 years of literature included in the study (Rodgers, 1989b, 1989c). Because *health policy* was found to be a relatively new concept, it was possible to trace its development from the superordinate concepts of public policy and social policy. In the early and mid-1970s the term *health policy* was used only rarely in the literature. The ultimate emergence of a distinct concept, along with increasing frequency in the use of the associated term, reflect the significance attached to this area of interest as it became a unique focus of inquiry and concern. Insight into current and emerging trends concerning the concept were gained by following the evolution of the concept over time. Because concepts are socially bound, exploring the social context and development of a concept can be an enlightening aspect of the analysis process.

Identifying Implications

Identification of directions for further inquiry is another important contribution of concept analysis. In fact, this heuristic function may be one of the most significant outcomes of this approach to analysis. The importance of this aspect is evident particularly in view of the philosophical foundation for this approach, which places emphasis on concept analysis as a basis for further inquiry and concept development, rather than as an end point itself.

Results of analysis of the concept of integration provide an example of the heuristic nature of this procedure (Westra & Rodgers, 1991). In this analysis, the four attributes of the concept were identified as process, combination, interaction, and unity. In other words, the concept of integration is characterized primarily as a process of combination in which two or more elements interact and form a new, unified entity (Westra & Rodgers, 1991).

Based on this analysis, a number of questions and areas for further research were identified. Field studies constitute one important area for research to evaluate the utility of the concept in actual nursing situations or to gather data for further clarification of the concept. This focus is consistent with the concept development procedure presented by Schwartz-Barcott and Kim (1986; see Chapter 9), which combines a literature-based analysis with a fieldwork phase. For the concept of integration, fieldwork might be conducted to determine the incidence of integration and its presence or applicability in actual nursing situations. Similarly, research could be designed to address questions concerning how people perceive their experiences in *integrating* various aspects of their fives, such as the combination of a previous sense of self with an altered self following some life change. Additional questions might be focused on newly acquired roles and relationships and the integration of a person with an altered functional status within an able society.

In addition to the many possibilities for productive fieldwork suggested by this analysis, further research may be facilitated by hypotheses derived from the analysis. Hypotheses could be developed regarding a variety of factors associated with integration, and these could be tested using a variety of research designs. Such research could include the development and testing of nursing interventions designed to promote integration. Similarly, for integration, criteria can be identified to assess the presence of integration as an outcome of nursing care or as a means for instrument development (Westra & Rodgers, 1991).

These types of research might be conducted without a prior analysis of the concept. Nevertheless, an initial analysis can enhance research by providing a solid conceptual foundation for further study. As a part of this process, it also provides a mechanism for systematic review of a large volume of literature. Finally, concept analysis can serve as a strong basis for substantiating the need for a particular study, particularly in regard to hypotheses and significant gaps in knowledge that are identified as a result of the analysis.

CONCLUSION

Concept analysis has an important role in the development of the knowledge base of nursing. However, there are numerous approaches to analysis, each with its own philosophical foundation. A philosophical foundation is implicit in many instances, yet has a profound effect on the conduct of the analysis and the interpretation and utilization of results.

The evolutionary approach to analysis is based on current philosophical thought regarding concepts and their role in knowledge development (Ryle, 1971; Toulmin, 1972; Wittgenstein, 1953/1968). This foundation emphasizes the dynamic nature of concepts, as concepts change with both time and context. In addition, it is consistent with the idea that vast interrelationships exist among phenomena and among the concepts that are associated with them. In general, this approach represents the philosophical rejection of essentialism and absolutism, which were prevalent in regard to concepts and knowledge during the first half of the twentieth century and which continue to pervade existing approaches to concept clarification. Instead, concepts are considered to change, grow, and develop (and need to be developed) in an evolutionary manner to enhance and maintain clarity and utility in the discipline. Concepts cannot be evaluated in regard to clear "boundaries" (Morse et al., 1996), but must be viewed with consideration of their usefulness and their position within a network of related (and also changing) concepts.

This philosophical basis, with all the attendant assumptions about conceptual change and the role of context, has significant implications for the actual method of concept analysis. Emphasis is placed especially on the conduct of a rigorous and systematic study. Specific considerations have been noted in regard to sample selection or literature review, an aspect of concept analysis that has not received adequate attention in the majority of discussions. Interpretation of the results of analysis is guided by this foundation as well, revealing the heuristic value of concept analysis. At present, this evolutionary view of concept analysis offers several advantages for the researcher doing the analysis, and provides a viable alternative to existing procedures. It has been used successfully with literature-based analyses of concepts as diverse as health policy (Rodgers, 1989b, 1989c); grief (Rodgers & Cowles, 1991; see Chapter 7); integration (Westra & Rodgers, 1991); family (Cook, 1990); strategic management (Galante, 1990); managed care (Kersbergen, 1997); caring (Sadler, 1995; see also Chapter 14); post-traumatic stress disorder (Symes, 1995); health promotion (Maben & Clark, 1995); quality (Attree, 1993); and mentoring (Stewart & Krueger, 1996), to name a few. I have encouraged, as well, analyses based on interview data rather than the usual literature approach. Cowles (1996; see Chapter 8) employed this approach using focus groups comprised of members of different cultures for further exploration of the concept of grief and as a means to identify cultural variations in constructions of the concept. This technique promises to be particularly valuable in clarification of cultural differences and to capture lay perspectives concerning the concept of interest as additional contexts for exploration.

Concept analysis can be a powerful heuristic to promote understanding and further growth of knowledge in nursing. Analysis can be carried out from a variety of perspectives, using diverse types of data, to reveal individual and group constructions of important concepts. Results of analysis and clarification subsequently can be applied and evaluated for their effectiveness and usefulness. Inquiry must be ongoing to ensure the continuing development of the concepts of interest in nursing.

REFERENCES

Attree, M. (1993). An analysis of the concept "quality" as it relates to contemporary nursing care. *International Journal of Nursing Studies, 30,* 355–369.

Barsalou, L. W., & Medin, D. L. (1986). Concepts: Static definitions or context-dependent representations? *Cahiers de Psychologie Cognitive, 6,* 187-202.

Boyd, C. (1985). Toward an understanding of mother-daughter identification using concept analysis. *Advances in Nursing Science, 7*(3), 78-86.

Brubaker, B. H., (1983). Health promotion: A linguistic analysis. *Advances in Nursing Science, 5*(3), 1-14.

Chinn, P. L., & Jacobs, M. K. (1983). *Theory and nursing: A systematic approach.* St. Louis: C. V. Mosby.

Chinn, P. L., & Jacobs, M. K. (1991). *Theory and nursing: A systematic approach* (2nd ed.). St. Louis: C. V. Mosby.

Chinn, P. L., & Kramer, M. (1991). *Theory and nursing: A systematic approach* (3rd ed.). St. Louis: C. V. Mosby.

Cook, A. (1990). The concept of family. Unpublished manuscript.

Cowles, K. V. (1996). Cultural perspectives of grief: An expanded concept analysis. *Journal of Advanced Nursing, 23,* 287-294.

Evans, S. K. (1979). Descriptive criteria for the concept of depleted health potential. *Advances in Nursing Science, 1*(3), 67-74.

Fehr, B. (1988). Prototype analysis of the concepts of love and commitment. *Journal of Personality and Social Psychology, 55,* 557-579.

Forsyth, G. L. (1980). Analysis of the concept of empathy: Illustration of one approach. *Advances in Nursing Science, 2*(2), 33-42.

Galante, C. (1990). Strategic management in nursing: A concept analysis. Unpublished doctoral dissertation, George Mason University, Fairfax, Virginia.

Johnson, D. E. (1968). Theory in nursing: Borrowed or unique? *Nursing Research, 17,* 206-209.

Kersbergen, A. L. (1997). Defining managed care in an evolving health care environment. Doctoral dissertation, University of Wisconsin-Milwaukee, 1996. *Dissertation Abstracts International, B 57/12,* 7450. (AAC#9717140)

Lincoln, Y. S., & Guba, E. (1985). *Naturalistic inquiry.* Beverly Hills: Sage.

Maben, J., & Clark, J. (1995). Health promotion: A concept analysis. *Journal of Advanced Nursing, 22,* 1158-1165.

Matteson, P., & Hawkins, J. W. (1990). Concept analysis of decision-making. *Nursing Forum, 25*(2), 4-10.

McCloskey, M. E., & Glucksberg, S. (1978). Natural categories: Well defined or fuzzy sets? *Memory & Cognition, 6,* 462-472.

Medin, D. L., & Bettger, J. G. (1994). Presentation order and recognition of categorically related examples. *Psychonomic Bulletin and Review, 1,* 250-254.

Meize-Grochowski, R. (1984). An analysis of the concept of trust. *Journal of Advanced Nursing, 9,* 563-572.

Morse, J. M., Mitcham, C., Hupcey, J. E., & Tason, M. C. (1996). Criteria for concept evaluation. *Journal of Advanced Nursing, 24,* 385-390.

Price, H. H. (1953). *Thinking and experience.* London: Hutchinson House.

Rew, L. (1986). Intuition: Concept analysis of a group phenomenon. *Advances in Nursing Science, 8*(2), 21-28.

Rodgers, B. L. (1989a). Concepts, analysis, and the development of nursing knowledge: The evolutionary cycle. *Journal of Advanced Nursing, 14,* 330-335.

Rodgers, B. L. (1989b). Exploring health policy as a concept. *Western Journal of Nursing Research, 11,* 694-702.

Rodgers, B. L. (1989c). The use and applications of concepts in nursing: The case of health policy. Doctoral dissertation, University of Virginia, 1987. *Dissertation Abstracts International, 49-11B,* 4756.

Rodgers, B. L. (1993). Concept analysis: An evolutionary view. In B. L. Rodgers & K. A. Knafl (Eds.), *Concept development in nursing: Foundations, techniques, and applications* (pp. 73-92). Philadelphia: W. B. Saunders.

Rodgers, B. L., & Cowles, K. V. (1991). The concept of grief: An analysis of classical and contemporary thought. *Death Studies, 15,* 443-458.

Rodgers, B. L., & Cowles, K. V. (1993). The qualitative research audit trail: A complex collection of documentation. *Research in Nursing and Health, 16,* 219-226.

Ryle, G. (1971). *Collected papers* (Vols. 1-2). London: Hutchinson House.

Sadler, J. J. (1995). Analysis and observation of the concept of caring in nursing (doctoral dissertation, University of Wisconsin-Milwaukee.) *Dissertation Abstracts International, B 56/ 05,* 2564. (AAC#9528682)

Schwartz-Barcott, D., & Kim, H. S. (1986). A hybrid model for concept development. In P. L. Chinn (Ed.), *Nursing research methodology: Issues and implementation* (pp. 91-101). Rockville, MD: Aspen.

Simmons, S. J. (1989). Health: A concept analysis. *International Journal of Nursing Studies, 26,* 155-161.

Smith, J. A. (1981). The idea of health: A philosophical inquiry. *Advances in Nursing Science, 3*(3), 43-50.

Smith, E. E., & Medin, D. L. (1981). *Categories and concepts.* Cambridge, MA: Harvard University Press.

Stewart, B. M., & Krueger, L. E. (1996). An evolutionary concept analysis of mentoring in nursing. *Journal of Professional Nursing, 12,* 311-321.

Symes, L. (1995). Post traumatic stress disorder: An evolving concept. *Archives of Psychiatric Nursing, 9,* 195-202.

Toulmin, S. (1972). *Human understanding.* Princeton, NJ: Princeton University Press.

Walker, L. O., & Avant K. C. (1983). *Strategies for theory construction in nursing.* Norwalk, CT: Appleton & Lange.

Walker, L. O., & Avant K. C. (1988). *Strategies for theory construction in nursing* (2nd ed.). Norwalk, CT: Appleton & Lange.

Westra, B. L., & Rodgers, B. L. (1991). Integration: A concept for evaluating outcomes of nursing care. *Journal of Professional Nursing, 7,* 277-282.

Wilson, J. (1963). *Thinking with concepts.* London: Cambridge University Press.

Wittgenstein, L. (1968). *Philosophical investigations* (3rd ed.) (G. E. M. Anscombe, Trans.). Chicago: University of Chicago Press. (Original work published 1953)

The Concept of Grief: An Evolutionary Perspective

Kathleen V. Cowles and Beth L. Rodgers

The concept of grief has been of interest to both practitioners and researchers from a wide variety of disciplines for many years. It has been compared and contrasted with depression, it has been equated with "melancholia" (Freud, 1917/1957), and it has been variously defined as an adaptational response (Bowlby, 1973), as an acute crisis or a series of crises (Caplan, 1974; Lindemann, 1944), as an illness (Engel, 1961; Volkan, 1970), as a syndrome (Lindemann, 1944; Parkes, 1972), and as a human response (Kim et al., 1989). Psychologists, psychiatrists, general medical practitioners, nurses, sociologists, veterinarians, educators, and theologians have all written about grief and the importance of understanding this universal experience. Despite the agreement across disciplines regarding the significance of the phenomenon of grief and despite the proliferation of multidisciplinary professional literature describing instances of its occurrence, there continues to be evidence in the literature that the concept of grief is vague and ambiguous and that, in fact, there is little agreement either within or among disciplines on a conceptual definition of grief.

In 1989 we completed a concept analysis of grief that was designed to systematically identify a definition of the concept as it had been used in the literature of nursing and medicine (Cowles & Rodgers, 1991). In addition to identifying a definition of grief, we traced the historical and contextual development of the concept and determined the areas of agreement and disagreement concerning grief as it had been conceptualized in the literature of these two disciplines.

The analysis revealed that the concept of grief covered a wide range of responses and experiences. The authors seldom provided an actual definition of *grief;* instead, they typically discussed grief in relation to a multitude of common, observable, and reported symptoms. In addition, many authors used a variety of terms other than *grief* to express their individual concepts and often used qualifiers to indicate subtle variations in the concept.

Despite the wide variety of approaches to the discussion of grief in both the medical and nursing literature, it was possible to identify the predominant attributes of the concept. The identification of these attributes resulted in the definition of grief as a *dynamic, pervasive, highly individualized process with a strong normative component* (Rodgers & Cowles, 1991). Although this conceptualization offered a significant contribution to the development of a knowledge base concerning grief in medicine and nursing, we decided that further study and clarification were warranted, particularly in light of the numerous disciplinary references to sociology and psychology and to specific authors from these disciplines throughout the literature of nursing and medicine. Therefore, a second phase of the analysis was focused on the literature of sociology and psychology and was completed in 1990. The remainder of this chapter is devoted to a discussion of the method of concept analysis used in these investigations, the interdisciplinary comparison of the findings, and the merged results of these studies.

CONCEPT ANALYSIS METHOD

Rodgers (1987, 1989a, 1989b) advocated a method of concept analysis that is an inductive, descriptive means of inquiry used to clarify the current status of a concept by identifying a consensus, to examine the historical or evolutionary background of the concept, and to determine areas of agreement and disagreement in the use of the concept among diverse disciplines. We strictly adhered to this method throughout both phases of the study.

Sample Selection

The samples for both phases were selected from English language literature published in the respective fields of medicine, nursing, psychology, and sociology during the years 1985 through 1988. Initially the population of indexed literature was identified through a manual search of the *Index Medicus* and the *International Nursing Index* because these indexes represented important reference sources for these two disciplines. Medicine and nursing constituted the focus of the first phase of the study because of our primary interest in conceptualizations of grief in these two fields of study. The search was accomplished by identifying all literature indexed under the subject headings *grief* and *bereavement* because these two terms frequently are used interchangeably in the literature in this topic area. Cross-referencing between indexes was eliminated through a manual review of the total population identified in each field. A computer search could have been used to accomplish this task. However, a computer search based on major headings would have produced a list identical to that published in the indexes. Consequently, a manual search was considerably less costly to use in this investigation. We also knew that there would be a sizable volume of literature indexed under the major headings of *grief* and *bereavement;* thus, there was no need to expand the search by using keywords, an abstract search, or other means of literature retrieval.

This initial search uncovered 242 items in the *Index Medicus* and 159 in the nursing literature. For ease of sample selection and to maintain a master list of the literature, the relevant pages from each index were photocopied and each discipline was assigned a letter for differentiation of the populations. Each data base was treated as separate, and the articles listed were numbered sequentially in each population. A sample was selected from each discipline (nursing, n = 30; medicine, n = 44) using computer-generated random numbers. In determining the sample size, the investigators first selected 30 as the target number of items to be selected from the smaller data base of nursing. Experience had shown that 30 items was the minimum needed to facilitate a credible analysis (Rodgers, 1987, 1989a, 1989b). The investigators recognized that more articles could be added if needed to identify a consensus. Because this sample size constituted approximately 18 percent of the literature identified in nursing, a corresponding sample of 18 percent of the literature indexed in medicine was selected. This same procedure was used later in selecting the samples from sociology and psychology using the *Social Sciences Index* (N = 150, n = 30, 20 percent) and *Psychological Abstracts* (N = 547, n = 109, 20 percent).

A purposive sample of works considered to be landmark or classic was included as well. For this study, this sample was identified through a review of the citations in the articles selected from each discipline. The most frequently cited references were selected to comprise this sample of classics. This sample included works by Bowlby (1980), Engel (1964), Lindemann (1944), and Parkes (1972, 1975), along with a chapter on conceptualizations of grief drawn from psychology, psychoanalysis, pastoral care, and medicine (Switzer, 1970). It may be of interest to note that works by Kubler-Ross (1969) were not included in this selection of classics. Although these works were cited frequently in the nursing literature on grief, they did not appear in the reference lists for articles selected from other disciplines. In addition, Kubler-Ross focused her work on death and dying, and not on a discussion of grief or bereavement.

Literature Retrieval and Data Collection

After the sample was selected, we obtained the literature through local libraries and interlibrary loan services. Each item was read initially to identify the general tone and theme of the work. This step helped focus our attention on the task of data collection, to become immersed in the literature, and to become sensitized to the authors' uses of the concept of grief. Phrases, themes, and, when possible, verbatim passages were recorded onto coding sheets developed to organize the data. For example, a coding form with the heading "Definitions" was used to document all data relevant to the question, "What are the attributes of the concept of grief?" Similar coding forms were used to record data relevant to other aspects of data collection as well (antecedents, consequences, references, related concepts, and surrogate terms). A separate set of coding forms was used for each discipline represented in the study. As relevant data were noted on the appropriate form, the complete item number from which the data were extracted was noted as well. Page numbers also were included, which made it possible for us to return to the original source of the data if additional clarification was needed. We reviewed each others' data collection and recording processes at intervals throughout the study to ensure a consistent approach to the inquiry and as a form of peer review (Lincoln & Guba, 1985) to diminish potential bias in the investigation.

Occasionally during data collection, the data obtained in each discipline were reviewed and reorganized as some categories began to emerge. Analysis was limited until near the end of data collection, however, to avoid premature closure regarding the relevant aspects of the concept. Instead, the minimal analysis conducted throughout the study was done primarily to promote organization of the data, which also facilitated later, formal analysis.

Data Analysis

As the actual investigation was conducted in two stages, data analysis also was carried out in two phases. Analysis first was focused on the nursing and medical literature, with the data from each discipline analyzed separately. Then the results of these analyses were combined to reveal a working definition of the concept. As noted previously, this analysis led to the second phase focused on the disciplines of sociology and psychology. Data from sociology and psychology also were reviewed separately, and then combined with the results of the first-phase analysis to provide greater clarity and an expanded and more comprehensive definition of the concept. Finally, the data and findings were scrutinized to examine areas of agreement and disagreement among the four disciplines, and to examine conceptual change over time.

In this study, analysis was carried out in an inductive, thematic manner similar to content analysis. Data collected within each discipline were analyzed relevant to the major categories of information recorded. In other words, all data recorded under the heading "Definitions" for one discipline were analyzed to identify a definition (the attributes) of the concept of grief; this same procedure was followed for antecedents, consequences, references, surrogate terms, and related concepts. Data were organized and reorganized until a coherent system of categories emerged for each aspect of the concept. Word labels then were selected to provide clear descriptions of each aspect of the concept, using actual words obtained from the data when appropriate. The only exceptions to this process were the surrogate terms and related concepts. Because data under these headings typically were noted as one- or two-word expressions, rather than as general themes or phrases, there was no need for categorizing and labeling; these data were in a final form as collected on the coding sheets. However, frequency counts were used on a limited basis to describe the findings in these areas, and some analysis was conducted to clarify relationships among the concept of interest, surrogate terms, and other related concepts.

Consistent with this approach to concept analysis (Rodgers, 1987, 1989a, 1989b), the actual analysis was focused generally on identification of a consensus to reveal the "state of the art," or the current state of knowledge, concerning the concept. Consequently, some data noted on the coding sheets were not incorporated into the final category system, especially in regard to the definition or attributes of the concept. The utilization of every piece of data recorded constitutes one of the most frequent concerns or questions of persons conducting this type of inquiry. Undoubtedly, each investigator noted some information that, during the analysis, was found to shed little light on the characteristics of the concept. This occurrence is common particularly because of the guideline used in this type of analysis that if some information seems even potentially relevant, it is better to note it on the data collection sheet than to risk losing the data altogether. As commonly occurs, some of the data collected in this study ultimately were found to be irrelevant, especially as the concept became more clear through analysis.

Another common situation, which also emerged during this study, involved some small bits of data that did not fit the category system that was developed to incorporate the majority of the data. Yet, these data were too important to be discarded as irrelevant. Since the emphasis here was on consensus, the categories generally were developed to incorporate as much of the data as possible and, certainly, to capture the dominant ideology. The remaining data provided significant insights regarding the concept nonetheless. These "outliers" were found to represent the remnants of earlier ideas, ideas outside of the mainstream (e.g., frequent references in nursing to the stages of grief purportedly addressed by Kubler-Ross), or emerging trends. Focused attention on these data, such as by examining their context in the literature sources, reference citations, background of author, and relationship of these ideas to others found in the literature, helped in determining the significance of this information in reference to the current status of the concept and the cycle of concept development.

Throughout all aspects of the study, strategies relevant to qualitative research were used to enhance the credibility of the findings (Lincoln & Guba, 1985). Each investigator maintained a reflexive journal as a record of all methodological decisions and as documentation of impressions that emerged during data collection and analysis. In addition, the involvement of two researchers helped to decrease the influence of individual biases in the research. The absence of any hypotheses in the conduct of the study also enhanced neutrality in this investigation. Finally, the rigor of the study was supported through the use of a probability sample and an adequate sample size to enable convergence of the data.

FINDINGS

The first, and perhaps most obvious, finding of this study was the tremendous variety of ways in which the concept of grief commonly was used. We had sufficient evidence prior to the study to document vagueness and ambiguity and the need for clarification and further development of the concept of grief. Yet, this investigation revealed a striking array of uses and interpretations of this concept.

Few authors provided an actual definition of *grief;* instead, grief was commonly discussed in regard to symptoms and interventions. In addition, the term *grief* frequently was interchanged with a variety of surrogate terms, most often *mourning* and *bereavement.* These terms also were defined only rarely by the authors of the literature examined. Finally, grief commonly was used in conjunction with a variety of modifiers, including *complicated, pathological,* and *dysfunctional* grief; *normal* or *typical* grief; and *anticipatory, atypical,* and *disenfranchised* grief.

Attributes of Grief

Even with this wide variety of approaches to grief, there was some consensus on the concept. Analysis of the literature in the disciplines of nursing and medicine resulted in the definition of the concept of grief as a dynamic, pervasive, highly individualized process with a strong normative component (Rodgers & Cowles, 1991). This listing of attributes—dynamic, process, individualized, pervasive, and normative—

was consistent throughout the literature in sociology and psychology as well. In fact, the "labels" selected for the attributes often were found in the literature examined in the second part of this investigation. Before the second phase, we put much thought into selecting appropriate descriptors for the attributes and into choosing labels that would best capture the nature of the attribute. On examination of the sociology and psychology literature, some of the actual terms selected to describe the attributes were found, particularly the terms *pervasive* and *dynamic*. The term *process* was used in some of the literature in all four disciplines, although less frequently in nursing. *Normative* was derived on the basis of numerous authors' discussions of *normal* or *typical* grief and of acceptable or appropriate grief responses in addition to some limited reference to cultural variations in regard to grief.

Dynamic. Most discussions of grief presented this concept as representing a nonlinear, fluctuating complex of emotions, thoughts, and behaviors. Although grief commonly was regarded as having distinct phases, there were many different descriptions of the nature of these phases. Some authors (Green & Goldberg, 1986; Zisook & DeVaul, 1985) did refer to grief as characterized by certain "steps" and a linear progression. However, these authors typically relied on older references as the sources for this idea. The more current use of the concept provided evidence of an increasing conceptualization of grief as constantly changing and, thus, dynamic in nature.

Also significant in regard to this attribute was an interdisciplinary difference noted as a part of this analysis. Frequent references to the work of Kubler-Ross (1969) and her portrayal of the stages of the *dying* process, which was used as a means to understand both dying and grieving, created a skew in the nursing literature away from the more contemporary idea of grief as dynamic and nonlinear. Rarely did references to Kubler-Ross appear in the literature of medicine, and they were not found at all in discussions of grief in the literature from sociology and psychology that was examined in this study.

Process. The attribute *process* is closely related to the attribute *dynamic*. The frequent reference to grief as characterized by phases or clusters of activity in movement toward some goal revealed the process aspect of this concept. A similar major idea expressed in the literature concerned grief as "work" (Clark, 1984; Elde, 1986; Martocchio, 1985; Worden, 1985). The work of grief consisted of a variety of tasks related to reconciliation of a loss or progression to get beyond the impact and effects of the loss. There was considerable disagreement about the amount of time needed for a person to complete the work of grief. Earlier ideas presented the grief process as approximately six months to two years in duration. Nevertheless, there was an emerging, and increasing, consensus that grief is potentially without any time limit. The enduring nature of grief is particularly evident in discussions of how significant events and other reminders of a loss serve to revive aspects of grief for many years (Paterson, 1987; Zisook & DeVaul, 1985).

Individualized. Authors of the literature reviewed presented a tremendous variety of both objective and subjective experiences associated with the occurrence of grief. The specific combination of experiences was thought to differ among individuals, with the particular experiences of a person affected by numerous factors including the relationship between the grieving person and the lost being or object, the nature of the loss (e.g., traumatic, acute, predicted), and existing support systems. Other factors, such as the individual's previous experience with loss and grief, culture, and religious beliefs also were presented as having a strong effect on grief. Overall, it was clear that the concept of grief is highly individualized, and manifested in many different ways from one person to the next. Some authors did attempt to provide a list of symptoms common to all persons experiencing grief (Lesher & Bergey, 1988; Norris & Murrell, 1987), and in fact, such symptoms often were advocated as definitive in nature. This analysis, however, clearly revealed that there was little agreement on any specific set of symptoms associated with grief. The general consensus was that grief is highly individualized in nature.

Pervasive. In addition to being highly individualized, the concept of grief also was considered to be pervasive, having the potential to affect every aspect of a person's existence. Grief may manifest in ways that can be classified as psychological, social, physical, cognitive, behavioral, spiritual, and emotional or affective. This tremendous range of possible experiences and manifestations associated with grief provides evidence of the pervasive attribute of this concept. Almost any combination, magnitude, or duration of manifestations is possible as a part of the concept of grief; more often than not, multiple aspects of a grieving person's existence are affected.

Normative. Although there was a consensus that grief is highly variable, there was a tremendous tendency on the part of the authors of the literature examined to identify what constituted *normal* grief. Authors frequently used terms such as *typical, uncomplicated,* and *healthy* grief, in addition to *normal*, to differentiate an expected or acceptable response from one that might be considered *complicated, pathological,* or *atypical*. Although there was not universal agreement as to what constituted *normal* grief, there was a clear consensus that there are limits beyond which grief becomes unacceptable or inappropriate. These limits commonly were discussed as being socially or culturally ascribed. The argument was made often that an individual essentially learns how to grieve as a part of socialization and enculturation processes.

Antecedents

All the literature examined revealed that the primary antecedent, or situation preceding an instance of the concept of grief, was some form of loss. We were not surprised to find that the type of loss most frequently addressed was the death of a significant other, especially a family member. There was, however, a considerable variety of losses discussed by the authors of the works included in this study. Some of these other losses associated with grief were relatively tangible in nature, such as physical dysfunction or impairment, the loss of a pet, or the loss of some significant object. Other losses were more abstract, such as the loss of independence or control; losses associated with aging or a change in lifestyle or residence and, less frequently noted in the literature, divorce, menopause, retirement; the loss of an idealized child (through infertility or birth defects); and loss of employment.

Some of these losses actually were described by authors in terms of *change,* such as a change in residence or employment or changes experienced in conjunction with aging. The emphasis on change in the literature was sufficient for us to consider it as another antecedent of the concept of grief. Nevertheless, further analysis revealed that change, alone, was not the antecedent; rather, it was the losses associated with change that may lead to grief. Consequently, the antecedent of loss subsumed all of the antecedents presented in the literature. By far, the antecedent most often discussed involved the death of a loved one.

Consequences

The consequences of grief, or situations that follow an instance of the concept, were difficult to discern in this analysis. Problems with this aspect of the inquiry were related to an interesting characteristic of the literature on grief, specifically the tendency of authors to refer to specific symptoms of grief as the outcomes or consequences. For example, authors frequently indicated that grief "results" in sadness, crying, loss of concentration, and a variety of somatic disturbances. However, for purposes of this analysis, attention was focused on the more long-range outcomes of grief. These other "results" of grief are more properly considered as symptoms or manifestations. These symptoms occur while the individual is grieving. Thus, they do not answer the question concerning what happens to a person as a result of a grief experience; in other words, what happens to someone who has made considerable movement through the grief process.

Two consequences of grief were identified: the development of a new identity and the establishment of a new reality. Typically, as a consequence of grief, a new personal and social identity emerge as the grieving individual reconceptualizes the self without the lost object (or person). Alterations in roles, activities, and routines, along with changes in social relationships, frequently occur. Ultimately, "life is never the same" (Karl, 1987, p. 645) for the person who has experienced grief, an expression that illustrates clearly the magnitude and extent of the outcome of grief in altering the person's identity and reality.

The consequences of grief were discussed most often in reference to effects on the grieving person. Nevertheless, the analysis demonstrated that a grief experience may have an effect beyond the impact on the persons actually grieving. Particularly, grief was noted by a few authors (Beckley et al., 1985; Kowalski, 1985) to have an effect on health care systems and professional care providers. Interestingly, however, this position was identified only in the nursing literature. Authors occasionally pointed out that health care delivery may be changed somewhat as a result of a grief experience in a setting and may include new interventions to assist grieving persons. Physical structures may be altered, for example, the development of privacy rooms for grieving family members on nursing units. Significantly, nurse authors also noted that health care personnel may be affected by an experience with grief either by the self or by others in the work setting, especially clients. An encounter with grief may contribute to feelings of inadequacy or helplessness, and may lead to questioning of personal beliefs, faith, and individual well-being and mortality in persons associated with a grieving individual.

Related Concepts

As noted previously, various terms were used interchangeably to express the concept of grief. Some of these terms actually were found to express related concepts, in addition to functioning as surrogate terms for *grief*. This determination was made based on an analysis that revealed sometimes subtle differences in expressions as well as authors who provided more precise definitions of alternate terms. For example, *bereavement* was defined as "the state of having experienced the death of a significant other" (Demi & Miles, 1986, p. 105). Similarly, *mourning,* another term frequently used interchangeably with *grief,* has been used specifically to refer to the rituals and practices that serve as a public display of grief (Parkes, 1985). Bereavement and mourning thus bear a close relationship to grief, yet could be used effectively to refer to specific aspects of a grief experience. Although such terms were presented frequently as surrogates, there was a distinct difference in the attributes of each associated concept. This interchange of terms not only adds to confusion in this area, but undermines the effectiveness of these various ways of characterizing unique aspects of a grief experience.

THE EVOLUTION OF GRIEF AS A CONCEPT

In addition to addressing common aspects of concept analysis, as well as interdisciplinary variations, we also examined changes that had occurred in the concept of grief over time. The purposive sample of landmark works utilized for this aspect of the analysis included six classic publications selected on the basis of frequency of citation as references in the contemporary literature. Analysis for this aspect of the study revealed that there has been little change in the concept of grief over time. Tremendous variation in discussions of grief was evident, and rarely was a definition of grief provided. Symptoms of grief provided the primary focus for authors of much of the classic literature, and terms were interchanged freely, both of which were apparent in contemporary writings as well.

Some subtle tendencies were noted in this aspect of the analysis, however, including a gradually expanding view of the duration and antecedents of grief. Although there was not uniform agreement among authors on the subject, there was some evidence that the time involved for resolution of grief is being viewed as less restrictive (for example, potentially limitless rather than persisting for only six months or so, after which grief may be "pathological"). Similarly, there has been a gradual increase in attention to grief in response to a variety of losses, rather than death of a significant other alone, although the primary emphasis continues to be on loss associated with death. Overall, there has been little progress in abilities to conceptualize grief clearly in development of a consensus and, particularly, in the ability to recognize or identify grief and differentiate grief from other related responses.

IMPLICATIONS

The lack of progress concerning the concept of grief, despite many years of inquiry, is one of the best indicators of the need for this analysis. The results of this study provide a foundation for the additional development of the concept that is needed. Particularly, these findings offer not only some of the needed clarity but serve a heuristic purpose in facilitating productive inquiry.

The definition of the concept of grief that was derived through this analysis may help providers who need to identify grief and differentiate it from related responses. One of the most significant outcomes of this analysis was the observation that grief cannot be identified on the basis of symptoms alone. Although symptomatology has been a focus in discussions of grief for many years, essentially there was no agreement on symptoms commonly or properly associated with grief. The highly variable and individualized nature of grief indicates that recognition of this response is best based on an individual's antecedent loss and the person's own description of his or her experience as *grief.* Grief is quite complex and varied such that an emphasis on symptoms alone is inadequate to enable identification of this response.

This finding obviously has implications for the development of nursing diagnoses concerning grief and related responses. Undoubtedly, determining a discrete set of defining characteristics is complicated by the myriad and highly individualized forms of grief. Furthermore, without a clear conceptualization of grief, it is difficult, and premature as well, to label or identify cases as "anticipatory" or "dysfunctional" grief. These existing diagnoses are vague and demonstrate considerable overlap, both of which limit their usefulness in clinical situations. Further research is needed before valid diagnostic statements can be developed and implemented.

Research using interviews is needed to enhance knowledge of appropriate interventions for grief. Currently, there is a sizable body of literature that is focused on counseling and other therapeutic activities for grieving persons. Nevertheless, there is minimal agreement on the interventions that are warranted, on the timing for implementation, and, in fact, on the appropriateness of any interventions in situations of grief. Interview-based research also may be helpful in clarifying the normative aspect of grief. Cross-cultural studies particularly are needed to shed light on cultural norms and to expand the currently limited knowledge on this topic.

In spite of the significance of interview-based research in expanding understanding of grief, other aspects of this analysis generated hypotheses and other directives to promote additional forms of inquiry. The identification of loss as the primary antecedent points to the need for research regarding grief responses in association with various types of loss. Although there is some research that suggests grief may vary in relation to the acuity or prior knowledge of an impending loss, less information is available regarding specific differences in response to losses other than the death of a significant other. Losses associated with the institutionalization of a loved one, the loss of a significant object, and more abstract losses including the loss of a previous sense of self, independence, and personal functions have been studied to a much lesser extent. Because the concept of grief was found in this analysis to be highly individualized, research to uncover some of the factors that influence individual variations is needed.

The consequences of grief identified through this analysis provide direction for additional research as well. In addition to their potential use in assessing progression through the grief process, these consequences offer a reconceptualization and a basis for evaluation of grief outcomes. Previously, research on the outcomes, or consequences, of grief had been limited primarily to a focus on symptom resolution. Research to develop means that are more precise to address changes in individual identity and reality ultimately would increase understanding of the dynamic nature of progression through a grief experience.

Attention needs also to be focused on the variety of related concepts and surrogate terms identified through this analysis. The frequent interchange of terms has contributed substantially to the existing confusion and ambiguity concerning the concept of grief. Similarly, it has created difficulties in synthesizing the results of research due to vast conceptual differences in studies of grief. It is important to recognize as well that many of these terms can be used effectively to address specific and important aspects of a response to loss. Clarification of terminology and associated concepts, especially the concepts of mourning and bereavement, would be a major step in advancing knowledge of grief. In addition, there is a need for attention to related concepts that refer to various types of grief, such as pathological or complicated. Analysis of these concepts, along with empirical research focused on grief experiences, can promote differentiation of these concepts and contribute to a broader knowledge base and, certainly, more useful and relevant concepts overall.

A prior analysis of the concept is not essential in conducting research along any of these lines. Nevertheless, analysis of the concept of grief was helpful in identifying the "state of the art," so to speak, in determining aspects of the concept that particularly need refining and in providing clear directions for inquiry. Ultimately, such an analysis enables additional research to be conducted with a strong conceptual foundation and to be potentially more productive as the inquiry is focused on specific deficiencies in knowledge. The method used in this investigation particularly strengthens future research efforts through its systematic approach to sample selection and literature review, attention to the evolution of the concept, and a focus on interdisciplinary analyses and comparisons. These factors contribute to a rigorous study and a multitude of useful outcomes.

Still, the results of this analysis do not specifically answer questions about what grief *is*. Indeed, the philosophical basis for the approach used in this study rejects the idea that any one definitive answer could exist. Concepts are not timeless, acontextual entities, but reflect a changing world and continuing alterations in their use. The method used in this analysis of the concept of grief differs from other approaches by emphasizing this philosophical assumption and by focusing on the current use of the concept. This method serves to clarify the current status of the concept and thus promotes the concept's more effective use and application. Further analyses are needed to clarify the array of related concepts to expand knowledge of this broad area of interest. Equally important, however, is the need for continuing research and development of the concept of grief to maintain a concept that is clear, useful, and relevant. This analysis can be considered a starting point for additional productive inquiry.

REFERENCES

Beckley, R. D., Price, R. A., Okerson, M., & Riley, K. W. (1985). Development of a perinatal grief checklist. *Journal of Obstretric, Gynecologic and Neonatal Nursing, 14,* 194-199.

Bowlby, J. (1973). *Attachment and loss: Vol. 2. Separation, anxiety and anger.* New York: Basic Books.

Bowlby, J. (1980). *Attachment and Loss: Vol. 3. Loss.* New York: Basic Books.

Caplan, G. (1974). Foreword. In I. Glick, R. Weiss, & C. Parkes (Eds.), *The first year of bereavement* (pp. vi-xi). New York: Wiley.

Clark, M. D. (1984). Healthy and unhealthy grief behaviors. *Occupational Health Nursing, 32,* 633-635.

Cowles, K. V., & Rodgers, B. L. (1991). The concept of grief: A foundation for nursing practice and research. *Research in Nursing and Health, 14,* 119-127.

Demi, A. S., & Miles, M. G. (1986). Bereavement. *Annual Review of Nursing Research, 4,* 105-123.

Elde, C. (1986). The use of multiple group therapy in support groups for grieving families. *American Journal of Hospice Care, 3*(6), 27-31.

Engel, G. L. (1961). Is grief a disease: A challenge for medical research. *Psychosomatic Medicine, 23,* 18-22.

Engel, G. L. (1964). Grief and grieving. *American Journal of Nursing, 64,* 93-98.

Freud, S. (1957). Mourning and melancholia. In J. Strachey (Ed. and Trans.), *The standard edition of the complete psychological works of Sigmund Freud* (Vol. 14, pp. 243-258). London: Hogarth. (Original work published 1917)

Green, S. A., & Goldberg, R. L. (1986). Management of acute grief. *American Family Physician, 33,* 185-190.

Karl, G. R. (1987). A new look at grief. *Journal of Advanced Nursing, 12,* 641-645.

Kim, M. J., McFarland, G. K., & McLane, A. M. (1989). *Pocket guide to nursing diagnoses* (3rd ed.). St. Louis: C. V. Mosby.

Kowalski, K. (1985). The impact of chronic grief. *American Journal of Nursing, 85,* 398-399.

Kubler-Ross, E. (1969). *On death and dying.* New York: Macmillan.

Lesher, E. L., & Bergey K. J. (1988). Bereaved elderly mothers: Changes in health, functional activities and family cohesion, and psychological well-being. *International Journal of Aging and Human Development, 26,* 81-90.

Lincoln, Y. S., & Guba E. (1985). *Naturalistic inquiry.* Beverly Hills: Sage.

Lindemann, E. (1944). Symptomatology and management of acute grief. *American Journal of Psychiatry, 101,* 141-148.

Martocchio, B. C. (1985). Grief and bereavement. *Nursing Clinics of North America, 20,* 327-341.

Norris, F. H., & Murrell, S. A. (1987). Older adult family stress and adaptation before and after bereavement. *Journal of Gerontology, 42,* 606-612.

Parkes, C. M. (1972). *Bereavement: Studies of grief in adult life.* New York: International Universities.

Parkes, C. M. (1975). Determinants of outcome following bereavement. *Omega, 6,* 303-323.

Parkes, C. M. (1985). Bereavement. *British Journal of Psychiatry, 146,* 11-17.

Paterson, G. W. (1987). Managing grief and bereavement. *Primary Care, 14,* 403-415.

Rodgers, B. L. (1987). *The use and applicaton of concepts in nursing.* Unpublished doctoral dissertation, University of Virginia, Charlottesville.

Rodgers, B. L. (1989a). Concepts, analysis, and the development of nursing knowledge: The evolutionary cycle. *Journal of Advanced Nursing, 14,* 330-335.

Rodgers, B. L. (1989b). Exploring health policy as a concept. *Western Journal of Nursing Research, 11,* 694-702.

Rodgers, B. L., & Cowles, K. V. (1991). The concept of grief: An analysis of classical and contemporary thought. *Death Studies, 15,* 443-458.

Switzer, D. K. (1970). *The dynamics of grief.* New York: Abingdon.

Volkan, V. (1970). Typical findings in pathological grief. *Psychiatric Quarterly, 44,* 231-250.

Worden, J. W. (1985). Bereavement. *Seminars in Oncology, 12,* 472-475.

Zisook, S., & DeVaul, R. (1985). Unresolved grief. *American Journal of Psychoanalysis, 45,* 370-379.

8

Grief in a Cultural Context: Expanding Concept Analysis Beyond the Professional Literature

Kathleen V. Cowles

oncepts are identified, discussed, described, defined, reduced to attributes, merged, expanded, and compared with other concepts throughout the professional literature by authors who, for a variety of reasons, are considered to be experts in a particular domain. In nursing, as in other practice disciplines, these experts draw their understanding of a concept predominantly from observations of others' experiences and from comparing and contrasting these observations with those of other experts. These activities are essential to the development of knowledge as they promote awareness of the existence of a concept, encourage conceptual refinement, and explore instances of how a concept may be used across numerous settings and in a variety of circumstances. However, as a concept becomes more widely discussed, its literary use may be expanded to the point where it becomes vague and its characteristics confused with those of other similar concepts.

It is often at this point, when ambiguity regarding a concept becomes increasingly evident in the literature, that researchers begin work to systematically analyze the concept, searching for clarity and consensus. Drawing on the professional literature, and thus on the observations of experts, researchers identify attributes most commonly ascribed to the concept and thereby arrive at a definition with associated antecedents and consequences. These analyses, like the early identification and literary discussions of the concept, are essential heuristic pursuits in the process of building knowledge. They serve as foundations without which theory generation and further investigation of conceptual relationships would have no starting point. Despite the importance of concept analysis and development as typically pursued through the literature, the outcomes of these endeavors remain abstract in the sense that they are derived through observations of others' experiences. Essentially, their relevance to, and application in, practice are only hypothetical.

The advancement of knowledge for actual use in nursing practice demands not only the identification and subsequent clarification of concepts by experts, but the validation and evaluation of the findings of these activities by those whose experience the concept is supposed to depict. As both Rodgers (1989; 1993b) and Schwartz-Barcott and Kim (1986; 1993) noted, if concepts and the findings of concept analyses are to serve as basic components of clinical nursing practice, empirical data from those who are recipients of nursing care need to be generated and compared with what has been presented in the literature. The perspectives of individuals for whom a concept, in its abstract form, represents a personal experience provide validation and/or further refinement of the work of understanding through conceptual clarity begun by professionals.

In the early 1990s, the author and her colleague, Dr. Beth Rodgers, completed an extensive concept analysis of grief based on current professional literature from nursing, medicine, and the social sciences (Cowles & Rodgers, 1991; Rodgers & Cowles, 1991). The primary goal of this initial analysis was the identification of a current conceptual definition of grief as it was used in the professional literature to promote understanding, clarity, and consistency. The impetus for this study was the author's long-standing work in the area of loss, grief, and bereavement during which she experienced an escalating frustration both with the synonymous use of the terms *grief, bereavement,* and *mourning* in the literature and the inconsistent definition and application of grief. The results of the analysis—a conceptual definition, identified antecedents and consequences of grief, and a variety of surrogate terms, related concepts, and references—were disseminated widely. Thus the primary goal of the research was met and a foundation for future knowledge generation regarding grief was laid. However, it was clear that the findings were only foundational; many questions remained, the most important of which was would this conceptual definition be useful when applied in practice? That is, was this definition that had been derived from the work of professional experts consistent with the personal definition that might be used by those experiencing grief?

Another related question arose from the researchers' observations of the authorship of the articles analyzed for the initial study. Although many questions have been raised regarding the potential for cultural differences in the experience of grief, the large majority of articles randomly selected for the concept analysis were authored by people of Anglo heritage. Thus, another question became important: Was the derived conceptual definition sufficiently culturally sensitive to make it generally acceptable for use in nursing practice and future research?

In order to answer these questions, a second study, an expansion of the concept analysis was conducted (Cowles, 1996). The purposes of this study were to discover how individuals from various broadly defined cultural groups who had experienced grief defined the concept, its antecedents, and its consequences, and to compare these findings with those of the initial concept analysis in which the professional literature had been the data source.

METHODS

The methods employed in this study were adapted from those developed by Rodgers (1989, 1993a, 1993b; see also Chapter 6) for concept analysis, and those that are generally employed by qualitative researchers for thematic analysis (Lofland, 1971; Bogdan & Biklen, 1982; Lincoln & Guba, 1985). Strategies for the conduct of, and data analysis for, focus group research (Basch, 1987; Carey & Smith, 1994; Kingry et al., 1990; Morgan, 1988; Ramirez & Shepperd, 1988; Stewart & Shamdasani, 1990) also were used. More specific details of the sampling strategies, informed consent procedures, and data collection methods can be found in Cowles (1996). However, it is important to note that the interview questions asked of each of the focus groups specifically reflected the six categories of data (concept attributes, antecedents, consequences, surrogate terms, related concepts, and references) that had been extracted from the professional literature in the initial concept analysis.

Following the thematic analysis using these six categories plus an additional category for perceived cultural influences of grief, analytic comparisons between the themes generated from the focus groups and those generated from the original concept analysis were made. It was through these comparisons that the researcher attempted to discover how consistent the perceptions of those who have experienced grief were with those of the experts, as well as to begin to address the cultural sensitivity of the conceptual definition derived from the original study.

FINDINGS

The findings of this expansion of the concept analysis of grief indicated that the intrapersonal experience of grief, or that which is individually believed, felt, and described as grief, was very similar across the cultural groups used in the study. As an African-American male stated, "I believe we all grieve the same. Any cultural group would probably use different words, but they all mean the same thing." The analysis also revealed that the participants, who had drawn their knowledge of grief primarily from their own personal experiences, defined grief in much the same way as the definition derived from the original concept analysis (Cowles, 1996). However, despite the many similarities noted in the conceptual definition, the study findings provided additional descriptive clarity for each of the attributes of the concept as well as for the antecedents originally identified. Perhaps more important, the comparison between the perceptions of those who described their own personal experiences with grief with those of the experts also revealed one very significant difference.

Clarifying the Attributes of Grief

The conceptual definition derived from the original study (Cowles & Rodgers, 1991; Rodgers & Cowles, 1991) consisted of five attributes; grief was defined as *a dynamic, pervasive, highly individualized process with a strong normative component*. While agreeing with contemporary experts that grief does not consist of a rigid, linear progression, and therefore can be defined as *dynamic*, the participants clarified further by particularly noting the many personal changes experienced by the grieving person over time and how unpredictable these changes can be. As one African-American participant stated, "Way in the back of your heart, way in back, it's still there. And it can always flare back up to the front."

The *pervasiveness* of grief, or its potential to affect every aspect of a person's existence, also was reflected in the participants' descriptions. One of them noted, "Grief is like the end of the world." A particular focus of many of the participants' experiences was on the persistent search for an understanding of why things happened as they did, a search that affected each of them psychologically, emotionally, and spiritually.

In describing the pervasiveness of their individual grief experiences, the participants also discussed the unique combinations of emotional, psychological, spiritual, physical, and social aspects that account for the *highly individualized* nature of grief. Of particular importance, there was no consensus either within or across focus groups as to what type of relationship loss, e.g., loss of a child, loss of a spouse, etc., was responsible for the most intense or prolonged grief. This lack of consensus, although consistent with the literature as a whole, contrasted with a number of individual authors who have suggested that grief resulting from one or another particular type of loss is usually the most intense and/or prolonged. As with the many manifestations of grief described by the participants, the impetus for grief too was viewed as highly individualized. In the words of one participant, "It (grief) has to go in proportion to the relationship."

Grief as a *process* was described by the participants most similarly to what has been discussed in the contemporary professional literature. Consistently characterized as work that occurs over time, grief also was described as phases of activity or feeling that were neither linear nor having a particular end point. Although some of the earlier classic professional literature indicated a sequential, linear progression of grief, the large majority of contemporary authors' works analyzed for the initial concept analysis indicated, as did the participants in this study, a process without sequential stages or rigid boundaries.

Although the analysis of the findings of this study did not uncover additional insights into grief as a process, the words of the participants did provide descriptive clarity. For example, although several authors have equated grief, either metaphorically or in actuality, with the process of wound healing, there has been little evidence that using this example in practice would assist persons experiencing grief to better understand their experiences as a process. However, several participants in this study, from varying cultural heritages, spontaneously described grief as similar to the healing of a wound. In addition, whenever this descriptor was used, other members of the focus group would verbally acknowledge an understanding of and agreement with this idea, and in some instances, would add to the description. An Asian-American male offered this description: "I tend to believe that grief is similar to a wound. It can be hurt, and at a certain time it may heal...but it's still there, it's not gone. Once you hit it again, the pain comes back." Several moments later, another member of the focus group, also an Asian-American male, stated, "Somebody was using the word wound healing. I think that the process of grieving is self-healing. . . . So I think that nature takes its course by healing that."

The most notable, and potentially most significant, distinction between the findings of the initial concept analysis and those of the expanded study was the virtual absence of any discussion of a *normative component* of grief by the focus group participants. While clearly acknowledging differences between cultures, the participants spoke only of differences in the associated traditions, rituals, and behavioral expressions as they understood them, not in the intrapersonal experience of grief. Unlike authors of the professional literature, the study participants placed no temporal or behavioral boundaries on grief, nor did any of them indicate that they would judge another's grief experience or expression as inappropriate or abnormal.

A woman of Chinese heritage, having recently observed some Anglo-

Americans grieving the death of a loved one, stated, "I find it very, very different." She went on to explain what she perceived to be cultural differences without giving any indication of either judging or questioning these differences. She simply stated that she found them to be "interesting."

The most striking example of the absence of a *normative component* in the participants' definition of grief came as a group of Native Americans openly demonstrated their nonjudgmental approach to another's grieving during the course of the study interview. As this group described some of their personal experiences, one member became distraught. Crying almost uncontrollably, she apologized to the others, noting that although her mother died years earlier, she could not "get over it." The group spontaneously broke away from the focus group format to acknowledge this woman's grief and support her as she cried. One of them reassured her, "There's nothing wrong with grieving." It was clear to the investigator that the entire group placed no limits on what they considered to be "normal grief."

Clarifying the Antecedents of Grief

The long and varied list of the possible antecedents of grief generated by the focus groups strongly indicated a general agreement with professional authors that "grief may be preceded by any situation in which there is a perceived loss, including separation from any object of attachment . . . an abstract personal need, or a physical object in which an individual has invested interest or importance. . . . " (Cowles & Rodgers, 1991). In addition, the focus group participants, like the authors of the professional literature, associated grief most often with loss occurring as the result of the death of another. However, they also provided convincing evidence, thus adding clarity to an understanding of grief, that despite death being the most frequent antecedent of grief, it is not necessarily the one engendering the most enduring or painful response. This evidence arose during several long, spontaneous discussions by some of the groups of marital divorce and its relationship to grief.

Several participants referred to their grief following a divorce as more intense and prolonged than that which they had experienced following the death of a significant other. A woman of Puerto Rican heritage noted, "Divorce hit me harder," while another woman of Anglo heritage explained that "divorce is worse than death" because of the associated "bitterness" and sense of personal failure.

Throughout the study interviews, although the majority of discussions centered on death as an antecedent to grief, it was clear that all participants recognized that other perceived losses might also stimulate a grief response. It is helpful for practitioners to know that, in general, many individuals can and do associate grief with a variety of personal losses because it is difficult, at best, to offer support or intervention when a loss is not acknowledged, or perhaps not even recognized, as a possible stimulus for an individual's distress.

DISCUSSION

Basing their descriptions of grief, its antecedents, and consequences on their own personal experiences and observations, the participants in this expanded study provided strong validation for four of the five attributes of grief identified in the original concept analysis. In addition, while clearly not representing all cultural or ethnic groups, nor even the many subcultures within the groups chosen for this study, the participants provided beginning evidence that a definition comprised of these four attributes is generally culturally sensitive, and therefore, acceptable for use in nursing practice and future research. Finally, the descriptive clarity found in the participants' words can both affirm and add significant insight into how professionals conceptualize and apply this definition of grief.

The comparative analysis did, however, also raise one very important question, which by itself serves as strong justification for pursuing concept analysis beyond the professional literature. As noted previously, whereas professionals wrote extensively about a normative component of grief, thereby supporting the notion that grief has, at least, temporal and behavioral boundaries beyond which it no longer may be considered as normal, the participants in this study gave no evidence that the normative component attribute was included in their definitions of grief. This discrepancy has significant implications both from a theoretical and conceptual perspective and from a clinical application perspective.

From the more theoretical perspective, questions arise concerning the origins and purpose of the attribute of grief identified by the experts as the *normative component*. Given that individuals often question whether their own experiences of grief are "normal," particularly when acute symptoms seem overwhelming, it is possible that the origins of this observation are in the acute intrapersonal experience, rather than in societal or cultural expectations. Currently, the focus of much of the literature describing a normative component of grief centers on the experts' observations of what is considered in the therapeutic realm as expected behaviors and duration of grief, not on individuals' expectations and/or concerns regarding their own grief. Should the origin of the normative component lie more exclusively within the grieving person, strategies to assist individuals with their personal expectations, fears, and concerns about their experience would be a primary focus of therapeutic intervention. Clearly, further study is warranted to explore whether the normative component should be addressed from the perspective of how persons view their own grief, as opposed to how others portray the grieving person.

Conceptually, one might question whether the discrepancy between the experts' definitions of grief and those of the study participants lies primarily in the lack of clarity in the literature regarding the differences between grief and mourning. As was clear from the study participants, mourning rituals and behaviors differ in a variety of ways both between and within cultures, while the experience of grief does not. If the term mourning is used interchangeably with the term grief by some of the experts, it is possible that the normative component ascribed to grief might be more accurately a characteristic of mourning.

Finally, from a clinical applications perspective, the discrepancy may suggest that professionals, whose traditional focus has been on active intervention, have more need than do the people they serve to norm the experience of grief by setting temporal and/or behavioral limits. Again, there is a need for additional research to attempt to uncover the origin and purpose of the normative component of grief so often portrayed in the literature, but not even mentioned by the participants in this study who described their own grief.

CONCLUSIONS

Concepts held, and used, by nurses must be not only clear, but relevant to the patient populations for whom care is provided. As Rodgers (1993b) pointed out, situational, individual, and cultural factors can be significant influences in the construction of concepts. Therefore, it is important to identify the relevance of concepts not only for potential patients or clients in general, but for groups of particular cultural backgrounds. The clarification and development of concepts useful in nursing can be enhanced substantially through collection of data from groups of laypersons and others outside the discipline of nursing. In this study, a focus group technique was successful in capturing the perspectives and conceptualizations of members of diverse cultural groups. The collection of such "real world" data is an important step in determining the "fit" and utility of the concept, and provides a substantive basis for further development of the concept.

REFERENCES

Basch, C. E. (1987). Focus group interviews: An underutilized research technique for improving theory and practice in health education. *Health Education Quarterly, 14,* 411–448.

Bogdan, R. C., & Biklen, S. K. (1982). *Qualitative research for education.* Boston: Allyn & Bacon.

Carey, M. A., & Smith, M. W. (1994). Capturing the group effect in focus groups: A special concern in analysis. *Qualitative Health Research, 4*, 123-127.

Cowles, K. V. (1996). Cultural perspectives of grief: An expanded concept analysis. *Journal of Advanced Nursing, 23*, 287-294.

Cowles, K. V., & Rodgers, B. L. (1991). The concept of grief: A foundation for nursing practice and research. *Research in Nursing and Health, 14*, 119-127.

Kingry, M. J., Tiedje, L. B., & Friedman, L. L. (1990). Focus groups: A research technique for nursing. *Nursing Research, 39*, 124-125.

Lincoln, Y. S., & Guba, E. G. (1985). *Naturalistic inquiry*. Thousand Oaks, CA: Sage.

Lofland, J. (1971). *Analyzing social settings*. Belmont, CA: Wadsworth.

Morgan, D. L. (1988). *Focus groups as qualitative research* (Sage University Paper Series on Qualitative Research Methods, Vol. 16). Newbury Park, CA: Sage.

Ramirez, A. G., & Shepperd, J. (1988). The use of focus groups in health research. *Scandinavian Journal of Primary Health Care (Suppl.), 1*, 81-90.

Rodgers, B. L. (1989). Concepts, analysis and the development of nursing knowledge: The evolutionary cycle. *Journal of Advanced Nursing, 14*, 330-335.

Rodgers, B. L. (1993a). Concept analysis: An evolutionary view. In B. L. Rodgers & K. A. Knafl (Eds.), *Concept development in nursing: Foundations, techniques, and applications* (pp. 73-92). Philadelphia: W. B. Saunders.

Rodgers, B. L. (1993b). Philosophical foundations of concept development. In B. L. Rodgers & K. A. Knafl (Eds.), *Concept development in nursing: Foundations, techniques, and applications* (pp. 7-34). Philadelphia: W. B. Saunders.

Rodgers, B. L., & Cowles, K. V. (1991). The concept of grief: An analysis of classical and contemporary thought. *Death Studies, 15*, 443-458.

Schwartz-Barcott, D., & Kim, H. S. (1986). A hybrid model for concept development. In P. L. Chinn (Ed.), *Nursing research methodology: Issues and implementation* (pp. 91-101). Rockville, MD: Aspen.

Schwartz-Barcott, D., & Kim, H. S. (1993). An expansion and elaboration of the Hybrid Model for Concept Development. In B. L. Rodgers & K. A. Knafl (Eds.), *Concept development in nursing: Foundations, techniques, and applications* (pp. 107-133). Philadelphia: W. B. Saunders.

Stewart, D. W., & Shamdasani, P. N. (1990). *Focus groups: theory and practice*. Newbury Park, CA: Sage.

An Expansion and Elaboration of the Hybrid Model of Concept Development*

Donna Schwartz-Barcott and Hesook Suzie Kim

Early in the 1970s, theory development became established as a national goal in nursing (Meleis, 1985). By 1975, 11 distinct nursing theories had been published (Walker & Avant, 1988). Simultaneously, nursing educators began experimenting with the incorporation of theories in undergraduate and graduate curricula. The National League for Nursing (1972) passed a new criterion requiring that curriculum plans be based on conceptual frameworks. The demand for nurses who could teach these theories, the increasing number of nursing theories, as well as the number of related non-nursing theories (e.g., stress, communication, coping, systems, and crises theories) already in the nursing literature, made the creation of courses specific to theory and its application in nursing practice inevitable.

The hybrid model emerged in response to the excitement, exigencies, and hidden complexities surrounding the development of one such course. The course that was created at the University of Rhode Island combined a three-credit theory component with a three-credit practicum. The focus of the practicum was on selecting, developing, and

*This chapter is a revised and expanded version of: A hybrid model for conceptual development. In P. L. Chinn (Ed.), Nursing research methodology: Issues and implementation (pp. 91–101), 1986. Reprinted with permission of Aspen Publishers, Inc. The authors would like to thank Dr. Jacqueline Fortin for her in-depth reading of the earlier chapter, discriminating use of the model, and invaluable comments and suggestions for the present chapter.

129

applying concepts and theoretical frameworks in specific clinical nursing situations. It quickly became apparent that the excitement over the use of theories in nursing was not accompanied by an equally developed arsenal of methods for applying them. There was little, if any, discussion in the nursing literature of how one was to select from among the various concepts or theories given a particular clinical problem or situation, or of the possible boundaries or time parameters for applying any one concept or theory. Each theory was seen as appropriate for any nursing care situation or setting. In fact, there seemed to be a rather universal assumption at the time that simply having knowledge of a particular theory was sufficient for its unending application.

An additional difficulty with these early theories was their high degree of abstractness and vagueness. It was not unusual to discover that the central concepts of a theory were lacking adequate definitions or measurements. One manageable way to address these difficulties was to focus attention on the analysis and refinement of individual concepts because they form the basic building blocks of a theory. In so doing, we began looking for an approach that would help ensure that:

1. The concepts selected for analysis would be integral to nursing practice.
2. The literature reviewed would be broad enough to capture the commonalities and extremes in conceptualization and usage of the concept across the disciplines.
3. The focus of analysis would be on the essential aspects of definition and measurement.
4. Analysis from the literature review would be tightly integrated with the empirical data being collected in the clinical practice.

No single approach or literature base addressed all these concerns; thus, an approach (now referred to as the hybrid model of concept development) was created based on knowledge from three bodies of literature, each of which approached concept development in a slightly different manner. These included literature from the philosophy of science (Hempel, 1952; Kaplan, 1964; Nagel, 1961), the sociology of theory construction (Blalock, 1969; Dubin, 1969; Gibbs, 1972; Hage, 1972; Reynolds, 1971), and writings on participant observation—more frequently referred to today as field research (Bogdan & Taylor, 1975; McCall & Simmons, 1969; Pelto, 1970; Schatzman & Strauss, 1973).

The model that was developed interfaces theoretical analysis and empirical observation, with a focus on the essential aspects of definition and measurement. The model involves steps used to identify, analyze, and refine concepts in the initial stage of theory development and is most applicable to applied sciences in general and to nursing specifically. Because the approach draws heavily on insights generated in clinical practice, it is especially useful in studying significant and central phenomena in nursing. Theoretical development based on this model at the initial stage thus can include concepts having both analytical and empirical foundations. The model was first described in Chinn's 1986 edition of *Nursing Research Methodology*. Some of our experience in using the model was presented later in that same year at the Third Annual Nursing Science Colloquium at Boston University (Schwartz-Barcott, 1986). The purpose of this chapter is to integrate these earlier writings with the additions and refinements that have been made to the model to date.

THE HYBRID MODEL

Figure 9-1 presents the major components of the hybrid model. It is composed of three phases: an initial, theoretical phase; a fieldwork phase; and a final, analytical phase. As the label denotes, the initial phase is largely theoretical in nature, although drawing directly on an experience from clinical practice. This experience is used to select a concept integral to nursing and draft a tentative definition. Once the concept has been selected, Reynold's (1971) approach is used to begin searching the literature, comparing and contrasting existing definitions with one's tentative definition, and moving toward the selection or creation of a working definition with which to begin the fieldwork. Reynold's approach is especially appropriate at this point because of its heavy emphasis on the essential nature of a concept rather than on the defining attributes, properties, antecedents, or consequences of a concept that are of more use after the essential aspect of a concept has been identified.

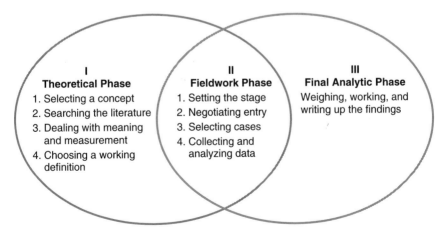

Figure 9–1   Major components of the hybrid model.

The second or fieldwork phase, which overlaps in time with the first phase, emphasizes the empirical component of the process. In this phase, methods from fieldwork are utilized to collect qualitative data for further analysis of the selected concept. The literature review begun in phase one is continued in phase two. Additionally, the literature review serves as an ongoing basis for comparison with data being collected in the field. Schatzman and Strauss' (1973) guide to field research is used directly for the overall structuring and sequencing of steps in this phase. Reynold's analytical approach helps undergird the collection and analysis of data. Wilson's (1969) analytical approach is brought forth as potentially useful for selecting cases and collecting and analyzing data in the second phase.

The third phase includes the final step in interfacing the initial theoretical analysis with insights gained from the empirical observations and writing up the findings. Here again Reynold's (1971) and Wilson's (1969) analytical approaches help in finalizing the analysis and suggesting possible alterations for refinements of the concept.

The above diagram emphasizes the intertwining of theoretical and fieldwork phases. Although it is possible to separate these phases, we have found the model is most useful when one enters the field at about the same time as one begins to search the literature. This helps one maintain a questioning frame of mind regarding the empirical relevance and nature of the selected concept. When one enters the field having already completed a comprehensive review of the literature and thus fully committed to the development of a particular concept, it is more difficult to deeply question and reflect on the appropriateness and meaning of the concept in the fieldwork phase. In such a case, the process often becomes focused on validating an existing definition rather than on probing and questioning the essential nature of the concept in a particular setting.

The following discussion of each step in the model is not meant to provide a cookbook approach to concept development. The intent is to describe the general aim and thinking underlying each step and to give a sense of options or ways one might think through concept development. We have tried to emphasize the importance of probing, reflecting, and taking time to think in place of the doing aspects of the model.

THE THEORETICAL PHASE

The principal focus in this phase is on developing a foundation for the later phases of in-depth analysis and concept refinement. This includes selecting and drafting an initial, very loose definition, beginning the literature review, and starting to map out the essential elements of definition and measurement. It ends as one identifies a working definition for the fieldwork phase.

Selecting a Concept

The selection of a concept for study has been approached by nursing scholars in various ways. Some authors, such as Brownell (1984), Hogue (1985), Panzarine (1985), and Reed and Leonard (1990), have drawn directly from existing concepts in other disciplines. Others, such as Leininger (1985), Norris (1982), and Rew and Barrow (1987), have drawn on identified but underdeveloped concepts from the nursing literature. Additionally, scholars using grounded theory have generated new concepts directly out of nursing practice or research (Atwood, 1978; Chenitz & Swanson, 1986; Wilson, 1986). Whatever the approach taken, some initial consideration needs to be given to ways of enhancing the probability of selecting a concept relevant to nursing.

To date, the most productive uses of the hybrid model have been those that begin by using an encounter drawn directly from clinical practice. This encounter is used then as a basis for selecting a concept, one that is closely linked to empirical reality. Some of the best encounters are those that are unexpected and leave the nurse feeling frustrated, horrified, angry, embarrassed, or bewildered. For example, a graduate student who was visiting an elderly client in a nursing home for the first time had the following experience:

> The foyer of the new, modern nursing home was filled with residents. At first glance it seemed to be full of potential hostesses, appropriately attired and positioned to offer a warm welcome to incoming visitors. But, as she entered a step further, moved toward one or two, to nod or smile— expecting in part to be ushered in or at least directed to her client—she discovered distant looks, vacuous smiles, and aimless muttering.

The student was surprised to discover that the initial image of social activity and animation among the elderly in the foyer was only a mirage. What was particularly disconcerting and saddening was the lack of human interaction among a group of individuals who appeared to need such interaction.

By filling in details related to the setting, the people involved, and the words exchanged, the investigator can use such an encounter to begin to ferret out a relevant concept. An emphasis on describing the encounter, rather than on trying to explain it, can help avoid premature interpretation. For example, much of the value of the early observations of the elderly group of residents in the foyer of the nursing home would have been lost if the word *senile* had been inserted before elderly. *Confusing mutterings* is much more descriptive of the encounter than the single term *confused*, which tends to imply that these individuals were always confused or spent most of their time in a state of confusion. This interpretation would have been erroneous given later observations.

Given a relatively full recording of the encounter, it can be reexamined for possible concepts to be used for labeling, and it can further understanding of the unexpected or problematic aspect of the encounter. The following questions can be used to focus attention on the existing pool of potentially relevant concepts from other disciplines and nursing, thus drawing on two of the approaches mentioned earlier for concept selection. What might be happening here? Is there a single concept, such as withdrawal or noncompliance, that provides a relatively accurate label of the focus of concern? How might a sociologist or anthropologist describe this encounter? What term might a physiologist or psychologist use to identify this same focus of concern? What language might other nurses use?

It is not necessary to strike on a single concept immediately. Initially, it is important to consider the wide range of possible scientific concepts or explanations that might help to illuminate this particular encounter. In the encounter with the elderly, one scholar may see indications of disorientation, withdrawal, or some combination of these in the faces and actions of the elderly. Another might see evidence of senility, sensory deprivation, or disengagement. It is not unusual, at this point, to be confronted with a number, even an overabundance, of potential concepts for further examination. In the case just mentioned, five potentially relevant concepts were identified.

There are additional steps that can be taken to focus on a single concept. First, the investigator can begin to delineate concepts that may be more useful as independent variables than as dependent variables. At this point, it is easy to confuse descriptive and explanatory uses of a concept. For example, in the case just mentioned, senility, sensory deprivation, and disengagement were being used primarily as concepts to explain the behavior observed among the elderly in the foyer. Second, the remaining concepts can be arranged by degree of plausibility. The investigator may want to refer back to the initial encounter to review the details in light of the concepts being considered at this point. Once one has a single concept in mind, it is time to try drafting a loose definition. This may simply consist of one or two phrases. In the above example the phrase *lack of human interaction* was used to begin defining withdrawal. One expects this definition to change, but this initial draft helps in keeping sight of the underlying phenomenon of interest and gives a point for comparison and contrast as one starts searching the literature for more formalized definitions.

In some cases, however, the investigator still may not be able to draw on any one or two existing concepts directly. Instead, a series of concepts may be identified, none of which seems to capture fully the image of reality that is of interest. In one situation, for example, a nurse was feeling harassed by the picayune, seemingly illogical, and endless demands of a patient who had chronic obstructive lung disease. These demands often were accompanied by abusive language. The patient had a lengthy history of admissions related to his disease and was well known to the staff. No amount of effort on the part of the nursing staff seemed to increase the patient's satisfaction or comfort. As one nurse described it:

> In cleaning up the bedside table—I moved the Kleenex box—he demanded it be replaced—he wanted it moved another quarter of an inch to the right. The bell would ring once or twice every fifteen minutes. The level of H_2O connected to the O_2 tank was down one-quarter inch, one inch above the level for refill. Mr. J. wanted the water refilled. The function and operation of the water apparatus were explained. Mr. J. nodded in seeming agreement. In five minutes the bell rang again. Mr. J. wanted the H_2O refilled.

It was not clear whether the nurse was dealing with forgetfulness, autocratism, manipulative behavior, hostility, fear, neurosis, a sense of helplessness, or just open, interpersonal conflict between patient and nurse. All of these concepts seemed to capture an important "reality" in this situation, but at the same time, none seemed to reflect its essence or fullness.

Given this kind of situation, it may be best to go ahead and create a new concept as a basis for tentative exploration in the field setting. Then, later, if an appropriate existing concept emerges, the investigator can simply discard the initial one. It is highly likely that the initial analysis and field data will be useful in examining and refining the existing concept.

Searching the Literature

As noted earlier, the search of the literature begins in this phase and then is continued and expanded in the fieldwork phase. Ultimately, the goal is to gain comprehensive command of the literature dealing with the concept and to acquire a deep grasp and understanding of it as it has been used across disciplines and over time. Such an understanding requires a broad systematic, cross-disciplinary search directed first at understanding the meaning of the concept and secondly, at the various ways it has been or might be measured. The following set of questions has been useful in providing an initial direction for this search. What is the essential nature of a concept? How can its essence be defined clearly? How can it be fleshed out so as to enhance its measurability? As these questions suggest, the initial review of the literature needs to be focused on central questions of definition and measurement. The aim is to capture the extremes in conceptualization and usage of the selected concept across disciplines. Later, after the investigator is well into the fieldwork phase, the focus will shift to more subtle elements of definition and measurement. References on integrative research reviews (Cooper, 1984; Ganong, 1987) may be helpful, although their emphasis is often on explanatory relationships derived from empirical research, rather than on definition and measurement of individual concepts across theoretical and empirical literature bases.

Dealing with Meaning and Measurement

Once a few definitions are in hand, it is helpful to look for major points of contrast and similarity. With a concept such as creativity, the investigator will be confronted with a variety of definitions. For some scholars, creativity is an aspect of cognitive functioning, a way of thinking. For others, it is an intrapersonal and interpersonal process. May (1972) speaks of creativity as an encounter between an intensively conscious human being with his or her world. But for Rogers (1972), creativity is a "novel relational product growing out of the uniqueness of the individual on the one hand and the materials, events, people or circumstances of his life on the other" (p. 5). Creativity, as a concept, thus is considered as a process of interaction between a person and his or her environment, as a product of interaction, or as an interpersonal process. This type of comparison gives the investigator some idea of the degree of consensus among users of a particular concept and leads to an understanding of what Reynolds (1971) refers to as the degree of intersubjectivity of meaning.

In the above sample, definitions of creativity were relatively abundant. It is not infrequent, however, to find that there are few explicit definitions for the concept one has chosen for study. In such a situation, it helps to look to see if there is a definition implied in the author's writings. Sometimes this is revealed in examples that the author has used in discussing the concept. Likewise, it is not uncommon to find authors using an instrument to measure a particular concept, without providing a definition for the concept. We have found the format in Table 9-1 helpful in beginning to organize and analyze readings from the literature in regard to defining and measuring a particular concept.

Choosing a Working Definition

Once major points of agreement and disagreement among existing definitions and between these and one's initial definition have become apparent, a definition is selected or generated for further detailed examination. Selecting a definition that seems congruent with one's initial

Table 9-1 Sample Format for Organizing and Analyzing Definitions

Reference	Explicit	Implicit	Examples	Comments

thoughts will help to maintain a nursing perspective; however, maintaining a tentative posture with respect to a selected definition is necessary if the investigator is to be open-minded in the refinement process.

FIELDWORK PHASE

The fieldwork phase is aimed at corroborating and refining a concept by extending and integrating the analysis begun in phase one with ongoing empirical observations initiated in this phase. The approach presented here is a modification of classic participant observation. It includes the basic steps found in any qualitative research that draws heavily on participant observation; setting the stage, negotiating entry, selecting cases, and collecting and analyzing data (Bernard, 1988; Chenitz & Swanson, 1986; Fetterman, 1989; Leininger, 1985; Lofland, 1976; Pelto & Pelto, 1984; Werner & Schoepfle, 1987). The steps in the fieldwork phase, however, differ in scope, focus, and time frame. Classic participant observation studies begin with a broad topical area. Often, the research question itself is not identified until the investigator is well into data collection. The focus generally involves the identification, description, and explanation of several concepts, and the minimum time frame for data collection is usually 1 year (Bernard, 1988; Keith, 1988; Messerschmidt, 1981; Whyte, 1984). In the hybrid model the focus is on a single concept, identified before the initiation of fieldwork, and on definition and measurement rather than explanation. The minimum time frame for data collection is 2½ to 3 months.

Schatzman and Strauss (1973) provide an excellent overview of each of the basic steps outlined in Figure 9-1, in *Field Research: Strategies for a Natural Sociology.* The proposed model represents the adaptation of these methods of field research for concept development in nursing. The following discussion highlights techniques that can be used in each step for maintaining the focus on definition and measurement and for incorporating the nursing perspective.

Setting the Stage

The focus in this step is on the selection of a fieldwork site and identification of major questions to guide the fieldwork phase. The selection of a site is somewhat critical to assuring a nursing perspective. By listing the potential range of patient populations or patient care situations in which the concept is expected to be relevant, the investigator can clarify core elements of the concept as well as increase the likely generalizability of the concept within nursing.

For example, in an initial literature review, Testa (1980) found that withdrawal was repeatedly and explicitly linked with elderly people and those who were mentally ill (see Chapter 10). Earlier observations of elderly in nursing homes suggested that withdrawal might occur with considerable frequency in almost any long-term institutionalized patient population. In addition, withdrawal seemed to be more common than indicated in the research on the elderly and the mentally ill populations. At times, it seemed like an almost normal phase—one that most patients pass through in trying to cope with any illness. It appeared, then, that withdrawal may be present with some frequency in a variety of institutional settings, ranging from prisons, mental hospitals, and nursing homes to extended ambulatory care centers and hospices. Withdrawal also may be experienced relatively frequently among the chronically ill and the elderly in noninstitutionalized settings.

Three essential criteria should guide the selection of a population and a setting: (a) the likelihood of frequent observations of the phenomenon under study; (b) the appropriateness of participant observation as a method of gathering empirical data; and (c) the likelihood that the researcher will be able to create and sustain a participant-observation role in the setting. In contrast to earlier and subsequent phases of this model, extensive familiarity with a specific site can act as a strong deterrent in sustaining the participant-observer role. This is depicted well in Benner's (1975) description of her experiences as a nurse-researcher who attempted participant observation in an intensive care unit in which she had previously worked as a staff nurse. She portrayed graphically the difficulties encountered in moving from participant to an observer role in a setting with which the researcher is very familiar. First, for Benner, her nurse's uniform evoked certain expectations from patients and families but, most importantly, from herself. In one bed, there was a man struggling with a urinal underneath his breakfast tray. Across the hall was an anxious-looking young woman, standing at the foot of the bed of a comatose patient—her eyes searching for help. No other nurses were in sight. Secondly, there were internal pressures she had to accept: the desire to be integrated into the group, the immense discomfort of being treated as an outsider—"the one who does not know the ways of the ICU" (p. 108).

One or two major questions can be used to link the concept with a specific patient population or a setting. For example, the investigator might be interested in the presence of withdrawal among elderly individuals, especially with regard to whether there is a progressive nature to withdrawal. At the same time, it is necessary to deal with the ambiguities inherent in trying to identify any one patient as being *withdrawn*. Questions guiding the fieldwork phase should address (a) the essential defining elements of a concept; (b) the differentiating elements that separate the central concept from similar concepts; and (c) the measurement criteria that may be developed for the concept.

Negotiating Entry

It is easy to disregard the subtleties of gaining access and legitimation to the selected population or setting demands until it is too late. In *Field Research*, Schatzman and Strauss (1973) cover the intricacy and complexity of this type of negotiation in much detail—especially as it applies to formal and highly complex organizations, such as a hospital. Many additional discussions of entry-level issues and techniques can be found in the large volume of writings that are currently available on the relational and personal processes of fieldwork (e.g., Agar, 1980; Ellen, 1984; Emerson, 1983; Wax, 1986; Whyte, 1984; Zola, 1983 in the sociological and anthropological literature, and Davis, 1986; Evaneshko, 1985; Field, 1989; Wilson, 1982 in the nursing literature).

Selecting Cases

Decisions regarding with whom the investigator should speak and how to focus observations in the field depend on the unit of analysis under study and the degree of clarity and intersubjectivity found in the initial review of literature. The unit of analysis depends on the concept. It most likely would be at the individual level for a study of withdrawal among the elderly or at the dyad level for a study of the use of touch among couples attending Lamaze classes. Other concepts that may be studied at the dyad level include empathy, attraction, and anger. Empathy and anger are also illustrative of concepts that may be studied at multiple levels. A small group could be a unit of analysis, if the investigator focused on empathetic interaction among group members. An entire unit, such as a floor in a nursing home, might be the unit of analysis if the presence of multiple patient roles and their patterns of interaction were of interest. As the investigator moves from a small group to a larger unit of analysis, however, more time is needed in order to gain adequate baseline knowledge of and familiarity with the group or unit under study.

A large number of cases is unnecessary and undesirable with this model of concept development. Three to six individuals, three or four dyads, one or two groups, and one floor or ward are more appropriate, because this enhances the possibility of frequent, repeated contact. Single encounters do not allow sufficient time for reflecting and probing. The selection of any one individual, couple, group, or floor will depend on the degree of definitional clarity gained in the theoretical phase. If the essential features of the concept are relatively clear, one or two indicators can serve as a basis for selection.

If the essential features of the concept are not clear and no indicators are apparent, Wilson's (1969) typology for concept analysis can be used as a basis for selection. This typology begins with the *model* case—one that absolutely reflects an instance of the concept. As Wilson notes, this is an instance in which we hear ourselves saying, "Well, if that isn't an example of so-and-so, then nothing is" (p. 28). Second is the *contrary* case, which according to Wilson represents a case that is absolutely not an instance of the concept: "Well, whatever so-and-so is, that certainly isn't an instance of it" (p. 29). Third is the *borderline* case. It appears as the "odd or queer" case (p. 31) and it helps highlight elements that make for a "true" case. The typology ends with the *related* case, which helps to clarify the central concept by identifying the criteria for a related concept.

The following excerpt from St. Angelo's (1983) observations of patient-nurse interactions in an emergency room (ER) provides an example of a model case of bonding. St. Angelo wondered if the concept of bonding (taken from the infant-mother bonding literature) might also be relevant to certain, rather "special" adult-nurse encounters that sometimes occur in the ER.

The model case. The emergency room doors opened. The rescue workers brought in a 55-year-old man with gasoline burns on his face, neck and chest. His lawnmower had exploded. He was conscious and had a saline-soaked drape on his face to cool the burns. Sue, the nurse, immediately took Mr. G.'s hand and told him her name and that she would be taking care of him. "I'm going to leave the drape on your face to cool the burns. Your chest is burned and I need to get these clothes off of you. Do you mind if I cut them?" Mr. G. replied, "Honey, you do anything you have to." Sue went on to tell Mr. G. that she was also going to have to draw some blood, start an intravenous, and that the doctor would be putting a Foley catheter into his bladder because of the need to monitor all the fluids going in and out of his body. Mr. G. jokingly said to Sue: "OK, but tell the doctor to cover me up—I'm shy." Sue told Bob not to worry as she drew the curtains around him and "whenever we aren't working on you we'll keep you covered. There's only me, another nurse and the doctor here."

Sue began to do the procedures necessary, explaining everything to Mr. G. as she went along. He asked her questions about the extent of his burns and about the other people at the scene. She answered as she worked. At one point Mr. G. jokingly said: "Hey Sue, what does my face look like? I hope I'm not going to be an ugly duckling." Sue came to the bedside, took his hand and spoke quietly at Mr. G.'s ear level: "Bob, you have some blisters on your face and I'm leaving the wet drape on so it will cool the area. Your eyelids might swell a little but it will go down in a couple of days. We have an excellent plastic surgeon coming in and he will debride the burns and start cleaning them with a special cream. You should have minimal to no scarring." In a more serious tone Mr. G. responded: "Well, I was just wondering...I have a heavy date with my wife for New Year's Eve."

The plastic surgeon was delayed in getting to the ER so there was a long waiting period. Sue stayed with Mr. G. during this time doing paper work at his bedside. She contacted family, offered pain medication prn and fed Mr. G. ice chips. The drape remained on Mr. G.'s face the entire time. When Sue transferred Mr. G. to a room on the surgical unit, Sue placed her hand on Mr. G.'s forehead and jokingly said: "Well, you took so much of my time today, Bob, that it's almost time for me to go home." Mr. G. responded: "Well, you turned out to be a swell date, Sue. We'll have to do this again sometime. Maybe next time I'll at least be able to see your face."

Next Saturday morning Sue went up on the floor to visit Mr. G. He was sitting up eating breakfast. His face had silvadene cream on it but his eyes were exposed. His lids were slightly swollen but they were open. Sue went into the room, smiled and said hello to Bob. He said hello but appeared hesitant as if he didn't know her. Sue went to the bedside and said: "Bob, my name is Sue. I took care of you in the emergency department on Thursday." Bob took Sue's hand and smiled: "Honey, I don't recognize you but I'd know that voice anywhere." (pp. 10–11)

Later, another excerpt from St. Angelo's (1983) observation was selected as a contrary case. Whatever was going on between this nurse and patient, it clearly was not an instance of bonding.

The contrary case. An 87-year-old man was wheeled into the ER. He had come from a local nursing home. On his right shoulder and scapular area was a large abscess. He was to meet his private physician for an incision and drainage of the abscess. The nurse, Peter, introduced himself to Mr. E, who was hard of hearing. Mr. E. was oriented to person and place but displayed some confusion as to time. Peter took Mr. E.'s vital signs and tried to obtain a patient history but Mr. E. was a poor historian. Peter sat at the desk and obtained the needed information from the transfer record. He returned to Mr. E. to make sure he was warm and safe. Peter then went about his other duties while waiting for the private physician to arrive. He periodically checked back with Mr. E. to see if there was anything he needed and to reassure him that the doctor would be coming. Mr. E. never asked for anything but always acknowledged Peter's orientation as to why he was waiting. The doctor arrived one hour later without apology. Peter immediately began to set up the anticipated equipment. He helped Mr. E. turn on his side. Peter then bent over, looked Mr. E. in the eyes and explained what would happen. "The doctor is going to wash your back with medicine and then he's going to put some medicine in your upper back to make it numb. You have to hold still." Mr. E. acknowledged Peter's comments with an "OK." The doctor proceeded with the procedure while Peter assisted. When the incision was made, a large amount of foul smelling drainage escaped. Everyone in the immediate area made facial expressions which indicated their awareness of the offensive odor. Mr. E. never said a word. Peter occasionally bent over to look at Mr. E. to ask how he was doing. Mr. E. would always respond, "OK." The incision was packed by the doctor and Peter applied a bulky dressing. Peter asked Mr. E. if he had any pain. Mr. E. did not comment. Peter asked again but a little louder. This time Mr. E. said "a little." Peter said he would get him some pain medication.

Later, Peter returned with the medication. He told Mr. E. that he would call the ambulance to take Mr. E. back to the nursing home. Peter called the home to review all the doctor's orders with the nurse who would be caring for Mr. E. He later found out that the ambulance would be delayed. He called the kitchen and ordered a lunch tray for Mr. E. Peter explained the situation to Mr. E. and assisted him with the lunch tray. (pp. 1914-1915)

Both of these encounters were selected for more intensive case work. Later, during the analysis phase, the cases were used to help identify essential aspects of bonding by eliminating the unessential features.

Collecting and Analyzing the Data

Schatzman and Strauss' (1973) notation system for collecting, recording, and analyzing fieldwork data is particularly well suited for concept analysis and refinement. This system utilizes a combination of participant observation augmented with periodic in-depth interviews. It facilitates multiple observations and in-depth reflections as well as probing dialogue with participants over time. Although there are several more recent publications on analyzing qualitative data (Bernard, 1988; Miles & Huberman, 1984; Strauss, 1987), this system is especially helpful in defining and measuring single concepts. More recent techniques tend to focus on the development of theoretical hypotheses or propositions, which often shifts the focus from definition and measurement to explanation.

The notation system includes observational notes (ON), theoretical notes (TN), and methodological notes (MN) that guide the researcher into possible analytic distinctions at the point of recording. The ON "are statements bearing upon events experienced principally through watching and listening. They contain as little interpretation as possible, and are as reliable as the observer can construct them" (Schatzman & Strauss, 1973, pp. 94–108). This is the who, what, when, where, and how of the phenomenon and identifies who said or did what under what circumstances. Quotation marks can be used to identify the exact words, phrases, or sentences that occurred in any one conversation. Otherwise, an apostrophe can be used for less accurate quoting or for simply paraphrasing. The TN is used to go beyond the "facts." The investigator can consciously interpret, infer, or speculate about the possible meaning of the observations. In the hybrid model, one can use the TN for bringing in definitions and measurements from the literature for comparing and contrasting with the data just described in the ON. The investigator's instructions to himself of herself are included under MN. This notation system encourages free-flowing yet systematic recording and organizing of the data. It makes for easy retrieval of key observations and is conducive to continual analysis and reflection.

Analyzing the Data

As is apparent from the notation system, data collection plunges the investigator into the analysis phase. Collection and analysis of data go on concurrently with every other step under the rubric of the TN. Nevertheless, about one half to three fourths of the way through the fieldwork phase, the investigator needs to begin to pull out and organize the data that are most relevant to the concept. Wilson's (1969) typology of cases can be helpful here. This can then serve as a basis for refocusing ongoing field observations and for more focused, in-depth probing as one moves through the latter half of this phase.

Mr. G. was the *model* case described earlier. He came in to the ER with face, neck, and chest burns from a lawnmower accident. St. Angelo (1983) first compared the behavioral indicators of bonding (e.g., nonprocedural touch; frequent, sustained eye contact; a "caring" tone of voice) that had emerged in the literature review of mother-infant bonding, with her own field observations:

> In this case, I saw indicators of touch. Hand-holding and gentle touch during the procedure were common. Also, when we brought Bob to his room, Sue put her hand on Bob's forehead as if to soothe him. There was absolutely no eye contact during this encounter which took about 5½ hours. Sue's tone of voice was very different from what I would have anticipated. Yet, it seemed to be very effective. She used a calm, confident tone of voice mixed with a joking attitude. There was indirect acknowledgement of but almost no direct reflection of Sue's or the patient's feelings. The patient's voice was initially shaky, then mixed with a joking attitude. (p. 14)

Touch, either procedural or nonprocedural, may reflect an essential element in patient-nurse bonding just as it does in mother-infant bonding. Sustained eye contact was not possible in this case because of the nature of the patient's injury. However, contrary to the literature, the lack of eye contact suggested that bonding can take place in the absence of such contact. Additionally, measurement problems became abundantly clear. St. Angelo struggled to judge whether a nurse's tone of voice demonstrating a *caring* quality.

Next, the data are reexamined to see if there are any *contrary* cases. These can be compared with model cases to highlight that which is distinctive to the latter. The following is an excerpt from St. Angelo's (1983) analysis of the contrary case presented earlier between the ER nurse, Peter, and Mr. E., an 87-year-old resident of a local nursing home who had come to the ER with a large abscess on his shoulder.

> I noticed that Peter did not use touch at any time other than to carry out a procedure. Yet, his touch was gentle, purposeful and appeared therapeutic. At first I interpreted this negatively but further searching of the literature suggested another possible view. I was interpreting touch (significant touch) to be anything other than procedural touch, but is that true? Peter's touch during procedures was always gentle. I began to equate this with the mother-infant literature and my own life experiences. After all, a mother's touch during diaper change is considered to be loving and caring. Sundeen, Stuart, Rankin, and Cohen (1976) state that the "use of touch in nursing goes beyond that which is necessary to attend to the client's personal physical needs. The manner in which the person is touched and the attitude of the nurse who is touching can convey a message of caring while physical needs are met" (p. 103). This literature changed my entire focus on Peter's care. Still I did not feel that this reflected "bonding." Instead, I would call it "caring." (pp. 23–24)

Earlier the term *bonding* was used to describe the special binding relationship that emerged between Sue and Bob. It seems completely missing in the encounter between Peter and Mr. E., even though Peter's touch denotes an element of caring. Thus, it may be that caring can occur without bonding taking place. In fact, there may be two separate or intertwining concepts in these situations: caring and bonding. Caring may be a separate but closely related concept. At the same time, this stage of analysis suggested the need to refocus attention on what is it that seems so unique to adult bonding. How can this kind of special interpersonal exchange in which each individual somehow becomes wedded to the other be "put into words?"

In the *borderline case*, it is not clear whether the concept applies. As Wilson (1969) notes, "by seeing what makes these cases 'odd or queer,' we come to see why the 'true' cases are not odd or queer" (p. 31) or, in other words, what makes them true cases. An example of a borderline case was not encountered in St. Angelo's (1983) field observations of bonding. A borderline case was present, however, in Roberts' (1982) field study of empathy among members in a sharing and caring group, namely, the Compassionate Friends, a group composed mainly of bereaved parents.

> At the December meeting, the group discussion centered around the upcoming holidays. A discussion about holiday tradition revealed a similarity between Pat and Betty; following that a significant interchange between these two women occurred. Pat was discussing her feelings regarding Christmas without her son. Betty, who appeared to have been listening intently, responded by talking about her own emotional experiences and feelings regarding the holiday. As Betty spoke, Pat remained seated on the edge of her chair, leaning towards Betty and maintaining eye contact. When Betty paused, Pat proceeded to finish the

story she had previously started, her voice revealing the intensity of her feelings. This "conversation" continued as both women verbally expressed their feelings. Neither one of them responded to the feelings expressed by the other, but instead focused on their own emotional experience which seemed similar. The rest of the group remained attentive and seemingly involved with the dialogue. I sensed a feeling of closeness between Pat and Betty following this interaction. (pp. 13-14)

Pat and Betty were intensely engaged in conversation in this example. Yet, neither one acknowledged or responded directly to the specifics of what the other said. At the same time, however, both women seemed to experience the interaction as positive and helpful. What made this case "odd or queer," in terms of empathy, was the failure of either party to react to the specific feelings being expressed by the other, although each responded to the other by sharing a similar experience or feeling. This analysis later led Roberts (1982) to propose three different degrees or levels of empathy:

> *Level one.* Individuals respond to each other by sharing a similar experience or emotion, but do not react to the specific feelings being expressed by the other.
>
> *Level two.* One individual (the empathizer) recognizes that the feelings being expressed belong to the other. The empathizer may begin to respond to the feelings being expressed by the other.
>
> *Level three.* The empathizer begins to feel, think, and act like the other, mirroring his or her emotion. At the same time, however, he or she maintains a clear sense of self and personal identity. (pp. 15-16)

Here, the odd case actually became incorporated within the concept as a minimal level indicator of empathy. Secondly, in constructing these levels, Roberts was able to move the measurement of empathy from a nominal to an ordinal level.

Another way of analyzing the data is to look for what Wilson (1969) called the *related* case: one that reflects a concept similar to the one under study. Often, this kind of case appears serendipitously. Sometimes, the investigator can be looking at a focal concept and discover another concept. Wilson suggests that the investigator can clarify the criteria for applying the related concept and may, in turn, be able to "get clear" more easily about the original concept. Here is an example from St. Angelo's (1983) study on patient-nurse bonding in an ER setting.

> A 36-year-old female was wheeled into the ER by the triage nurse. She was obese and stated that she had MS (multiple sclerosis). She was presently having urological problems for which the physician inserted a Foley catheter until further testing and possible surgery could be done. The Foley catheter had fallen out and the client wanted the catheter replaced. The nurse helped undress the client and inserted the catheter. During this time, the client shared that she had once weighed about 500 lbs and now

weighed 350 lbs. She attributed the excessive weight gain to prednisone which she took for the MS. The client had poor personal hygiene and the body odor was difficult to deal with in such close quarters. Her perineal area was also in need of good hygiene. During the actual insertion of the catheter, the nurse never looked at the client; however, she maintained the conversation throughout the procedure. The nurse spoke with inflections and a tone of voice which demonstrated warmth and caring. She utilized therapeutic reflective communication techniques and seemed to have a good understanding of the client's situation and feelings. At one point the client commented that she really hoped the catheter would be taken out soon and that the doctor would take care of this problem. The nurse responded: "You really feel gypped, don't you?" To this, the client paused and then said: "Yeah—I'm supposed to be getting married soon and this is making things hard on me—pause—I don't want to be left out." The nurse commented: "And I suppose your doctor really doesn't understand that." The client ended this exchange with, "Well, I guess not"—pause—"the tests will be done soon to see if I have a blockage."

In this example, there was no eye contact, no touching other than procedural or purposeful, but the tone of voice was unique. The nurse used a concerned tone of voice with a lot of inflections and excellent reflective techniques. St. Angelo interpreted the nurse's communications as a taking in, digesting and giving back of an understanding of the client, which the client validated in her responses. The nurse was attempting to communicate to the client that her ideas, feelings, and so on, were the ones that are important, not those of the nurses or others.

As the nurse mentioned in the staff conference, she had some difficulty maintaining her professionalism because of the body odor. St. Angelo saw a lot of energy being used in this case. It took energy to maintain professionalism in a difficult situation. It took energy to care for someone the nurse found to be offensive and still utilize a therapeutic communication. Also, it is not clear why the nurse did not look at the client during her care. Were there some personal feelings related to the client's age (close to the nurse's) and her pending marriage in spite of her obesity and her disease, that were affecting the nurse? Obese women with crippling disease and urinary tract problems in our society are not usually portrayed as sexual beings. Yet, the nurse was able to overcome most of these aspects to the best of her ability by providing the client with what might most accurately be called empathy. (pp. 16–17)

Thus, in looking for evidence of bonding, St. Angelo uncovered empathy. The bonding indicator of touch was not present, although the student saw a "caring" quality in the tone of voice. But, more important in this analysis was the description of the nurse's inherent dislike of the patient. It took a lot of energy and concentration for the nurse to keep this element from interfering with the care she felt the patient needed. It would seem, then, that a mutual liking and attraction needs to emerge between the patient and the nurse, in the context of the nurse's touch and caring, in order for bonding to take place. And, it is perhaps this special mutual attraction that best characterizes the unique aspect of a bonding relationship.

FINAL ANALYTICAL PHASE

During the analytical phase, the investigator steps back from the intensity and details of the fieldwork and reexamines the findings in light of the initial focus of interest. The following questions may be asked in this phase:

1. How much is the concept applicable and important to nursing?
2. Does the initial selection of the concept seem justified?
3. To what extent do the review of literature, theoretical analysis, and empirical findings support the presence and frequency of this concept within the population selected for empirical study?

For example, Testa's (1980) fieldwork with withdrawal tended to support the presence and importance of psychosocial withdrawal among residents in a nursing home setting. At the same time, the fieldwork suggested that, although the phenomenon existed frequently, withdrawal was not necessarily inherent in the adjustment process. In addition, the review of the literature and empirical findings altered an earlier perception of withdrawal as a predominantly negative process. It became apparent that withdrawal can be a positive factor by providing a "time-out" period for energy renewal and in maintaining one's self-dignity as well as gaining some control over the immediate environment, even when that environment reflects the dictates of a total institution.

At other times, the investigator may be less convinced of the relevance of a concept after fieldwork than he or she was before. Sometimes it is not so much that the findings do not support the existence of a particular concept as it is that a new concept or reformulation of the initial idea emerges out of the empirical observations and analysis. For example, Hassma (1979) was surprised to find little empirical support for the presence and importance of denial among repeat heart attack victims. She had expected to encounter a high level of denial among patients who showed a substantial lag period between the appearance of symptoms and hospitalization. Instead, Hassma found that difficulties in the process of "differential diagnosis," by patients, families, and in some cases physicians, were more a factor in producing a significant lag period than was the denial of symptoms.

Sometimes, it is not so much that the findings do not support the existence of a particular concept as it is that a new concept or reformulation of the initial idea emerges out of the empirical observations and analysis. For example, Janicki (1981) began fieldwork with a focus on the "mental suffering" of patients in the terminal phase of an illness, usually cancer. As she became more and more precise in the description of these patients' sufferings, the term *anguish* began to emerge as a more accurate label of the phenomenon she was observing.

If the importance of the initial concept was supported, then the next step is to reconsider the findings in light of the concept's definition and measurability. The investigator may want to begin by going back to the initial, tentative definitions and the listing of key elements in, and the analysis of, these definitions. At this stage, the investigator is asking, How do the definitions compare and contrast with the empirical findings? It may be that, at this point, one definition stands out as more useful than another. For example, Reilly (1982) found that creativity, in the context of nursing home residents, was far more an "active life process," involving one's entire being, than it was predominantly an activity of the mind. She also began to see an association between an individual's level of adjustment and the person's level of creativity. Those who adjusted exceedingly well seemed to actively remold the nursing home. Sometimes this remolding included the rearrangement of furniture in their rooms. Other times it occurred on a larger scale, such as the negotiation of a new role—that is, mailman or gardener— within the institutional setting. Whichever the case, for those who did very well, the adjustment was not simply passive acceptance of a given environment but a seeking out and revamping of that environment.

In another case, the empirical findings may lead to a redefinition of a concept or refinements in an existing definition. Testa (1980) concluded that psychosocial withdrawal needed to be separated explicitly from physical withdrawal. Also, the former concept needed to be redefined in terms of a process rather than as simply a symptom of something else or as a solitary state. Additionally, withdrawal needed to be reconceived as a social-psychological process that could range along a continuum of normality and not be limited to an abnormal, purely intrapsychic experience.

Yet, in other cases, it may be a matter of making explicit what has been implicit in the literature. Roberts (1982) defined *empathy* as an active process in which an individual senses another's emotional state, identifies with this state unconsciously or consciously, and reacts to the state, which results in a sharing of feelings. The importance of this definition was in making the implicit explicit. Additionally, in defining empathy in this way, it became possible to differentiate empathy from imitative behavior—an important distinction not included in earlier definitions.

Empirical findings also may lead to the recommendation of a new way of measuring a concept or to suggestions for refinements in existing measures. For example, Testa (1980) was able to begin operationalizing *withdrawal* by identifying a complex of physical, social, and emotional indicators. And, differing levels of severity were identified, which allowed for measurement at the categorical level. Her empirical findings lend support to these beginning efforts at measuring withdrawal.

Sometimes, the empirical findings may simply raise the need for different indicators, given the lack of support for existing ones. To some extent, this was one of the results of St. Angelo's (1983) work on adult bonding. The indicators from the mother-infant bonding literature (continuous eye contact, nonprocedural touch, and tone of voice) were just not comprehensive or germane enough to adult-adult relationships of this nature. Instead, it seemed that the investigator needed to look more closely at some form of subjective indicator, or a mixture of these more objective ones, with one or two more subjective indicators.

Writing Up the Findings

Reporting the results of a hybrid model analysis requires the integration of two separate writing traditions: concept analysis and fieldwork. The best single approach to integrating these traditions, to date, has been to frame the introduction and initial review of the literature in accord with the classic format of concept analysis and then draw on writing styles used in fieldwork to present and integrate the empirical observations with the literature review.

Textbooks and writings on concept development in the social sciences and in nursing seldom address the various techniques and formats used to write up a concept analysis (Bulmer, 1984; Chinn & Jacobs, 1983; Norris, 1982; Sartori, 1984; Walker & Avant, 1988; Wilson, 1969). In general, the author must use examples, such as those provided by Norris (1982), Kim (1983), Bertman and Krant (1977), and Gardner (1979). Kim presented two examples of minianalyses of the concepts of restlessness and compliance that aligned well with the emphasis on definition and measurement found in the hybrid model. In each analysis, Kim moved from a discussion of definitions across diverse bodies of literature to differentiation of the concept from other similar concepts (like Wilson's borderline or related concepts), to operationalization, and lastly to possible relationships with other concepts. In addition there is a need to begin with a discussion of the importance and relevance of the concept in nursing.

In writing up the empirical findings, the investigator has to consider the same questions facing any researcher in reporting a study involving fieldwork data: Who will the audience, or reader, be? What should the timing and pacing of the writing process be? How long should the manuscript be? Which details of methodology should be included? How should credibility be established? What facts or interpretations can ethically be made public? Early textbooks on participant observation addressed these issues in detail (e.g., Bogdan & Taylor, 1975; Lofland & Lofland, 1984: McCall & Simmons, 1969; Schatzman & Strauss, 1973). In addition, Taylor and Bogdan (1984) identified seven basic points of methodology (e.g., time and length of study and researcher's frame of mind) that serve as a useful checklist of content not to be forgotten. Lofland and Lofland's (1984) depiction of the necessary stages involved in writing a fieldwork report (from withdrawal and contemplation to the agony of omitting material and the creating of a serious outline) help the author anticipate the time and skills necessary for this type of writing.

More recent writings on participant observation have suggested that the presentation also needs to reflect the underlying purpose and the particular fieldwork approach taken in the study, for example, Lofland's (1976) strategic interaction orientation, Spradley's (1980) ethnographic approach, and Glaser's (1978) and Strauss' (1987) grounded theory methodology. Perhaps the model most closely approximating the kind of participant observation used in the hybrid model is grounded theory. The investigator, however, must keep in mind that the focus in grounded theory is on categorizing key concepts and explicating theoretical relationships, rather than on defining and measuring these concepts. On the horizon, investigators can expect to find an even wider range of considerations and styles for writing up fieldwork, as the recent debates and efforts of anthropologists to incorporate more humanistic and reflexive aspects of fieldwork into the reports themselves become known (e.g., Danforth, 1989; Denzin, 1989; Geertz, 1988; Van Maanen, 1988).

USES OF THE HYBRID MODEL TO DATE

To date the hybrid model has been used to examine a wide variety and range of concepts. Examples of some of these are shown in Tables 9–2 and 9–3 according to client, client-nurse, and practice domains in nursing (Kim, 1987).

Concepts related to the client domain are shown in Table 9–2. Kim's (1987) scheme for categorizing phenomena in the client domain provides a beginning basis for clustering the concepts. The three relevant categories in this scheme include: (a) essentialist concepts that refer to phenomena present in the client as essential characteristics and processes of human nature; (b) problematic concepts that refer to phenomena present in human beings as pathological or abnormal deviations from normal patternings; and (c) health care experiential concepts that refer to phenomena that arise from people's experiences in the health care system.

Examples of concepts that relate to client-nurse and practice domains are given in Table 9–3. Under the client-nurse domain are concepts that characterize in some way the nature of client-nurse interactions. The concepts seemed to form into certain clusters. For example, some, such as caring, mutuality, bonding, and friendship, tend to reflect more the quality of an interaction than the fundamental process or the central

Table 9–2   Client Domain

Essentialist Concepts

Relaxation	Fatalism
Dying	Control
Creativity	Self-care
Independence	Territoriality
Coping	Personal space
Regroup	Self-esteem
Problem solving	Body image
Information seeking	Connectedness
Decision making	Autonomy
Definition of the situation	Social support
Temperament	

Problematic Concepts

Fatigue	Chronic sorrow
Restlessness	Helplessness
Dyspnea	Panic
Suffering	Boredom
Memory loss	Loneliness
Obesity	Loss
Delayed recovery	Submission
Homelessness	Withdrawal
Masking behavior	Isolation
Denial	Anomie
Fear	Alienation
Anguish	Negligence
	Stigmatization

Health Care Experiential Concepts

Noncompliance
Stigma
Separation anxiety

focus of an interaction. In contrast, concepts of power and exchange relate to central processes of the interaction itself. And concepts such as presence, touch, empathy, and advocacy are more narrowly focused on the quality of the nurse's action.

The practice domain includes phenomena particular to the nurse who is engaged in delivering nursing care. It refers to the cognitive, behavioral, and social aspects of professional actions taken by a nurse in addressing client problems. The examples given here are predominantly cognitive in nature.

To date, the model has been useful in five ways. First, it has been helpful in giving some initial idea about the existence, frequency, and potential importance of any one concept in a given patient care setting. Each time we have used the model we have come away with a rather solid notion of the adequacy or inadequacy of existing definitions and possible approaches to measurability. For example, the results of one

Table 9–3   Client-Nurse and Practice Domains

	Client-Nurse Domain	
Concepts Reflecting the Character of an Interaction	*Concepts Characterizing Subprocesses Underlying or Forming the Focus of an Interaction*	
Mutuality	Central Process	
Bonding	Power	
Therapeutic alliance	Exchange	
Mutual participation	Subprocesses	
Negotiation	Independence/dependence/interdependence	
Attachment	Information seeking	
Friendship	Decision making	
	Self-disclosure	
	Trust	
	Empowerment	
	Concepts Reflecting Some Aspects of Actions of Nurse	
	Presence	
	Touch	
	Affective sensitivity	
	Empathy	
	Advocacy	
	Practice Domain	
Decision making	Vigilance	Compassion
Critical thinking	Making a case	Knowledge utilization
Validation	Home visiting	Commitment

study suggested that the concept of independence may be unduly limited to an individual's physical ability to carry out a manual task. For example, given current definitions, the following two individuals would be considered extremely dependent—a notion we found difficult to comprehend: (a) a paralyzed elderly client capable of orchestrating an array of personal services to maintain her living quarters in a private apartment complex; and (b) a kidney dialysis patient able to supervise, instruct, and support his wife's performance of the daily dialysis routines.

Secondly, the shortened time frame of the hybrid model has facilitated multiple analyses of single concepts. These additional analyses have been especially helpful in (a) examining a concept's relevancy and centrality across nursing settings and client populations and (b) separating the essential aspects of a concept from those that systematically vary across clinical settings and client populations. For example, in the fieldwork phases of three analyses, we found fear to be a constantly important and frequent phenomenon. This is in marked contrast to the heavy emphasis placed on anxiety in the nursing literature. The fieldwork phases of these analyses dealt with the fear experienced by women in anticipation of labor and delivery (Hightower, 1979), patients waiting for hospitalization for cardiac surgery (Seidler, 1984), and by myocardial infarction patients during hospital and posthospital phases of recovery (Amato-Vealy, 1987). In each setting, the essential quality of fear as an emotional response to a consciously recognized and external threat of danger and its distinctiveness from anxiety was confirmed. At the same time, the specific content, timing, and duration of the fear varied according to the event around which the fear centered. Brown's (1993, 1995, 1997) work with the concept of respect among health care providers and patients in a multicultural outpatient clinic in a U.S. hospital and in a Cree-Ojibway First Nations Community in Western Canada represents another example of the value of studying a concept across settings and client populations.

Additionally, multiple analyses have helped to identify situations where nurses may mistakenly be using a single concept (e.g., withdrawal) to label what are actually two distinct phenomena, such as psychosocial withdrawal as opposed to physical, or substance, withdrawal. A similar situation seems to be occurring with the concept of empathy. Nurses may need to consider separating clinical empathy, as a conscious and cognitive-based nursing intervention, from the more spontaneous and experientially based empathy seen among patients, such as that described earlier in Roberts' (1982) work with two self-help groups (Dalton, 1989).

A third and unintentional outcome of the fieldwork phase of the model has been the illumination of both problematic and nonproblematic consequences of a given phenomenon. A good example of this is seen in DeNuccio and Schwartz-Barcott's (2000) work on withdrawal, which is presented in the next chapter. Studies such as this provide important baseline information for developing nursing diagnoses.

A fourth unexpected result of many of the concept analyses completed to date has been the identification of clusters of concepts that appear to be interrelated (e.g., problem solving, decision making and compliance, or isolation, loneliness, and social support). This has prompted work on a second model (The Concept Differentiation Model), which is currently being developed by the authors. It is aimed at identifying the relationships among a small cluster of concepts as a step toward explanation and the identification of relational statements.

Lastly, the hybrid model has served as an initial step toward dissertation research and the building of programs of research that closely link theory development with the realities of practice. For example, Byrd's (1995a, 1995b) concept analysis of home visiting and Patterson's (1992, 1995, 1997) on social support led to the identification and beginning corroboration of these concepts as processes and an initial depiction of the major steps involved in each process. Subsequent dissertation research was used to more fully map out each process and begin to identify antecedents, consequences, and factors influencing these processes in a particular nursing care setting (Byrd, 1996, 1997). In another example, O'Neill's (1992, 1994a, 1994b) use of the hybrid model provided an initial understanding of clinical decision making in home care that later helped inform and refine the content she used to develop a set of clinical inference vignettes that were used in her dissertation to examine home health nurses' use of base rate information in diagnostic reasoning. For others, this first step has led to reexamination of a known concept, for example, Williams' (1995) focus on transcendence, to the linkage with an existing theory, for example, Lusardi's (1993, 1996) work linking the making of meaning of ICU patients with neurophysiological and symbolic interaction theoretical perspectives and, sometimes, to whole new ways of addressing an area of inquiry, as in Dluhy's (1993, 1995) research with chronic illness.

REFERENCES

Agar, M. (1980). *The professional stranger: An informal introduction to ethnography.* New York: Academic.

Amato-Vealy, E. (1987). *A concept analysis of fear as experienced by myocardial infarct patients.* Unpublished manuscript, University of Rhode Island, Kingston, RI.

Atwood, J. R. (1978). The phenomenon of selective neglect. In E. Bauwens (Ed.), *The anthropology of health* (pp. 192–200). St. Louis: Mosby.

Beck, C. T. (1996). A concept analysis of panic. *Archives of Psychiatric Nursing, 10*(5), 265–275.

Benner, P. (1975). Nurses in the intensive care unit. In M. Z. Davis, M. Kramer, & A. L. Strauss (Eds.), *Nurses in practice: A perspective on work environments* (pp. 106–128). St. Louis: Mosby.

Bernard, R. H. (1988). *Research methods in cultural anthropology.* Newbury Park, CA: Sage.

Bertman, S., & Krant, M. J. (1977). To know of suffering and the teaching of empathy. *Social Science and Medicine, 1,* 53–61.

Blalock, H. M. (1969). *Theory construction: From verbal to mathematical formulations.* Englewood Cliffs, NJ: Prentice Hall.

Bogdan, R., & Taylor, S. J. (1975). *Introduction to qualitative research methods.* New York: John Wiley & Sons.

Brown, A. (1993). A conceptual clarification of respect. *Journal of Advanced Nursing, 18,* 211–217.

Brown, A. (1995). The meaning of respect: A First Nations perspective. *Canadian Journal of Nursing Research, 27*(4), 95–109.

Brown, A. (1997). A concept analysis of respect applying the hybrid model in cross-cultural settings. *Western Journal of Nursing Research, 19*(6), 752–780.

Brownell, M. J. (1984). The concept of crisis: Its utility for nursing. *Advances in Nursing Science, 6*(4), 10–21.

Bulmer, M. (1984). Concepts in the analysis of qualitative data. In M. Bulmer

(Ed.), *Sociological research methods* (pp. 241-262). New Brunswick, NJ: Transaction Books.

Byrd, M. E. (1995a). A concept analysis of home visiting. *Journal of Public Health Nursing, 12*(3), 80-86.

Byrd, M. E. (1995b). The home visiting process in the contexts of the voluntary versus required visit. *Journal of Public Health Nursing, 12*(3), 196-202.

Byrd, M. E. (1996). Making maternal-child home visits: A field research investigation. (Doctoral dissertation, University of Rhode Island, 1996). *Dissertation Abstracts International, 57*(08), 4974B.

Byrd, M. E. (1997). Child-focused single home visiting. *Public Health Nursing, 14*(5), 313-322.

Chenitz, W. C., & Swanson, J. M. (1986). *From practice to grounded theory: Qualitative research in nursing.* Reading, MA: Addison-Wesley.

Chinn, P. L. (1986). *Nursing research methodology: Issues and implementations.* Rockville, MD: Aspen.

Chinn, P. L., & Jacobs, M. K. (1983). *Theory and nursing: A systematic approach.* St. Louis: Mosby.

Cooper, H. M. (1984). *The integrative research review: A systematic approach.* Beverly Hills: Sage.

Dalton, J. (1989). *Empathy, social support and caring: A cluster analysis.* Unpublished manuscript, University of Rhode Island, Kingston, RI.

Danforth, L. M. (1989). *Firewalking and religious healing.* Princeton, NJ: Princeton University Press.

Davis, M. Z. (1986). Observation in natural settings. In W. C. Chenitz & J. M. Swanson (Eds.), *From practice to grounded theory: Qualitative research in nursing* (pp. 48-65). Reading, MA: Addison-Wesley.

DeNuccio, G., & Schwartz-Barcott, D. (2000). A concept analysis of withdrawal: Application of the hybrid model of concept development. In B. L. Rodgers & K. A. Knafl (Eds.), *Concept development in nursing. Foundations, techniques, and applications* (2nd ed.) (Chapter 10). Philadelphia: W. B. Saunders.

Denzin, N. (1989). Review symposium on field methods. *Journal of Contemporary Ethnography, 18*(1), 89-109.

Dluhy, N. M. (1994). Metatheoretical blueprint for cumulating nursing knowledge: A reconstructed theory of chronic illness. (Doctoral dissertation, University of Rhode Island, 1993.) *Dissertation Abstracts International, 54*(7), 3550B.

Dluhy, N. M. (1995). Mapping out knowledge in chronic illness. *Journal of Advanced Nursing, 21,* 1051-1058.

Dubin, R. (1969). *Theory building: A practical guide to the construction and testing of theoretical models.* New York: Free Press.

Ellen, R. F. (1984). *Ethnographic research: A guide to general conduct.* New York: Academic Press.

Emerson, R. M. (1983). *Contemporary field research: A collection of readings.* Boston: Little, Brown.

Evaneshko, V. (1985). Entrée strategies for nursing field research studies. In M. M. Leininger (Ed.), *Qualitative research methods in nursing* (pp. 133-148). New York: Grune & Stratton.

Fetterman, D. M. (1989). *Ethnography: Step by step.* Newbury Park, CA: Sage.

Field, P. A. (1989). Doing fieldwork in your own culture. In J. M. Morse

(Ed.), *Qualitative nursing research: A contemporary dialogue* (pp. 79-91). Rockville, MD: Aspen.

Ganong, L. H. (1987). Integrative reviews of nursing research. *Research in Nursing and Health, 10,* 1-11.

Gardner, K. (1979). Supportive nursing: A critical review of the literature. *Journal of Psychiatric Nursing and Mental Health Services, 17*(10), 10-16.

Geertz, C. (1988). *Works and lives: The anthropologist as author.* Palo Alto, CA: Stanford University Press.

Gibbs, J. (1972). *Sociological theory construction.* Hinsdale, IL: Dryden Press.

Gibson, C. H. (1993). A study of empowerment in mothers of chronically ill children. (Doctoral dissertation, Boston College, 1993). *Dissertation Abstracts International, 94,* 02789.

Gibson, C. H. (1995). The process of empowerment in mothers of chronically ill children. *Journal of Advanced Nursing, 21*(6), 1201-1210.

Glaser, B. G. (1978). *Theoretical sensitivity: Advances in the methodology of grounded theory.* Mill Valley, CA: The Sociology Press.

Hage, J. (1972). *Techniques and problems of theory construction in sociology.* New York: John Wiley & Sons.

Hassma, J. (1979). *A concept analysis of denial.* Unpublished manuscript, University of Rhode Island, Kingston, RI.

Hempel, C. G. (1952). *Fundamentals of concept formation in empirical science.* Chicago: University of Chicago Press.

Hightower, A. (1979). *A concept analysis of fear in the context of childbirth.* Unpublished manuscript, University of Rhode Island, Kingston, RI.

Hogue, C. (1985). Social support. In J. Hall & B. Weaver (Eds.), *Distributive nursing practice: A systems approach to community health* (2nd ed.) (pp. 58-81). Philadelphia: J. B. Lippincott.

Janicki, J. (1981). *Anguish: A concept analysis.* Unpublished manuscript, University of Rhode Island, Kingston, RI.

Kaplan, A. (1964). *The conduct of inquiry: Methodology for behavioral science.* New York: Chandler.

Keith, J. (1988). Participant observation. In K. Schaie, R. Campbell, W. Meredith, & S. Rawlings (Eds.), *Methodological issues in aging research* (pp. 211-230). New York: Springer.

Kim, H. S. (1983). *The nature of theoretical thinking in nursing.* Norwalk, CT: Appleton-Century-Crofts.

Kim, H. S. (1987). Structuring the nursing knowledge system: A typology of four domains. *Scholarly Inquiry for Nursing Practice: An International Journal, 1*(2), 99-110.

Leininger, M. M. (1985). Ethnography and ethnonursing: Models and modes of qualitative data analysis. In M. M. Leininger (Ed.), *Qualitative research methods in nursing* (pp. 33-71). New York: Grune & Stratton.

Lofland, J. (1976). *Doing social life.* New York: John Wiley & Sons.

Lofland, J., & Lofland, L. H. (1984). *Analyzing research settings: A guide to qualitative observation and analysis.* Belmont, CA: Wadsworth.

Lusardi, P., & Schwartz-Barcott, D. (1996). Making sense of it: A neuro-interactional model of meaning emergence in critically ill ventilated patients. *Journal of Advanced Nursing, 23,* 896-903.

Lusardi, P. T. (1994). Making sense of it: The ICU experience. A participant observation—Patient centered study (Volumes I & II). (Doctoral dissertation,

University of Rhode Island, 1993). *Dissertation Abstracts International, 54*(7), 3351B.

Madden, B. P. (1990). The hybrid model for concept development: Its value for the study of therapeutic alliance. *Advances in Nursing Science, 12*(3), 75-87.

May, R. (1972). The nature of creativity. In H. H. Anderson (Ed.), *Interdisciplinary symposia on creativity* (pp. 55-68). New York: Harper & Row.

McCall, G. J., & Simmons, J. L. (1969). *Issues in participant observation: A text and reader.* Reading, MA: Addison-Wesley.

Meleis, A. I. (1985). *Theoretical nursing: Development and progress.* Philadelphia: J. B. Lippincott.

Messerschmidt, D. A. (1981). *Anthropologists at home in North America: Methods and issues in the study of one's own society.* New York: Cambridge University Press.

Miles, M. B., & Huberman, A. M. (1984). *Qualitative data analysis.* Beverly Hills: Sage.

Nagel, E. (1961). *The structure of science.* New York: Harcourt, Brace & World.

National League for Nursing. (1972). *Criteria for the appraisal of baccalaureate and higher degree programs in nursing.* New York: Author.

Norris, C. M. (1982). *Concept clarification in nursing.* Rockville, MD: Aspen.

O'Neill, E. S. (1993). Forms of knowledge and the use of the representativeness heuristic in clinical inferencing tasks of community health nurses. (Doctoral dissertation, University of Rhode Island, 1992.) *Dissertation Abstracts International, 53*(8), 4033B.

O'Neill, E. S. (1994a). Home health nurses' use of base rate information in diagnostic reasoning. *Advances in Nursing Science, 17*(2), 77-85.

O'Neill, E. S. (1994b). The use of similarity in the clinical inferencing tasks of community health nurses. *Scholarly Inquiry for Nursing Practice, 8,* 261-271.

O'Neill, E. S. (1996). Clinical decision making in community health nursing. *Home Healthcare Nurse, 14,* 363-368.

Panzarine, S. (1985). Coping: Conceptual and methodological issues. *Advances in Nursing Science, 7*(4), 49-58.

Patterson, B. (1993). Social support: A fieldwork study of adjusting to life in a nursing home. (Doctoral dissertation, University of Rhode Island, 1992.) *Dissertation Abstracts International, 53*(8), 4034B.

Patterson, B. (1995). The process of social support: Adjusting to life in a nursing home. *Journal of Advanced Nursing, 21,* 682-689.

Patterson, B. (1997). Catalysts and barriers to social support in a nursing home. *Health in Later Life, 2*(2), 73-84.

Pelto, P. J. (1970). *Anthropological research: The structure of inquiry.* New York: Cambridge University.

Pelto, P. J., & Pelto, G. H. (1984). *Anthropologist research: The structure of inquiry* (2nd ed.). New York: Cambridge University.

Phillips, M. (1992). Chronic sorrow in mothers of chronically ill and disabled children. *Issues in Comprehensive Pediatric Nursing, 14,* 34-77.

Reed, P. G., & Leonard, V. E. (1990). An analysis of the concept of self-neglect. *Advances in Nursing Science, 12*(1), 39-53.

Reilly, H. A. (1982). *A concept analysis of creativity.* Unpublished manuscript, University of Rhode Island, Kingston, RI.

Rew, L., & Barrow, E. M. (1987). Intuition: A neglected hallmark of nursing knowledge. *Advances in Nursing Science, 10*(1), 49–62.

Reynolds, P. D. (1971). *A primer in theory construction.* New York: Bobbs-Merrill.

Roberts, N. (1982). *An analysis of the concept of empathy.* Unpublished manuscript, University of Rhode Island, Kingston, RI.

Rogers, R. (1972). Toward a theory of creativity. In H. H. Anderson (Ed.), *Interdisciplinary symposia on creativity* (pp. 69–82). New York: Harper & Row.

St. Angelo, L. (1983). *The concept of bonding.* Unpublished manuscript, University of Rhode Island, Kingston, RI.

Sartori, G. (1984). *Social science concepts: A systematic analysis.* Beverly Hills: Sage.

Schatzman, L., & Strauss, A. L. (1973). *Field research: Strategies for a natural sociology.* Englewood Cliffs, NJ: Prentice Hall.

Schwartz-Barcott, D. (1986, April). Conceptualization: Concept formation. In N. Wells & C. Bridges (Eds.), *Strategies for theory development in nursing III* (pp. 19–35). Proceedings of the Third Annual Nursing Science Colloquium. Boston University, Boston, MA.

Schwartz-Barcott, D., & Kim, H. S. (1986). A hybrid model for concept development. In P. L. Chinn (Ed.), *Nursing research methodology: Issues and implementations.* Rockville, MD: Aspen.

Seidler, S. (1984). *Fear in the patient undergoing a coronary artery bypass graft.* Unpublished manuscript, University of Rhode Island, Kingston, RI.

Spradley, J. P. (1980). *Participant observation.* New York: Holt, Rinehart and Winston.

Strauss, A. L. (1987). *Qualitative analysis for social scientists.* New York: Cambridge University Press.

Sundeen, S. J., Stuart, G. W., Rankin, E. A., & Cohen, S. A. (1976). *Nurse-client interaction: Implementing the nursing process.* St. Louis: Mosby.

Taylor, S. J., & Bogdan, R. (1984). *Introduction to qualitative research methods: The search for meanings* (2nd ed.). New York: John Wiley & Sons.

Testa, G. (1980). *A participant observation study of the concept of psychosocial withdrawal in the aged nursing home resident.* Unpublished manuscript, University of Rhode Island, Kingston, RI.

Van Maanen, J. (1988). *Tales of the field: On writing ethnography.* Chicago: University of Chicago Press.

Walker, L. O., & Avant, K. C. (1988). *Strategies for theory construction in nursing.* Norwalk, CT: Appleton & Lange.

Wax, R. H. (1986). *Doing fieldwork: Warnings and advice.* Chicago: University of Chicago Press.

Werner, O., & Schoepfle, G. M. (1987). *Foundations of ethnography and interviewing* (Vol. 1). Beverly Hills: Sage.

Whyte, W. F. (1984). *Learning from the field: A guide from experience.* Beverly Hills: Sage.

Williams, J. (1996). Transcendence as a human response to life-threatening illness: Description and understanding through narratives. (Doctoral dissertation, University of Rhode Island, 1995). *Dissertation Abstracts International, 56*(9), 4819.

Wilson, H. S. (1982). *Deinstitutionalized residential approaches for the se-*

verely and mentally disordered patient: The Soteria House approach. New York: Grune & Stratton.

Wilson, H. S. (1986). Presencing—social control of schizophrenics in an antipsychiatric community: Doing grounded theory. In P. Munhall & C. Oiler (Eds.), *Nursing research: A qualitative perspective* (pp. 131–144). Norwalk, CT: Appleton-Century-Crofts.

Wilson, J. (1969). *Thinking with concepts.* London: Cambridge University Press.

Zola, I. K. (1983). *Socio-medical inquiries: Recollections, reflections and reconsiderations.* Philadelphia: Temple University Press.

A Concept Analysis of Withdrawal: Application of the Hybrid Model*

Geraldine DeNuccio and Donna Schwartz-Barcott

> *I recall a man who no one seemed to like; at least no one was ever visiting him. Each day, rain or shine, he would sit on the porch, his head hung low. He would stare at the screen door with a faraway look in his eyes. He never seemed to notice when I walked by. Once I sat next to him. I thought he would like some company. But, he didn't notice. He didn't look at me or talk to me. The next day I asked a nurse about him. "Can he talk, can he walk?" She said, "Yes, he can talk and walk, but he doesn't care to anymore, just sort of withdrawn into a world of his own."*
> *How sad, I thought. Why Mrs. S. and Miss B. who I visited each afternoon, they had not withdrawn.*

This impression of the man in the nursing home which I developed as a child of 8 stayed with me, first as a youth and then as an adult. During my initial years as a graduate nurse, I frequently drew on this image. When charting and talking with other nurses, I often would use the term withdrawn to describe a patient. "Withdrawn and apathetic." "Withdrawn, did not leave room today." "Withdrawn, did not engage in any conversation." Particularly, I remember my experience

---

*This work was initially undertaken in the early 1980s as part of master's level coursework. The principal author is Geraldine DeNuccio. The follow-up work, which included an update of the literature, is presented in this chapter, in collaboration with Donna Schwartz-Barcott.

with a young man with diabetes for whom I cared over a long period of time. As his disease progressed and renal problems developed, his response to these events changed. He stopped taking interest in his care; refused to give insulin injections; stopped talking to me; and spent most of his time in bed. I described his behavior as withdrawn, but what did this word mean? Was the same thing happening to him that happened to the elderly man in the nursing home so many years ago?

WITHDRAWAL: ITS USAGE IN NURSING

Withdrawal is a highly pervasive and, at the same time, a relatively underdeveloped concept in nursing. Nurses freely use the term in communicating, reporting, and writing. "Patient withdrawn." "Withdrawal noted." "Is more withdrawn today." In the nursing literature, withdrawal has been used to characterize the behavior of the mentally ill patient (Jasmin & Trygstad, 1979; Oden, 1963; Schmidt, 1981; Tudor, 1952) and the behavioral responses of patients to acute and chronic physical illness (Davis, 1975; Friedrick & Lively, 1981), as well as the responses of nurses in their interactions with patients and to situations of high anxiety and stress (Beland, 1980; Hutchinson, 1987; Jacobson, 1983; Kramer, 1974; Scully, 1980; Travelbee, 1971; Tudor, 1952). Yet, any attempt at greater understanding of this phenomenon is hindered by its lack of explication and development in nursing. For example, the term is not even cited as a subject in the *Cumulative Index to Nursing and Allied Health Literature*. Likewise, when it is used, it is often embedded in other phenomena, such as protective isolationism (Kramer, 1974), distancing (Beland, 1980; Jacobson, 1983; Scully, 1980), psychological immobilization (Friedrick & Lively, 1981), panic (Oden, 1963), anxiety (Peplau, 1963), and depression (Jasmin & Trygstad, 1979). Additionally, it is sometimes used as a behavioral indicator of related but different concepts, such as alienation, anomie, helplessness, hopelessness, and powerlessness. And most recently, it is being used in the nursing diagnosis literature as a defining characteristic for the diagnoses of fear, pain, social isolation, and spiritual distress (Kim et al., 1987). It seems that nurses operate with the assumption that the meaning of withdrawal is universally understood.

It is this evasive quality of withdrawal that leads one to question the underlying meaning of the phenomenon. The following concept analysis was undertaken in hopes of establishing a base for further theoretical and empirical understanding of this phenomenon in nursing. More specifically, the questions to be addressed are: To what extent is there a universal meaning and definition of withdrawal? Have there been any attempts at measuring withdrawal? If so, to what extent are these linked with existing definitions? To what extent can any of these definitions or measurements be applied, and if not, what refinements are needed?

In this paper, the authors attempt to answer these questions by using the hybrid model of concept development to further define and measure withdrawal. The subsequent section gives a review of behavioral, social science, and nursing literature where the concept has been partially defined and used with varying degrees of frequency. The focus of the review is first on existing definitions and secondly on measurements of withdrawal. These are used then as a basis for reexamining the concept of withdrawal among residents in a nursing home setting. Lastly, a refined definition and operationalization is proposed based on the above theoretical and empirical analysis of withdrawal.

DEFINING WITHDRAWAL

In its simplest form, withdrawal is a physical, defensive maneuver in which animals and humans engage to meet an actual or anticipated threat. The earliest impressions of withdrawal were obtained from observations of the defensive behavior of animals in their natural environments. This resulted in the elucidation of predator-prey interactions as a form of survival behavior (Edmunds, 1974). Withdrawal, also called the flight response, was described in terms of biological adaptation, an instinctive physical response (Coehlo et al., 1974).

Withdrawal as an Abnormal Behavior Pattern Indicating a Disturbance in Objective Reality

Withdrawal as a flight response was conceptualized in the field of psychiatry as an unconscious, intrapsychic process rather than a biological adaptation. Such a behavioral process, called a fugue, from the Latin word *fuga* meaning flight, included physical retreat or withdrawal as a dominant feature. Ziegler (1933) described a fugue as a pathological retreat from reality.

Within the field of psychiatry, withdrawal has been used to characterize several mental health problems including depression, personality disorders, neurotic syndromes, and the psychosis described as schizophrenia. In fact, Tudor (1952) suggested that the predominant characteristic of the mentally ill person is a physical and social withdrawal. In schizophrenia, withdrawal has been included as a significant component of the schizophrenic process. In the *Theory of Schizophrenic Negativism*, Bleuler (1912) defined autistic withdrawal as the "retreat of a person into his own phantasy world accompanied by a reduction in activity and a growing disinterest in his surroundings" (p. 2). As related by Grinker (1971), further description of the syndrome was provided by Kraepelin in 1919. In Kraepelin's classification of schizophrenia, catatonia was described as a form in which the person is withdrawn, mute, and immobile. Expanding on these ideas about schizophrenia,

Schmidt (1981), a psychiatric nurse, provided a broader definition of withdrawal in her work with schizophrenic patients. She defined withdrawal as:

> a behavioral pattern characterized by an individual's retreat from interpersonal relationships and contacts with the external environment . . . a reduced response to external stimuli and increased response to internal stimuli . . . withdrawal may be manifested in a wide variety of behaviors ranging from mild to severe based upon the individual's degree of personality disintegration. (p. 28)

Withdrawal as a Primary Defense Mechanism

Sigmund Freud's theory on human defense mechanisms included the concept of repression as an unconscious defense of the ego against anxiety. Within the concept of repression, the term *withdrawal* was described as a "refractory period in which nothing more is allowed to happen, no perception is registered and no action is performed" (Sprott, 1936, p. 55). Moving away from an emphasis on the unconscious, Sullivan stressed the conflict often associated with relationships, viewing withdrawal as a retreat from interpersonal contact in response to an emotionally painful relationship (Perry, 1962). Similarly, Horney (1937) referred to withdrawal as one of four principal mechanisms to protect a person from anxiety. Here, withdrawal is viewed as an emotional detachment. "If I withdraw, then nothing can hurt me" is the theme of this detachment (p. 99).

Withdrawal as a Behavioral Response

Other social scientists view withdrawal as a transient coping response or a continuous behavioral pattern that may be progressive. Their work illuminates the potential adaptive and maladaptive purpose of withdrawal. The adaptive function of withdrawal was highlighted empirically in a study by Hamburg and colleagues (1953), which explored patients' emotional recovery from life-threatening burns. They found that for those patients who used withdrawal as a coping response, it was a transient phenomenon lasting the first 2 weeks following injury. In none of the patients studied did withdrawal continue or progress. Sapirstein (1948) emphasized this idea also by suggesting that the temporary use of withdrawal as a defense against anxiety is useful. Furthermore, he depicted withdrawal as a transitory state for energy conservation to prepare for action and to reestablish a sense of equilibrium.

Ironside (1980) concluded that the concept of "conservation-withdrawal" is a universal feature of survivor behavior during disaster experiences. He defined conservation-withdrawal as a "biological threshold mechanism whereby survival of the organism is supported by processes of disengagement in activity from the external environment" (p. 163). Conservation-withdrawal is seen as adaptive, assisting the individual physically and psychologically to cope and prepare for "action-engagement" in order to face and meet environmental demands.

A similar depiction of withdrawal was made in the nursing literature by Beland and Passos (1975). These authors argued that withdrawal can help patients adjust psychologically and socially to illness. At the same time, they cautioned nurses not to allow the withdrawal to go too far, when energy conservation is no longer needed and patients should assume responsibility for meeting their own needs (p. 372).

In an explanatory study of the social withdrawal experiences of adults, Cochrane (1983) identified active withdrawal (lasting for brief moments to several hours) as a transient adaptive coping response to environmental stimuli overload. Social withdrawal was assumed to be a physical or psychological movement from other people and into self.

The notion of withdrawal as an adaptive process, indicating successful adjustment to aging, emerged emphatically in Disengagement Theory. Disengagement was conceived by Cumming and Henry (1961) as an inevitable, mutually satisfying process of withdrawal between the aged person and society in which a psychological withdrawal either precedes or accompanies a social withdrawal as an intrinsic, natural process. However, subsequent research in social gerontology has not fully supported disengagement as a desirable, inevitable process (Brehm, 1968; Burbank, 1986; Havinghurst, 1961; Lowenthal & Boler, 1965; Maddox, 1965).

The *maladaptive* response of withdrawal has been described in relation to the aged person who has not been successful in socially and psychologically adjusting to relocation in a nursing home environment (Chenitz, 1983). Withdrawal may also surface in this population, if the aged person does not possess the coping and social skills necessary for such an adjustment. If resources are not mobilized and social support made available, the person may continue to withdraw with a reactive type of depression accompanied by feelings of loneliness and boredom (Griffin, 1979; Wolk & Reingold, 1975).

Maladaptive withdrawal has also been described in institutionalized infants. The works of Escalona and Leitch (1949) and Spitz (1946) have provided highly poignant descriptions of withdrawal under extreme situations of stress. During an 18-month period of observation, Spitz described a syndrome called anaclitic depression in 19 of the 123 infants cared for in an institutional setting. This syndrome was characterized by progressive and profound withdrawal of the infants from their environment. In the following example, Spitz described the sudden withdrawal of a once friendly 7-month-old girl. The child began to show signs of apprehensiveness. Over the next two weeks, these became accentuated and accompanied by frequent crying. By four weeks:

> she could no longer be approached. No amount of persuasion helped. Whenever approached, she sat up and wailed. Two weeks later, she would lie on her face, indifferent to the outside world, not interested in the other children living in the same room. Only strong stimulation could get her out of her apathy. She would then sit up and stare at the observer wide-eyed, a tragic expression on her face, silent. She would not accept toys, in fact she withdrew from them into the farthest corner of her bed. (p. 315)

In another study, Escalona and Leitch (1949) observed the behavioral responses of infants to separation from their natural mothers after transfer to a child placement service institution. Approximately one third of the infants developed progressive withdrawal behavior characterized by lethargy and lack of excitability.

A common theme in these infant studies was the occurrence of withdrawal in response to prolonged separation from the infants' natural mothers and residence in an institutional setting. Also, the withdrawal was progressive and continued for a long period of time. Peplau (1952) described such infant syndromes as negative withdrawal, a behavioral response that occurs when needs are not met and feelings of satisfaction are denied.

The progressive nature of withdrawal was supported further by Cochrane (1983) in an explanatory study on social withdrawal experiences of adults. Three types of social withdrawal experiences were identified from the data: active, passive, and reactive. Passive withdrawal was described as an extreme form of reactive withdrawal indicative of a maladaptive coping response to stress lasting up to three months with a more prolonged period of immobilized activity.

Withdrawal as a Strategic Maneuver to Manage Stress

The notion of withdrawal as a control strategy used to exercise power in social situations was described by Sites (1973). Sites suggested that various degrees of withdrawal exist, starting with "fringe" membership and noninvolvement to complete physical withdrawal. Withdrawal is used in social situations where continued involvement is no longer rewarding or safety is threatened. According to Sites, withdrawal can be classified into three types: (a) ritual withdrawal in which the individual remains in the group and acts as though he/she is interested in the goals of the group, but is not; (b) physical withdrawal in which the individual or group completely leaves the interactional scene and removes him/herself to another place; and (c) disbanding of the group (p. 170).

Withdrawal as a *patient's* control strategy over nurses was presented by Glaser and Strauss (1965) in their trajectories of dying patients. They suggested that "withdrawal is the patient's most extreme control over the pace of interaction with nurses" (p. 208). Furthermore, this withdrawal is more than "giving up." It is an implicit message that the patient is finished with everything and everyone, including the nursing staff (p. 89).

Withdrawal also has been discussed as a *nursing* strategy to handle anxiety associated with clinical nursing problems (Hurteau, 1963). Kramer (1974) viewed withdrawing as one form of "protective isolationism," a strategy used to cope with stressful work environments. This included the new graduate nurses' withdrawal to bed, sleeping more hours than usual, and withdrawal to the night shift. In another nursing study, Hutchinson (1987) described withdrawal as a self-care strategy that nurses use to cope with job stress. Self-reports from hospital-based nurses indicated that withdrawal increased their emotional control and protected them from chronic emotional drain. Withdrawal behaviors were described as both physical and emotional in which physical withdrawal helped the nurse to withdraw emotionally. Examples of withdrawal behaviors included: leaving the unit, requesting that another nurse take on the patient, working the night shift, taking time out by eating alone or leaving during lunch, and resigning as an extreme form of withdrawal in a hopeless situation.

In a classic study of withdrawal, Tudor (1952) demonstrated that withdrawal or avoidance can be used by both the *nurse* and *patient*. In this exploratory study Tudor identified the problem of mutual withdrawal between nursing staff and schizophrenic patients. She argued that the nurses' social interaction pattern of avoidance reinforced the patients' withdrawal and was the dominant reason for the maintenance of the patients' mental illness. Later, Travelbee (1971) described withdrawal or avoidance being used as a strategy by *nurses and families*.

In 1975, Davis discussed the stratagem of withdrawal between chronically ill *patients* and *others* with respect to the patient as a part of the process in social isolation. In these instances, withdrawal was viewed as mutual and in most cases resulted in increased social isolation of the patient.

Lastly, in a case study, Leyn (1972) described the withdrawal exhibited by a young mother while dealing with her son's fatal illness of leukemia. Leyn observed the emergence of a pattern of emotional and physical withdrawal. It began as emotional aloofness and led to avoidance. The transient nature of withdrawal was evident in this case, inasmuch as within a short period of time, the mother was able to approach her dying son, providing comfort and emotional support to him.

In summary, the literature reviewed here illuminates the diverse use of withdrawal in behavioral, social, and nursing sciences. It has been used to characterize animal defensive behaviors, human responses to stress, ranging from severe deprivation to the more usual stresses of daily life, and as an active coping strategy. Additionally, withdrawal has been described as both an adaptive and maladaptive coping mechanism that at times may be progressive.

Yet, explicit definitions of withdrawal were seldom encountered. There was, implicitly, a moderate degree of agreement in the shared impressions and terms (e.g., flight, retreat, avoidance, detachment, disengagement, autism, and isolation) used to express the idea of withdrawal. Most fundamentally, withdrawal seems to entail some form of retreat. Earlier definitions refer to a physical action—a moving out of the immediate environment. Later, this physical action is associated with emotional inaction, rather than actual physical removal from the setting. Recently, the focus has been on retreat from social interaction. Thus, it appears that withdrawal includes three major dimensions: physical, emotional, and social.

Lastly, there is a scarcity of literature about withdrawal as a separate phenomenon. There is a need to distinguish withdrawal from other closely related concepts, such as avoidance, depression, and social isolation. In the process of defining withdrawal, one needs to define what is not withdrawal.

MEASURING WITHDRAWAL

The measurement of withdrawal, like its definition, remains relatively undeveloped. There is limited agreement on the approaches to be used in measuring the concept, and no reliable comprehensive instruments exist to date. Of those measures encountered, most have focused on the social dimensions of withdrawal. For example, Lowenthal and Boler (1965) examined social withdrawal among elderly community residents. In this longitudinal study, subjects were asked to identify their current level of social participation with family members, with others outside their family, and within social/community organizations. Withdrawal was measured as a reduction in participation within these three areas, and an index of social withdrawal was developed. Additionally, the authors identified two types of withdrawal: voluntary and involuntary. The findings supported the existence of both types.

Cochrane (1983) studied the subjective experiences of social withdrawal among students and faculty in a college setting. Subjects were asked to reexperience a situation of social withdrawal through a mental visualization technique. They were asked to describe the context, the particular events leading to, and the movement out of this experience.

Additionally, they were asked to compare this experience with earlier ones in relation to their overall meaning and function. Based on data analysis, three types of social withdrawal experiences were identified: active (a brief adaptive coping method), reactive (a frequent defensive coping mechanism), and passive (a more extreme form of reactive withdrawal that may be maladaptive). Clearly, this approach to the measurement of withdrawal emphasized the conscious, subjective recall of past experiences among well adults.

King (1956) explored withdrawal as a component of schizophrenia in which withdrawal was operationalized as behavior directed away from at least two types of environmental stimuli: people and things. Four measures of withdrawal were used in relation to these two behavioral processes in which staff reports of patients' participation in group therapy, ward activity, occupational therapy, and an operant conditioning program were used to measure withdrawal. King was especially interested in the extent to which "people withdrawal" always accompanied "thing withdrawal," in order to establish whether people and thing withdrawal form a single unity. The findings did not support an association between people and thing withdrawal and thus suggest the possibility of two types of withdrawal. However, it was unclear how King distinguished between a patient's withdrawal from things versus simply disinterest in a particular activity.

Frieswyk (1977) examined the emotional dimension of withdrawal through the evaluation of the effect of treatment on subjects with psychoses through the assessment of the relational disposition, "fantasy withdrawal," from Rorschach face sheet data. In this study, fantasy withdrawal was defined as:

> the degree in which the individual has withdrawn from human involvement in favor of the kind of self-absorption of his own thoughts, fantasies, wishes and somatic experiences to the relative exclusion of reality information and feedback from others and to which this has crystallized as the major organizing factor in the life adjustment of the individual. (p. 1133)

The significance of this study lies in its attention to the emotional dimension of withdrawal and in its measurement of the degree of withdrawal by rank ordering and quantifying several aspects of fantasy production.

In contrasting with the above studies, Schmidt (1981) tried to measure all three dimensions of withdrawal among a sample of schizophrenic patients. She generated a list of 24 behavioral indicators, along four categories: physical, verbal, affective, and disruption in reality. The level of measurement was nominal. Any one behavior was checked off as present or absent. The indicators and categories were not weighted. The presence of five or more indicators, irrespective of the category, constituted withdrawal. Although this study highlighted the diversity of potential behaviors in withdrawal, it did not raise the level of measurement above that of nominal.

Lastly, Pallister (1933) conducted a study to determine if a negative or withdrawal *attitude* can be seen as a personality trait. The researcher likened a withdrawal attitude to the concept of introversion in which there is a tendency to withdraw from direct contact with the environment. The sample included 209 college freshmen women taking courses in elementary psychology. An adjustment questionnaire, called the Individuality Record, was used as a measure of a withdrawal attitude. This instrument included 200 questions divided into eight categories of attitudes toward family, sex, cooperation, nervous symptoms, optimism, physical symptoms, social confidence, and work habits. Included in each of these categories were situational questions, requiring a yes or no response. Yes was measured as an approach response and no as an avoidance or negative response. The findings supported the existence of a withdrawal attitude as a personality trait. The measurement of withdrawal as an approach or avoidance response is consistent with other researchers such as King (1956). However, the empirical support of withdrawal as a personality trait is different from other research, which focused more on the behavioral processes of withdrawal rather than a fixed variable such as a personality trait. The significance of withdrawal as a personality trait suggests that certain individuals may be predisposed to withdraw, and measurement of this variable could be useful in predicting these individuals.

There appears to be potential for measuring withdrawal along three dimensions: physical, emotional, and social. Drawing on the efforts of Schmidt (1981) and other descriptions in the literature reviewed, a group of potential behavioral indicators of withdrawal, in terms of its physical, social, and emotional dimensions, were developed. These are presented in Table 10–1. However, it is clear also, from the table, that a number of questions still remain. For example, Spitz (1946) referred to the infant's averted face, rigid expression, and wide-opened eyes. Can the eye behavior of withdrawal be more precisely defined? Is there a difference between the wide-opened, faraway looking, or vacant looking eyes? Facial expressions may be useful as indicators because rigid, tense, and expressionless faces were a few of the descriptions encountered in the literature (Escalona & Leitch, 1949; Spitz, 1946; Weinstein et al., 1955). Additionally, one could observe body positions and sleep patterns. Social indicators of withdrawal could be measured by a reduction in social interaction, decrease in frequency of social contacts, and approach or avoidance responses to people and social situations.

More descriptive studies could help decipher the importance of any

Table 10-1 Indicators of Withdrawal

Physical Indicators

Fatigue	Diminished movement
Lethargy	Decreased fluency
Increased sleep pattern	Immobile
	Lack of muscle excitability
Flight	
	Meditative silence
Sad facial expression	Self-preoccupation
Frozen, rigid expression	Lowering of voice
Averted face	Use of monosyllables
Decrease in eye contact	Mutism
Sad look in eyes	
Vacant look in eyes	Staying in room
Wide open look in eyes	
Dazed look in eyes	
Far away look in eyes	

Social Indicators

Reduction in level of social interaction	Avoidance of people
Being late for and avoiding appointments	Avoidance of social interaction

Emotional Indicators

Aloofness	Autism
Apathy	Confusion
Indifference	Delusions/hallucinations

one indicator over another and potentially allow one to address degrees of withdrawal. Measurement of withdrawal at a higher level would advance knowledge in nursing science since more precise statements could be made concerning the relationship of withdrawal to other behavioral concepts.

FIELDWORK PHASE—WITHDRAWAL IN THE AGED NURSING HOME RESIDENT

Shortly after the review of the literature was initiated, a fieldwork phase was begun to examine withdrawal among residents in a nursing home setting. This population was selected for several reasons. Earlier experiences by the authors and colleagues suggested that withdrawal had been encountered rather frequently in this setting. In the initial literature review, withdrawal had been explicitly linked with the elderly. Additionally, it was anticipated that withdrawal would be highly frequent in the context of relocation to a nursing home and the stress associated with adjustment to this setting. And lastly, the nursing home setting was a feasible, practical, and not overly familiar environment in which one of the authors (DeNuccio) could undertake a three-month period of participant observation.

Method and Setting

To obtain a rich and full understanding of the dynamics involved in withdrawal, investigation was done through overt participant observation employing unstructured observation techniques during situational and casual conversation and incidental questioning, as forms of informal interviewing. Other sources of data included the use of medical records and discussions with the nursing staff, social workers, and activity directors. After a short period of familiarization with the setting, the focus of these observations centered on four residents, each of whom the researcher saw on the average of one hour a week over a 2½-month period. Journals and field notes were organized according to Schatzman and Strauss's (1973) notation system of observational, theoretical, and methodological notes.

The setting was a large, multilevel nursing care facility located in a suburban section of Rhode Island. Three levels of nursing care were provided, with geographic separation of patients depending on the required level of care. The physical structure consisted of a five-year-old brick building resembling an acute care hospital setting. There were six patient care units, each with a central dining and lounging area. Patients' rooms were small, semiprivate areas with bathroom facilities shared by two adjacent rooms. The third floor offered five available private rooms for those people who had sources of private payment rather than federal government-funded Medicare payment. The basement level housed specific patient services such as barber shop, beauty salon, gift shop, activity room, and physical and occupational therapy areas.

During the course of this study, one subject was followed after transfer to another nursing home. In contrast to the primary setting, this nursing home was smaller, had just one level, and was built a year prior to the initiation of the present study. The physical structure was that of a sprawling brick building situated in a rural area of Rhode Island. The physical appearance resembled that of a modern motel. It included two patient care units with a mixed population. There were central dining and activity rooms and similar patient services. The patients' rooms were all semiprivate with shared bathroom facilities. However, these rooms were larger, brighter, and more spacious than those in the other setting.

The vast majority of patients in both nursing homes were local residents of Canadian origin who spent their lives as laborers in the textile industry. French was the dominant language of these people, although over one half of the residents also spoke fluent English. The nursing staff in both facilities were cooperative, friendly, and receptive to the presence of the researcher, who had had no prior knowledge of or affiliation with either facility.

Initial Frame of Reference and Key Questions

Several questions acted as a guide to the fieldwork phase. These stemmed from the focus on definition and measurement found in the hybrid model for concept development and from the initial exploration of the literature on withdrawal.

1. Is there any evidence of the existence of withdrawal among residents in this setting?
2. If so, to what extent do existing definitions sufficiently capture the essential nature of this phenomenon?
3. What indicators best reflect the existence of withdrawal?
4. Is there any evidence of withdrawal becoming progressive?
5. If so, under what conditions does withdrawal become progressive?

These questions did not alter over time, but observations kept surfacing that influenced prior thoughts and perceptions of withdrawal. For example, two basic assumptions underlying the initiation of fieldwork were that men and women need and desire social activity and meaningful interaction and secondly, that withdrawal is maladaptive, in that it inhibits the meeting of these needs. During fieldwork, these beliefs were called into question repeatedly, as will be discussed later in the analysis and conclusions of the paper.

Selection of Subjects and Operationalizing Withdrawal

The following working definition was used as a basis for initiating the fieldwork phase. Withdrawal is a behavioral response of physical, emotional, and social detachment from the external environment that may be progressive and is manifested in a wide variety of behaviors. A decision was made to focus on patients who already appeared withdrawn and who had various lengths of residence in the nursing home environment, in order to examine possible changes in withdrawal over time. An additional aim was to select at least one patient who was a new admission in order to observe withdrawal from an adjustment perspective. At the beginning of the fieldwork, the nursing staff was asked to describe patients who were withdrawn. They mentioned several. However, upon further discussion, it became apparent that these patients included individuals who were bedridden, senile, dying from a terminal illness, diagnosed as depressed, or receiving large doses of medication. At this point, it was decided to place some restrictions on the patients selected for intensive observation, given the difficulty of deciphering withdrawal under these conditions. Thus, patients were not selected who had major physical or emotional disorders that would contribute overwhelmingly to withdrawal behavior. Examples provided to the staff were patients who were deaf, blind, aphasic, had a terminal progressive disease, or were being treated for a diagnosed psychiatric disorder. Patients who were receiving medications that had side effects of drowsiness, lassitude, or provided a change in emotional response were not eligible. Patients needed to be oriented to person, but not necessarily to place and time, and thus not in a continuous confused state. They also needed to be able to speak and understand English.

Furthermore, four broad indicators were identified as an initial basis for detecting the withdrawn patient. These reflected three dimensions (social, physical, and emotional) found in the working definition. Thus, potentially withdrawn patients were those who did not get involved in social activities or functions within the nursing home, even though they had the physical ability and health status to do so; rarely, if ever, talked to or interacted socially with other residents and staff, and spent the majority of time in their room and physically away from other residents; and generally appeared unhappy or not accepting of being in the nursing home.

The actual selection of four patients (three men and a woman) involved reviewing patients' records and talking with a potential list of patients provided by the nursing staff and one new admission suggested by the social worker. Many patients who were described as withdrawn by the staff and who were eligible did not appear withdrawn, given the above broad indicators. For example, several patients did not interact socially within the nursing home, but at the same time, they did not show any indication of emotional withdrawal, inasmuch as they were fairly accepting of the need to be in a nursing home. Others maintained a strong source of emotional and social attachment with friends or family outside of the nursing home environment, although not involved with people or activities in the nursing home. These patients maintained contact with this network and occasionally left the nursing home environment on daytime passes or leaves.

From the onset of this investigation, the researcher's relationship with the subjects was fairly open. They were aware that the researcher was a graduate student conducting a study on the patients' thoughts and feelings toward living in a nursing home. The term *withdrawal* was not mentioned. Patients never questioned the researcher's intentions and were able to engage in conversation. At some point in time and in the context of casual conversation, patients were asked to talk about their lives (e.g., family, friends, activities) before entering the nursing home. Also, what was life like for them in the home? Did they experience feelings of loneliness, boredom, or depression? These general questions were used to gain a greater sense of the psychosocial context out of which withdrawal was being observed.

In the following section, the fieldwork data are presented in relation to each of the four patients, here referred to anonymously as Mr. Cardeur, Mrs. Bianco, Mr. Charpentier, and Mr. DuBois. The data are presented in first person to give the reader a more vivid image of the context and the nature of the interaction between the patient and researcher.

INDIVIDUAL CASE PRESENTATIONS

Case 1—Mr. Cardeur

The nursing staff refers to Mr. Cardeur as a poor old man because he is always alone. A nurse's aide was saying, "Why he is so quiet that you almost forget he is here." The nurses' notes recorded repeatedly the statement, "withdrawn, keeps to himself"; "withdrawn, refuses to participate in activities or social events with other residents"; "withdrawn, spent the entire day in his room lying on bed." The nursing care plan listed the problem—withdrawal—with the goal of increasing socialization and encouraging participation in group activities.

Mr. Cardeur, who is around 78 years old, was transferred to the nursing home 1½ years ago from the acute hospital setting. He does not recall the events leading up this hospitalization, except that he must have passed out in his apartment. He was told that his landlord called the rescue department and that is how "this whole mess started." It seems that he had been taking aspirin for quite some time to relieve the pain from his arthritis. He realized that he had been failing lately, saying that he "couldn't walk as well since his legs had been bothering him too much." The doctor said that he had some type of internal bleeding A series of tests were done and some blood transfusions given while he was in the hospital. At this time the doctor and social worker felt he was too weak to return to his apartment and since he had no family, arrangements were made for him to be transferred to a nursing home. Mr. Cardeur felt, "that there was nothing he could do, no place else to go."

During the first week after being transferred to the nursing home, Mr. Cardeur refused to eat or drink anything. "I just wanted to die rather than be in a place like this." Being in a nursing home was like a "living death" to Mr. Cardeur. Mr. Cardeur referred to his "starvation attempts" as "useless, they stuck me with needles in my arms until I would start to eat." He said that there was "no choice or freedom for a person in a place like this so he started to eat, resigning himself to this useless life." Mr. Cardeur often said, "I might have to stay here, but I surely don't have to like it."

Much of Mr. Cardeur's time with me was spent talking about his past life, "the good old days." His mother died young and he had to fend for himself. Mr. Cardeur never married, saying, "I never took much of a fancy to women" and spent all of his adult life living alone. He referred to himself as a "loner in this world" who spent much of his leisure time hunting and fishing when he was not working in the mill. After his retirement, Mr. Cardeur lived in a local low-income housing development for the aged. He never bothered much with the other people who lived there, saying that he "never really had a gift of gab." He did meet one man whom he liked and spent some time with him. They would occasionally get together and play cards or take a stroll to a local tavern for a beer or two. This man died two years ago, and at his friend's funeral Mr. Cardeur met the funeral director and made arrangements for his own funeral. "I thought it was a good idea since without any family around you have to plan for these things yourself." Mr. Cardeur often said that he's "not afraid of death, better than being here in this living hell." About once a month the funeral director stops in to check on Mr. Cardeur just to see if he is all right and if he needs anything. "But what does a man need in a place like this" is Mr. Cardeur's response. I checked Mr. Cardeur's record and the funeral director is listed as the responsible person to be notified in case of emergency.

Frequently, Mr. Cardeur would talk about missing life in the open outdoors. "It's tough for a man like me to be cooped up in a place like this." I suggested that we might take a walk outdoors, but he would reject my offer saying, "What's the use, life just isn't the same any more. Can't do anything important like work, hunt, fish."

Mr. Cardeur would always avoid being near or with the other residents calling them "half-witted crazy people." He is glad he is not like them because at least he "has his mind." He purposefully avoids his roommate and plans his day so that they have no contact. "I think the man got the hint that I don't want to bother with him since he now spends most of his day outside with the other men smoking and talking." Mr. Cardeur is pleased with this arrangement since he practically has the room to himself with no one to bother him.

When he first came to the nursing home, the nurses would "pester" him to get out of his room and join in the activities. He flatly refused, feeling like these social events are a way of "forcing people together against their will." The nurses have seemed to get the hint and do not bother him too much anymore about getting out of his room.

Throughout the visits, Mr. Cardeur was not overly talkative. Much of the initiation of conversation was left to me; however, I did not have to direct or control its content once he started to speak. Rarely did Mr. Cardeur ever make eye contact with me. He never avoided me or missed scheduled appointments. I always found him sitting on the edge of his bed in his room. There was one recliner chair in the central lounge area in which Mr. Cardeur would occasionally sit. This chair was situated in a corner at the far end of the room. On one occasion, I did observe Mr. Cardeur sitting there when another resident began walking towards him. As the resident got closer, Mr. Cardeur got up, took his walker and returned to his room. Most of Mr. Cardeur's day was spent lying down and sleeping. He did make it a point to read the evening newspaper if possible. Most of the content of Mr. Cardeur's conversation was reminiscing about the "good old days." He did not consider himself to be depressed, bored, or lonely, but had "resigned himself to this useless life until the good Lord decided to take him."

A description of withdrawal in this case shows a conscious, intentional, voluntary behavioral pattern with no evidence of progression from the time of relocation to the nursing home through the 1½ years of residing in this environment. In regard to the notion of degree of withdrawal, there may exist a very low degree of withdrawal as evidenced by the behavioral indicators of long sleeping pattern, retreating to room, avoiding social contacts, and decreased eye contact. However, I would suggest that in this case withdrawal might have to be distinguished from the concept of aloneness, which may be considered to be a voluntary type of withdrawal characteristic of a life-long pattern of limited social interaction with the environment. From analysis of the data I have identified the factors influencing the development of withdrawal in this case to be: no input into the decision-making process concerning relocation to the nursing home with loss of control over environment (decision made by doctor and social worker, prior lifestyle as a loner), loss of significant other (only friend died two years ago), no remaining social support system (no living friends or relatives), loss of self-esteem (frequent reference to feelings of uselessness), inability to find a meaningful role within the nursing home environment (an outdoor man confined within a building), and not a highly sociable person (has no gift for gab).

Case 2—Mrs. Bianco

The nursing staff refers to Mrs. Bianco as "withdrawn, difficult, moody and unwilling to mix with other patients."

Mrs. Bianco, who has just turned 65, is an educated woman of middle- to upper-class Italian descent. Although she has never been employed, the majority of her adult life was spent caring for her aging parents. After her parents' death, she married a "lovely well-to-do gentleman." Her interest shifted to caring for their home and development of her "artistic ability of oil painting." She related a life-long history of social drinking, enjoying a good wine with her meals and an after-dinner drink. Four months prior to her entry to the nursing home, Mrs. Bianco's husband died suddenly of a heart attack. She describes her reaction as one of "panic, shock and total grief since they were so close particularly since there were no children." Most of their time was spent together and they never developed any close friends. After his death, Mrs. Bianco continued to live alone. She relates that at this time she began drinking heavily, losing interest in life and feeling very depressed. This pattern of drinking continued for a few months. She couldn't recall much towards the end, except that she must have been experiencing some "black out spells." Unexpectedly, her brother stopped by and found Mrs. Bianco in a stuporous condition, very weak, thin and untidy. "He must have called an ambulance and had me brought to the hospital, I really don't remember." The medical record states that she was treated in the hospital for "alcoholism and malnutrition."

"After my husband's death, no one cared about me. We really didn't have any close friends or family." The only family members are Mrs. Bianco's brother and sister, who she recalled never came to call or visit after the funeral. Mrs. Bianco described her relationship with her siblings as "full of strife and jealousy since childhood." She rarely saw her sister in her adult life and is not close to her brother, describing him as "cold as ice" towards her. Mrs. Bianco often spoke of resentful feelings towards her brother. While she was in the hospital in a weakened condition and not thinking too clearly, her brother just "up and took control of everything." Apparently he obtained legal and financial control of her estate, selling her home and furniture. Arrangements were made by her brother to have Mrs. Bianco transferred to a nursing home to gain strength, control her drinking, and receive physical therapy. "I felt like a victim, everything taken away from me and brought to a place like this."

During the early stages of Mrs. Bianco's entry to the nursing home, she spent most of her time sleeping, staying in bed, and skipping meals. The staff relates that she was very "resistant to their attempts to help her and was quite uncooperative." Initially, the nurses thought she was depressed and tried to help her adjust to the nursing home. One nurse said, "but she is such a difficult woman, everything we do here is wrong." The staff said that Mrs. Bianco would always complain about something, either the "noise, the food, or other patients." She found all of the patients irritating and annoying almost as though she was "different from and better than the other patients." Mrs. Bianco would often accuse the nursing staff and other patients of taking personal items from her drawers. While talking with Mrs. Bianco she told me, "it was unbearable to look at those other people, so pitiful, so sloppy and such poor table manners." She refused to eat in the central dining room with the other patients and would take her tray to her room. Her refusal to eat with the other patients seemed to annoy the nursing staff. Also, Mrs. Bianco had one of the private rooms on the third floor for "privacy," which also seemed to annoy the staff who commented among themselves about Mrs. Bianco feeling "superior" to the other residents.

Within a few months of being in the nursing home, Mrs. Bianco confronted her brother about getting out and regaining control of her finances. Although she had no intention of staying with him (he would never offer to take her), Mrs. Bianco was beginning to feel stronger and thought that she could care for herself with the help of a woman. The brother scorned her suggestions and offered a transfer to a local religious affiliated rest home. She rejected his offer, describing it as "going from the frying pan into the fire."

At the time of our first meeting, Mrs. Bianco had been in the nursing home for almost 1 year. She maintains weekly contact with her brother saying that he is her "only link to the outside world." Each Saturday afternoon, he picks her up and takes her out to lunch. Although she doesn't like her brother, Mrs. Bianco looks forward to each weekend because she is able to have a glass of wine with her lunch. She simply knows that things will change someday and that she will get out of the nursing home. She thinks that her brother "doesn't trust her, wants her to stay in the nursing home because he fears she will start drinking heavily and spend all her money." Mrs. Bianco is aware that the nursing staff does not approve of these weekly lunches, especially since she has a glass of wine. Although she tries to hide the smell of wine by sucking on mints, the nurses are aware since they have mentioned the situation to her brother and to the doctor. Mrs. Bianco resents being called an "alcoholic" and the staff's attempts to have her attend weekly AA meetings held in the nursing home. She does not admit to having a drinking problem and attributes the events leading to hospitalization to despair over her husband's death.

The nurses' notes continually describe Mrs. Bianco as withdrawn, always staying in her room with the door shut, not interacting with patients or staff and not attending any social activities within the nursing home. The only contact with the nursing staff is in the morning because Mrs. Bianco requires some assistance getting in and out of the bathtub. The only time Mrs. Bianco leaves her room is to smoke cigarettes in the designated "smoking area." Mrs. Bianco spoke often of the lack of privacy within the nursing home and the "ridiculous rules and regulations concerning smoking." She has purchased locks and bolts for her closet and drawers to prevent the staff from taking her belongings.

Mrs. Bianco feels that the activities within the nursing home are not interesting and she does not intend to socialize with the other patients. Recently, a volunteer art instructor from a local school has started weekly classes. Mrs. Bianco has attended a few of these classes and has learned to do charcoal sketches. I visited these classes and observed Mrs. Bianco talking to the instructor; however, she sat at a table by herself not interacting with the other five patients attending the class. On our journey back to her room, I observed Mrs. Bianco's reaction towards the other patients. As we passed the lounges and patient rooms, she would look straight ahead almost ignoring the existence of these people. Recently, another woman in her late 50s was admitted to the nursing home. Mrs. Bianco met her in the smoking area and occasionally sits with her. She describes this relationship as "superficial, just someone to pass the time with and have a cup of coffee with."

Our relationship never evolved to one of any type of intimacy. Mrs. Bianco would remain rather "aloof" and displayed little facial expression when we talked. She would physically distance herself from me and rarely make eye contact. It was apparent that she wanted to remain in control of the situation since she often placed restrictions on the time and length of our conversation. When we did meet, it was usually in her room. She would sit in a chair with the lights dim and curtains drawn. She was quite open and frank with me saying, "I would not talk to you at all, if I did not like the way you looked or acted." This indicated that for Mrs. Bianco to even engage in any conversation with me, I must have been socially and culturally acceptable to her. She admitted that she was not lonely or particularly bored, yet she was still a bit depressed. This depression seemed to be improving since she was sleeping less often during the daytime. Occasionally, she would reminisce about her marriage and fond memories of her husband. Towards the end of the study, she did share with me the charcoal sketches she had been working on in the art class. Although her future was "one big question mark," she did maintain some hope that things would change.

Description of withdrawal in this case shows a pattern of conscious, intentional, voluntary behavior with no evidence of progression during the year of nursing home residence. In regard to the notion of degree of withdrawal, there may have existed a higher degree of withdrawal during the earlier phase of adjustment as evidenced by long daytime sleeping behavior and depression. These behaviors have decreased during the length of institutionalization as Mrs. Bianco gained some hope of leaving the nursing home environment and began to find some meaningful pursuit (art classes) to occupy her time. The present behavioral indicators suggesting a low degree of withdrawal are: expressionless face, minimal eye contact, aloofness, physical distancing during interaction with me, avoiding social contact with other residents, staying in room most of the day and affective feeling of depression. The following factors influencing withdrawal are identified as: recent loss of significant other (husband's death), weak social network (ambivalent feelings toward brother), no input into decision-making process concerning relocation to nursing home ("a victim" decision made by brother), class in lifestyle imposed by nursing home environment (educated, social etiquette oriented to middle- to upperclass women in comparison to lower working class population in nursing home), age (65 compared with mean age of 77 in the nursing home), and depression (indicated by drawn curtains, dim lights, and admission from patient).

It is interesting to note that the only social contacts that Mrs. Bianco made were "not typical" of the aged nursing home population such as myself, the younger patient in her late 50s, and the volunteer art instructor. Although depression was clearly evidenced during the early adjustment period, explanation of the degree of withdrawal and its relationship to depression cannot be done from such qualitative data.

Case 3—Mr. Charpentier

The nursing staff refers to Mr. Charpentier as "withdrawn, refuses to walk or leave room, does not interact with other patients." "Withdrawn, sits in chair all day, forgetful, confused, occasionally uses foul language."

Mr. Charpentier had been residing in the nursing home for three years. He turned 90 years old this fall. The event leading to hospitalization and subsequent relocation to the nursing home was a fall at home resulting in a fractured hip. His wife died 10 years prior to the fall, and Mr. Charpentier had been living alone managing his own apartment. His only daughter does not maintain much contact with Mr. Charpentier. A decision was made by the physician and hospital social worker that it would be best for Mr. Charpentier to be transferred to a nursing home because it was not safe for him to be living alone.

On our initial meeting, Mr. Charpentier was sitting in a chair in the corner of his room. A blank look was on his face and eyes were partially closed. He did not notice my presence and he appeared preoccupied twiddling his thumbs in a repetitious movement while talking to himself. There existed much disagreement among the staff as to the level of orientation of Mr. Charpentier. Some felt he was confused while others strongly disagreed saying that he was "pretending to be confused so that people would not bother him or talk to him."

During subsequent visits, I would always find Mr. Charpentier in the same chair performing the same repetitious movements and often talking to himself. At first his self-dialogue seemed nonsensical, yet the content was about his past as if he was talking to people he once knew. He did not take notice of my presence and continued preoccupied with his conversation and hand movements. It was difficult to obtain an adequate behavioral description of Mr. Charpentier at the time of his admission three years ago. The nurses' notes were vague and the staff has changed. However, there did appear to be some agreement from the nurses' notes that he was "quiet, alert and oriented." He was able to recover from the hip fracture and could walk with the assistance of one person. I persisted with my visits, introducing myself, sitting next to him and repeating his name. Eventually, he took notice of my presence and stopped the repetitious hand movements and began talking about his past. He had a vacant look in his eyes and no expression on his face. He rambled on about his younger days as a bricklayer. He would talk about people in the past, foods he liked, and things he did. It was difficult to maintain a conversation with Mr. Charpentier because he did not talk about the present and between the flow of reminiscing, he would be silent most of the time. The few occasions in which I was able to move the conversation to focus on the nursing home environment were quite productive. Although he was oriented to person and place, he had lost track of the month and year. When I asked about his feelings about being in the nursing home, he often would ignore my questions and start talking about something in the past, usually about work and food. When I mentioned his daughter's name, he responded with negative comments saying she "didn't care and had no time for him." When I inquired as to friends in the nursing home, he replied that "he didn't have any friends here and that's the way he wants it." He said that he was not really that outgoing but he did have one friend, a man he worked with who died nearly five years ago.

As our sessions continued, Mr. Charpentier did not appear as confused. He remembered my name and asked if I brought some candy with me. Often, I would pass by his room before I entered and he would be talking to himself twiddling his thumbs. Whenever I talked about the nursing home, he would refer to such talk as a "waste of time since life is useless now, nothing to do, nowhere to go." Once he said, "the only way I'll ever get out of here is in a coffin."

Mr. Charpentier would get quite upset and swear if anyone changed the arrangement of anything in his room, especially his chair. It always had to be in the same corner facing away from the window. I offered to turn the chair towards the window so that he could look outdoors but he would comment, "why bother, I've seen everything there is to see in life." He referred to his corner as "his world now." He particularly got upset if his roommate's belongings or bedside table was moved to his side of the room. Occasionally, he would agree to take a walk in the hall with me but only if other patients were not around. On these excursions, he would sometimes peer into the other patients' rooms and make derogatory comments often telling them to "shut up." Frequently, he would comment about his roommate as a "foolish old man who told lies." He never would engage in any conversation with the man and avoided looking at him. It was not until the end of October that Mr. Charpentier began to acknowledge my presence. The repetitious hand movements continued, yet he would stop them once a flow of conversation began. The majority of his conversation was of a remininising nature with little desire or willingness to talk about the present situation of living in a nursing home. He did not feel lonely or bored but was just waiting his time out.

The description of withdrawal in this case shows a progressive behavioral pattern with a higher degree of withdrawal than the previous two cases. Although I was not able to obtain an adequate baseline description of Mr. Charpentier's behavior three years ago, there does seem to be some evidence to support the notion that the withdrawal may have progressed. Initially his behavior was described as quiet, alert and oriented. At the time of this study there were many pauses in his conversation, he seemed less alert and somewhat confused. The degree of withdrawal may be described by the high degree of self-preoccupation, possible confusion and beginning signs of autistic behavior (talking to himself and repetitive hand movements). Also, the extreme degree of retreat, one specific chair in one specific corner, may indicate a higher degree of withdrawal. However, it was apparent that in describing withdrawal there was an obvious voluntary nature to his behavior (avoiding contact with other residents, not looking at his roommate and not wanting any friends in the nursing home).

Other behavioral indicators descriptive of withdrawal are vacant look in eyes and expressionless face. The factors that I have identified as contributing to withdrawal are: no input into decision-making process concerning relocation to nursing home (advice of physician and social worker), age (90, higher than nursing home norm), length of institutionalization (three years), inability to find a meaningful role in the nursing home environment (always talking about past roles, particularly work role as a bricklayer), absent social network (wife and friend dead, daughter rarely visits), low self-esteem (life is useless), and physical variables of the environment itself leading to physical withdrawal (attempt to maintain personal space and territorial rights).

Case 4—Mr. DuBois

I initially met Mr. DuBois on the second day after his relocation to the nursing home. Prior to this time, he had been living with his son and his family. He had only been with them for a month when things were not going well. He spoke of conflict with his daughter-in-law and feeling as though he was always in the way. During the last year, his wife had died and he decided to give up his home and move in with his son. He was not happy about living in a nursing home, but realized that it was the best thing to do since he could not take care of himself. Mr. DuBois said that he "would try to make the best of it and just take things as they come." Also, he would see his son and grandchildren, which seemed to please him. When I entered the room, I observed Mr. DuBois lying on his bed staring at the ceiling. He looked relieved to see a friendly face. I introduced myself as a graduate nursing student interested in talking with new patients in the nursing home. He spoke of recent losses within the past year, his wife, his home, his driver's license, car, and health. Since his retirement at age 65 (he is now 83), the majority of his time was spent in leisurely activities such as gardening, woodworking, and puttering around the yard. These activities became more difficult since he has advancing osteoarthritis and has to wear a back brace most of the time. Losing his wife was the hardest. He misses her terribly. Throughout our conversation, he remained alert, oriented, made eye contact and displayed facial expression appropriate to the conversation (when he saw me he smiled, when he spoke of his wife he looked sad). When I got up to leave, he reached out to me and gently held my face between his hands proceeding to kiss me on each cheek. He hoped that I didn't take offense since this was a French custom, a gesture of liking someone common to his family.

Our next encounter was five days after relocation. I observed Mr. DuBois walking down the corridor in the nursing home. He appeared to be having trouble gaining his bearings and looked somewhat fearful of maneuvering within this environment. When he reached the patient lounge, he sat down in the first chair he found and immediately picked up a magazine leafing through the pages. I approached him and he smiled saying that he was "happy to see a familiar face." I shared my observations with him inquiring about his eyesight. He said that he could see fairly well with his glasses and attributed his hesitancy to "being unfamiliar with the place." He thought that with time he would get more comfortable and make out all right, since he was pretty much a sociable man. He was alert and oriented during our conversation, telling me that his son visited last evening and took him out to dinner.

The following week Mr. DuBois was transferred to another nursing home, a smaller one closer to his family, which was the original choice of the son. Two weeks had passed before I gained entry to this facility. When I saw Mr. DuBois he was sitting in a lounge by himself. At first he did not recognize me. He did not make eye contact when he talked. After a few minutes he remembered me, yet showed no expression in his face when we talked. He cut our visit short saying he was tired and wanted to lie down. As I observed him walking down the corridor, he appeared to have trouble finding his room. I followed him to his room and found him lying down on the bed with his face turned towards the wall.

Speaking to the nursing staff led to some unsettling thoughts. They described Mr. DuBois as a quiet, somewhat confused man who frequently gets lost wandering around the nursing home. Investigation into the nurses' notes led to comments such as "keeps to himself, sleeps often especially during the day, appears to be adjusting well to environment, potential for socialization not known at this time." I couldn't understand how these behaviors could be described as adjusting well! The next visit I found Mr. DuBois in his room lying on the bed. Although he recognized me, he was very quiet and asked to be left alone to sleep. The following encounter, I found Mr. DuBois sitting in the lounge alone. When I approached him, he got up to leave as though he was avoiding me. I followed him and he said that he was "going to lie down." He went outdoors and wandered around the yard, saying he was "looking for his room." I helped him get to his room and then he laid on the bed.

I was definitely observing a change in his behavior. Although my observations were supporting the notion of withdrawal as progressive, I couldn't passively stand by and observe further progression. That afternoon I approached Mr. DuBois to talk about his feelings and my observations. He was willing to talk. He admitted to feeling depressed and lonely. He had no interest to do anything and was bored. He just felt like sleeping and forgetting the whole situation. Although he saw his son, he had not become involved with any activities or people in the nursing home. After a lengthy conversation and exploring possible resources, I met with the nursing staff and activity director in an effort to mobilize resources and intervene with Mr. DuBois. Suggestions were shared with the staff to increase his familiarity with the nursing home environment and place some distinctive, colorful sign outside of the door to Mr. DuBois's room to lessen the chance of getting lost. The activity director spent extra time with Mr. DuBois and soon he joined a men's social hour. Opportunity for gardening and the development of woodworking shop was explored. The staff was helpful in spending extra time with Mr. DuBois to increase his awareness of and interest in the environment.

Over a period of time, these interventions led to improvement in Mr. DuBois's adjustment. He was spending less time sleeping, and began to socialize with other patients. During the following visits, I found Mr. DuBois sitting in the lounge talking with two other patients. He smiled when he saw me and made eye contact during our conversation. He discussed plans to visit his son's home over the holidays. He did not appear confused and had no difficulty finding his room.

During our subsequent interaction, he was open and friendly with me. Although he still felt somewhat depressed, he was not as lonely anymore. He spent time talking to his roommate and made a few friends at the social hour meetings. He particularly enjoyed speaking in French with the other men. On our last visit, I attended a holiday party with him. He got all dressed up with a bowtie on and referred to me "as his date."

Although intervention with Mr. DuBois did lead to a change in behavior, I can say with a strong degree of confidence that if I had passively stood by it is highly likely that his behavioral pattern would have progressed towards a higher degree of withdrawal.

A description of withdrawal in this case shows a progressive, behavioral pattern that emerged during the initial adjustment phase to the nursing home environment. The behavioral changes that were observed indicating a progressive development of withdrawal are the following: initially Mr. DuBois was friendly, outgoing, talkative, alert, displayed facial expression and made eye contact during conversation. Over approximately a six-week time frame, these behaviors changed to quietness, avoidance, indifference, wandering (could this be an attempt at flight?), prolonged daytime sleeping, silence, no facial expression, no eye contact, and confusion. The factors that I have identified negatively effecting Mr. DuBois's adjustment and influencing the emergence of withdrawal are: recent loss of significant other (wife died within the last year), compounded by other recent losses (house, car, health), a possible depression with inability to find a meaningful role within the nursing home environment.

CONCLUSIONS

In both the literature review and in the nursing home studied here, scholars and practitioners used the term *withdrawal* rather frequently to characterize patient behavior. In the field study, nurses almost automatically associated the term with patients who were alone, immobilized, confused, or depressed. This was not unlike what was found in the literature, where the term was embedded in similar phenomena such as isolation, immobilization, and depression. As in the literature, nurses in the field study saw this behavior as predominantly negative. Withdrawal was considered a nursing care problem to be intervened with by increasing socialization and encouraging participation in group activities.

The data from the fieldwork phase add empirical support to the occurrence and importance of withdrawal among nursing home patients. However, they do not fully support the idea that withdrawal is negative and necessarily requires intervention. Among the four patients followed, withdrawal appeared as both a response during adjustment and as a long-term control strategy that probably was not unique to the nursing home context. Some of the literature, and certainly this fieldwork, suggests that nurses may need to be more attentive to the inappropriate usage of withdrawal and the assumption that it is inherently problematic. Certainly, my original impression that all people desire and need social interaction for a healthy adjustment to the nursing home was seriously challenged by these data.

Although this fieldwork purposely excluded a focus on withdrawal as an aspect of mental illness, I believe that the progressive nature of withdrawal in the case of Mr. DuBois could have led to depression and further loss of touch with reality. Also, the borderline nature of withdrawal in Mr. Charpentier's case, with the degree of self-preoccupation and emergence of autistic behavior, supports the idea that at times withdrawal can be progressive and maladaptive.

The problem of mutual withdrawal between nursing staff and patients was clearly described by Tudor (1952). The present study did not focus on staff-patient interactions. However, incidental observations suggest that avoidance by the staff was a subtle, yet predominant interactional pattern of the staff that further reinforced at least one patient's withdrawal. After Mr. DuBois's transfer to the second nursing home in which the nursing staff described him as confused, the staff had limited interaction with him, and did not recognize his need for help in adjusting. Perhaps there was a mutual withdrawal operating that contributed to the sudden progression of this patient's withdrawal. I believe this study highlights the need to examine the possibility of mutual withdrawal between staff and nursing home patients. Further examination might support the idea that withdrawal is most significant as a nurse-patient related phenomenon and is best studied as an interactional concept.

In relation to definition, the fieldwork phase tended to validate earlier notions about withdrawal as a retreat, a movement away from people, things, and situations. It also added some support to the working definition of withdrawal as a "behavioral response of physical, emotional and social detachment from the external environment, which may be progressive, and is manifested in a wide variety of behaviors." Yet, further expansion and refinement of this definition is needed to better encompass the notion of withdrawal as a behavioral strategy and a response to stress. Specifically, the term *response* implies a passive reaction to a stimulus, rather than a more active strategy, which was the most frequent form of withdrawal encountered in the fieldwork phase. It might be more accurate to define withdrawal as a behavioral process of moving away from environmental and situational stressors. It includes physical, emotional, and social dimensions that can be both adaptive and maladaptive and at times may be progressive. It is evidenced by a variety of behavioral indicators. In this form, the definition of withdrawal is highly generalizable, reflects both the literature and the fieldwork findings, and is amenable to measurement through operationalization of the behavioral indicators.

Future field investigations need to separate out more clearly withdrawal from closely related concepts and examine their potential interactive effect. For example, immobilization was closely associated with the withdrawn patient. With the increasing attention in nursing being given to immobility among the elderly, an important empirical question is: To what extent are immobilization and withdrawal associated, and if so, under what conditions and with what consequences? Similarly, boredom, depression, and loneliness were three concepts that indirectly emerged during unstructured interviewing of these cases and originally were identified in the literature as potential consequences of poor adjustment of the nursing home patient. Patients' subjective reports of the presence or absence of these feelings begin to support an empirical generalization suggesting that loneliness, depression, and boredom may contribute to a form of withdrawal that is progressive and maladaptive. Also, data obtained in the description of withdrawal in Mr. DuBois strongly emphasize the need to distinguish between loneliness and aloneness of the elderly and their relationship to withdrawal. Lastly, the concept of social isolation seems most essential to delineate from withdrawal.

The measurement of withdrawal in the fieldwork phase adds empirical support to the relevance of the behavioral indicators presented in Table 10-1. No additional indicators became evident from the fieldwork data. The two indicators of avoidance of people, including avoidance of social situations and staying in one's room, were the strongest in all four cases. However, the indicators of self-preoccupation, confusion, and autistic behavior were more characteristic of a higher degree and potential progression of withdrawal. These findings support the need to further measure and weigh these behavioral indicators. Furthermore, drawing on the case analysis, descriptions of withdrawal gained in the fieldwork, and the literature review, further expansion in measurement and beginning exploration of degrees and progression of withdrawal can be presented as illustrated in Table 10-2.

Indicators of withdrawal in Class I are seen as conscious, purposeful behaviors indicating a strategic use of withdrawal that is either transient or a continuing control strategy. Class II behaviors suggest beginning progression and a higher degree of withdrawal indicating "at-risk" people in need of support to mobilize coping skills, facilitate adaptation, and prevent progression of withdrawal. However, indicators in Class III reflect an unconscious, involuntary progressive response with a higher degree of withdrawal suggesting low-level adaptation to stress or unsuccessful intervention in Class II.

Further explanation of withdrawal requires identification of factors

Table 10-2 Progression of Withdrawal

Class I	Class II	Class III
Expresses desire to be alone	Feelings of boredom, loneliness, and depression surface	Apathetic
Quiet affect	Self-preoccupation Confusion emerges	Autistic behavior
Avoidance of people Avoidance of social situations	Further retreat from people and social situations	Self-absorption Progression of confusion
Physically removes self to room	Stays in room Increase in sleep pattern	Delusions/hallucinations Immobile

that influence the use of withdrawal as a temporary or continuous strategy rather than a progressive long-term response to stress. The dramatic development of progressive withdrawal in the case of Mr. DuBois illuminates some of these factors contributing to the development of withdrawal as a response to the stress associated with relocation. He had recently lost his wife. Secondly, he had minimal social support to buffer the impact of stress associated with this change. Thirdly, he had no input into the decision-making process concerning relocation and subsequently experienced a loss of control. This loss of control and inability to find a meaningful role within the nursing home led to feelings of uselessness and a negative self-image. Lastly, he had difficulty adjusting to the physical layout of the environment. It seems that the characteristics of the environment had a negative effect contributing to and supporting the withdrawal.

The negative influence of these factors has been supported in the literature by Chenitz (1983). Furthermore, Chang (1978) suggests that the personality of the individual and characteristics of the nursing home environment are significant variables affecting the person's adjustment. Additionally, the environment with its close proximity to other residents can lead to inadequate personal space and the emergence of withdrawal as an attempt to secure privacy (Tate, 1980).

Although the first three cases, who presented with a nonprogressive strategic use of withdrawal, had similar factors of minimal social support, negative self-image, and loss of control, there were several other dissimilar factors between these cases and Mr. DuBois that are useful to explain the different processes of withdrawal. These dissimilar factors relate to the variables of lifestyle, personality, and affective response to the nursing home environment. Specifically, the first group (cases 1 to 3) perceived themselves as not sociable and preferring to be alone. They did not feel lonely or bored and spent their time with reminiscing and individual activities. However, Mr. DuBois referred to himself as outgoing, sociable, and enjoying company. Furthermore, he did admit to feelings of boredom, loneliness, and depression. These findings seem to support a relationship between the variables of preadmission social isolation, non–socially outgoing personality, and the conscious use of withdrawal as a strategic nonprogressive pattern. The avoidance of other residents and not participating in social activities as indicators of withdrawal may be explained by the following analysis. These individuals lacked the social skills to participate within a group because these activities were inconsistent with their prior lifestyle and personality. The nursing home with its emphasis on group activities and socialization was incongruent with their lifestyle and personalities and reinforced the withdrawal. The use of withdrawal was an intentional strategy to maintain control.

In contrast to these cases, Mr. DuBois had an active social support network, including his wife and son's family with whom he had lived. Yet, in a short time span he had lost his wife, moved out of his son's home to the first nursing home, and then moved to a second nursing home. The use of withdrawal surfaced as a response to these stressors and progressed as the feelings of loneliness, boredom, and depression developed.

The emergence of withdrawal in this situation of continued stress emphasizes the need to examine the potential for withdrawal in other populations. Other populations that merit inquiry include the chronically ill, long-term hospitalized, mentally ill, and the terminally ill client. Nurses could examine the stressors associated with illness and their impact on these populations, yet they could also examine the impact of stress associated with relocation such as hospital to hospice care, hospital to long-term care institution, and other situations of environmental change. For example, Slavinsky and Krauss (1980) believe that the problems associated with deinstitutionalization of the chronic mentally ill person can be explained by mutual withdrawal between these people and the communities in which they have relocated. Therefore, the focus of study could be at the patient level, the nurse-patient level, and the patient-community level to examine all potential processes of withdrawal. Further inquiry might discover that withdrawal is a central phenomenon in nursing common to most people as they attempt to deal with the anxiety associated with stressful situations. The crucial factor for nursing seems to be the discovery of when withdrawal is no longer useful and intervention is indicated.

REFERENCES

Beland, I. (1980). The burnout syndrome in nurses. In Werner-Beland, J. (Ed.), *Grief responses to long-term illness and disability: Manifestations and nursing interventions*. Reston, VA: Reston.

Beland, I. L., & Passos, J. Y. (1975). *Clinical nursing: Pathophysiological and psychosocial approaches* (3rd ed.). New York: Macmillan.

Bleuler, E. (1912). *The theory of schizophrenia negativism* (W. A. White, Trans.). New York: The Journal of Nervous and Mental Disease.

Brehm, H. P. (1968). Sociology and aging: Orientation and research. *Gerontologist, 8*, 24–31.

Burbank, P. M. (1986). Psychosocial theories of aging: A critical review. *Advances in Nursing Science, 9*(1), 73–86.

Chang, B. L. (1978). Generalized expectancy, situational perception and morale among institutionalized aged. *Nursing Research, 27*, 316–323.

Chenitz, C. E. (1983). Entry into a nursing home as status passage: A theory to guide nursing practice. *Geriatric Nursing, 4*, 92–97.

Cochrane, N. J. (1983). An explanatory study of social withdrawal experiences of adults. *Nursing Papers, 15*(2), 22–37.

Coelho, G. V., Hamburg, D. A., & Adams, J. E. (1974). *Coping and adaptation*. New York: Basic Books.

Cumming, E., & Henry, W. E. (1961). *Growing old—The process of disengagement.* New York: Basic Books.

Davis, M. Z. (1975). Social isolation as a process in chronic illness. In M. Z. Davis, M. Kramer, & A. L. Strauss (Eds.), *Nurses in practice: A perspective on work environments.* St. Louis: C. V. Mosby.

Edmunds, M. (1974). *Defenses in animals.* New York: Longman.

Escalona, S., & Leitch, M. (1949). The reactions of infants to stress. *Psychoanalytic Study of the Child, 3,* 121–140.

Friedrick, R. M., & Lively, S. I. (1981). Psychological immobilization. In L. K. Hart, J. L. Reese, & M. O. Fearing (Eds.), *Concepts common to acute illness: Identification and management.* St. Louis: C. V. Mosby.

Frieswyk, S. (1977). The assessment of a relational disposition, "fantasy withdrawal" from Rorschach face sheet data. *Journal of Clinical Psychology, 33,* 1132–1140.

Glaser, B. G., & Strauss, A. L. (1965). *Awareness of dying.* Chicago: Aldine.

Griffin, A. (1979). The loneliness of the elderly. *Canadian Nurse, 5,* 23–25.

Grinker, R. (1971). An essay on schizophrenia and science. In R. Cancro (Ed.), *This schizophrenic syndrome: An annual review* (pp. 53–92). New York: Brunner/Mazel.

Hamburg, D. A., Hamburg, B., & deGoza, J. (1953). Adaptive problems and mechanisms in severely burned patients. *Psychiatry, 16,* 1–21.

Havinghurst, R. J. (1961). Successful aging. *Gerontologist, 1,* 8–13.

Horney, K. (1937). *The neurotic personality of our time.* New York: W. W. Norton.

Hurteau, P. M. (1963). Disguised language: A clinical problem in nursing. In S. F. Burd & M. A. Marshall (Eds.), *Some clinical approaches to psychiatric nursing.* London: Macmillan.

Hutchinson, S. (1987). Self-care and job stress. *Image, 19*(4), 192–196.

Ironside, W. (1980). Conservation-withdrawal and action-engagement: On a theory of survivor behavior. *Psychosomatic Medicine, 42,* 163–175.

Jacobson, S. F. (1983). Burnout: A hazard in nursing. In S. F. Jacobsen & M. H. McGrath (Eds.), *Nurses under stress.* New York: John Wiley & Sons.

Jasmin, S., & Trygstad, L. N. (1979). *Behavioral concepts and the nursing process.* St. Louis: C. V. Mosby.

Kim, M. J., McFarland, G. K., & McLane, A. M. (1987). *Pocket guide to nursing diagnoses* (2nd ed.). St. Louis: C. V. Mosby.

King, G. F. (1956). Withdrawal as a dimension of schizophrenia: An exploratory study. *Journal of Clinical Psychology, 12,* 373–375.

Kramer, M. (1974). *Reality shock: Why nurses leave nursing.* St. Louis: C. V. Mosby.

Leyn, R. M. (1972). A mother's reaction to her son's fatal illness. *Maternal Child Nursing Journal, 13,* 231–241.

Lowenthal, M. F., & Boler, D. (1965). Voluntary vs. involuntary social withdrawal. *Journal of Gerontology, 20,* 363–371.

Maddox, G. L. (1965). Fact and artifact: Evidence bearing on disengagement theory from the Duke geriatrics project. *Human Development, 18,* 117–130.

Oden, G. (1963). Individual panic: Elements and patterns. In S. F. Burd & M. A. Marshall (Eds.), *Some clinical approaches to psychiatric nursing.* London: Macmillan.

Pallister, H. (1933). The negative or withdrawal attitude: A study in personality organization. *Archives of Psychology, 151,* 1–56.

Peplau, H. E. (1952). *Interpersonal relations in nursing.* New York: G. P. Putnam's Sons.

Peplau, H. E. (1963). A working definition of anxiety. In S. F. Burd & M. A. Marshall (Eds.), *Some clinical approaches to psychiatric nursing.* London: Macmillan.

Perry, H. S. (1962). *Harry Stack Sullivan: Schizophrenia as a human process.* New York: W. W. Norton.

Sapirstein, M. R. (1948). *Emotional security.* New York: Crown.

Schatzman, L., & Strauss, A. L. (1973). *Field research: Strategies for a natural science.* Englewood Cliffs, NJ: Prentice-Hall.

Schmidt, C. S. (1981). Withdrawal behavior of schizophrenics: Application of Roy's adaptation model. *Journal of Psychiatric Nursing and Mental Health Services, 19,* 26-33.

Scully, R. (1980). Stress in the nurse. *American Journal of Nursing, 80*(5), 912-915.

Sites, P. (1973). *Control: The basis for social order.* New York: Dunellen.

Slavinsky, A. T., & Krauss, J. B. (1980). Mutual withdrawal or Gwen Tudor revisited. *Perspectives in Psychiatric Care, 18*(5), 194-203.

Spitz, R. A. (1946). Anaclitic depression. *Psychoanalytical Study of the Child, 2,* 313-341.

Sprott, W. (1933). *New introductory lectures on psychoanalysis.* New York: W. W. Norton.

Tate, J. (1980). The need for personal space in institutions for the elderly. *Journal of Gerontological Nursing, 6,* 439-447.

Travelbee, J. (1971). *Interpersonal aspects of nursing.* Philadelphia: F. A. Davis.

Tudor, G. E. (1952). A sociopsychiatric nursing approach to intervention in a problem of mutual withdrawal on a mental hospital ward. *Psychiatry, 15,* 193-217.

Weinstein, E. A., Kahn, R. L., & Slote, W. H. (1955). Withdrawal, inattention and pain asymbolia. *AMA Archives of Neurology and Psychiatry, 74,* 235-248.

Wolk, R., & Reingold, J. (1975). The course of life for old people. *Journal of American Geriatrics Society, 23,* 376-380.

Ziegler, L. H. (1933). Hysterical fugues. *Journal of the American Medical Association, 101,* 571-576.

BIBLIOGRAPHY

Aldrich, E. K., & Mendkoff, E. (1963). Relocation of the aged and disabled: A mortality study. *Journal of American Geriatrics Society, 11,* 185-194.

Barrett, J. H. (Ed.). (1972). *Gerontological psychology.* Springfield, IL: Charles C. Thomas.

Barrie, J. (1980). Social isolation: How can we help? *Nursing Times, 1,* 208-210.

Benedict, R. (1959). *Patterns of culture.* Boston: Houghton-Mifflin.

Birren, J. E. (1964). *The psychology of aging.* New Jersey: Prentice-Hall.

Brown, M. I. (1968). Social theory in geriatric nursing. *Nursing Research, 17,* 213-217.

Bunker, H. A. (1945). "Repression" in pre-Freudian American psychiatry. *Psychoanalytical Quarterly, 14,* 469-477.

Busse, E. W. (1960). Psychoneurotic reactions and defense mechanisms in the aged. In P. H. Hock & J. Zubin (Eds.), *Psychopathology of aging.* New York: Grune & Stratton.

Caplan, G. (1955). *Emotional problems of early childhood*. New York: Basic Books.

Catman, M. (1983). *An application of general systems theory to the system problem of withdrawal in the terminally ill oncology patient*. Unpublished paper, University of Rhode Island, Kingston, RI.

Chapman, A. H., & Chapman, M. C. (1980). *Harry Stack Sullivan's concepts of personality development and psychiatric illness*. New York: Brunner/Mazel.

Chess, S. (1985). Temperament differences: A critical concept in child health care. *Pediatric Nursing, 11*(3), 167–171.

Chess, S., & Thomas, A. (1986). *Temperament in clinical practice*. New York: The Guilford Press.

Chodorkoff, B. (1954). Self-perception, perceptual defense and adjustment. *Journal of Abnormal Social Psychology, 49*, 508–512.

Cumming, E., Dean, J. R., Newell, D. S., & McCaffrey, I. (1960). Disengagement—a tentative theory of aging. *Sociometry, 23*, 23–35.

Dagenais, J. (1981). *Psychosocial withdrawal during adolescent pregnancy*. Unpublished manuscript, University of Rhode Island, Kingston, RI.

Davis, M. Z. (1973). *Living with multiple sclerosis: A social psychological analysis*. Springfield, IL: Charles C. Thomas.

Engel, G. L., & Reichsman, R. (1956). Spontaneous and experimentally induced depression in an infant with gastric fistula. *Journal of the American Psycho-analytical Association, 4*, 428–452.

Fox, D. L. (1982). *Fundamentals of research in nursing*. New York: Appleton-Century-Crofts.

Freud, S. (1936). *The problem of anxiety* (H. A. Bunker, Trans.). New York: W. W. Norton.

Furman, S., Rahe, D. F., & Hartup, W. W. (1979). Rehabilitation of socially withdrawn preschool children through mixed-age and same age socialization. *Child Development, 50*, 915–922.

Glaser, B. G., & Strauss, A. L. (1968). *Time for dying*. Chicago: Aldine.

Graham-McClowry, S. (1990). The relationship of temperament to pre- and post-hospitalization behavioral responses of school-age children. *Nursing Research, 39*(1), 30–35.

Granick, R., & Nahemow, L. (1961). Preadmission isolation as a factor in adjustment to an old age home. In P. H. Hock and J. Zubin (Eds.), *Psychopathology of aging* (pp. 285–301). New York: Grune & Stratton.

Haigh, G. (1949). Defensive behavior in client-centered therapy. *Journal of Consulting Psychologists, 13*, 181–189.

Hall, C. S., & Lindzey, G. (1970). *Theories of personality*. New York: John Wiley & Sons.

Hamburg, B. A. (1979). Early adolescence as a life stress. In S. Levine & H. Ursin (Eds.), *Coping and health* (pp. 121–141). New York: Plenum Press.

Jacox, A. (1974). Theory construction in nursing. *Nursing Research, 23*, 4–13.

Kahn, R., Pollock, M., & Goldfarb, A. (1961). Factors related to individual differences in mental status of the institutionalized aged. In P. H. Hock & J. Zubin (Eds.), *Psychopathology of aging* (pp. 104–113). New York: Grune & Stratton.

Kalish, R. A. (1972). Of social values and the dying: A defense of disengagement. *Family Coordinator, 22*, 18–94.

Kanner, L. (1944). Early infantile autism. *Journal of Pediatrics, 25*, 212–217.

Katz, L., Neal, M., & Simon, A. (1961). Observations on psychic mechanisms in organic psychoses of the aged. In P. H. Hock & J. Zubin (Eds.), *Psychopathology of aging* (pp. 160–181). New York: Grune & Stratton.

Kübler-Ross, E. (1969). *On death and dying*. New York: Macmillan.

Kutner, B. (1962). The social nature of aging. *Gerontologist, 2*, 5–8.

Levine, S. (1979). A coping model of mother-infant relationship. In S. Levine & H. Ursin (Eds.), *Coping and health* (pp. 87–99). New York: Plenum Press.

Liberman, M. A. (1961). Relationship of mortality rates to entrance in a home for the aged. *Geriatrics, 16*, 515–519.

Miller, S. (1979). When is a little information a dangerous thing? Coping with stressful events by monitoring versus blunting. In S. Levine & H. Ursin (Eds.), *Coping and health* (pp. 145–169). New York: Plenum Press.

Mullen, E. (1977). Relocation of the elderly: Implications for nursing. *Geriatric Nursing, 3*, 13–17.

Muus, R. E. (1968). *Theories of adolescence*. New York: Random House.

New Merriam-Webster dictionary, The (F. C. Mish (Editor-in-chief). (1989). Springfield, MA: Merriam-Webster.

Noyes, A., Camp, W., & VanSickel, M. (1964). *Psychiatric nursing*. New York: Macmillan.

Payne, R. (1960). Some theoretical approaches to the sociology of aging. *Social Forces, 38*, 359–363.

Peplau, H. E. (1973). *Basic explanatory concepts on withdrawal behavior*. PSF Productions Series 200: Tape No. 7.

Pie-Nie, P. (1979). *Schizophrenia disorders: Theory and treatment from a psychodynamic point of view*. New York: International Universities Press.

Polcina, A. (1979). Loneliness—the genesis of solitude, friendship and contemplation. *Hospital Progress, 8*, 61–65.

Polit, D., & Hungler, B. (1978). *Nursing research: Principles and methods*. Philadelphia: J. B. Lippincott.

Qualls, P. E., Justice, B., & Allen, R. (1980). Isolation and psycho-social functioning. *Psychological Reports, 46*, 279–285.

Reed, D. L. (1970). Social disengagement in chronically ill patients. *Nursing Research, 19*, 109–115.

Reynolds, P. D. (1971). *A primer in theory construction*. Indianapolis: Bobbs-Merrill.

Riley, M. W., Johnson, M., & Foner, A. (1972). *Aging and society*. New York: Russell Sage Foundation.

Roberts, S. L. (1978). *Behavioral concepts and nursing throughout the life-span*. Englewood Cliffs, NJ: Prentice-Hall.

Rodin, J. (1979). Managing the stress of aging: The role of control and coping. In S. Levine & H. Ursin (Eds.), *Coping and health*. New York: Plenum Press.

Roget's international thesaurus (4th ed.). (1977). New York: Harper & Row.

Rouslin, S. (1963). An antidote for alcoholism. In S. F. Burd & M. A. Marshall (Eds.), *Some clinical approaches to psychiatric nursing*. London: Macmillan.

Roy, C. (1976). Problems in self-ideal and expectancy: Powerlessness. In C. Roy (Ed.), *Nursing: An adaptation model*. Englewood Cliffs, NJ: Prentice-Hall.

Ruddy-Wallace, M. (1989). Temperament: A variable in children's pain management. *Pediatric Nursing, 15*(2), 118–121.

Sadowski, A., & Weinsaft, P. (1975). Behavioral disorders in the elderly. *Journal of the American Geriatrics Society, 23*, 86–92.

Sarma, D. E. (1953). The nature and history of Hinduism. In K. W. Morgan (Ed.), *The religion of the Hindus*. New York: Ronald Press.

Spotnitz, H., & Meadow, P. (1976). *Treatment of narcissistic neuroses*. New York: The Manhattan Center for Advanced Psychoanalytic Studies.

Strumpf, N. (1978). Aging—a progressive phenomena. *Journal of Gerontological Nursing, 4*, 17–23.

Sullivan, H. S. (1927). The onset of schizophrenia. *American Journal of Psychiatry, 7*, 105–134.

Sullivan, H. S. (1929). Research in schizophrenia. *American Journal of Psychiatry, 9*, 553–568.

Testa, G. (1980). *A participant observation study of the concept psycho-social withdrawal in the aged nursing home resident*. Unpublished manuscript, University of Rhode Island, Kingston, RI.

Testa, G. (1980). *An analysis of the concept psycho-social withdrawal*. Unpublished manuscript, University of Rhode Island, Kingston, RI.

Thomas, A., & Chess, S. (1984). Genesis and evolution of behavioral disorders: From infancy to early adult life. *American Journal of Psychiatry, 1441*(1), 1–9.

Tobin, S., & Lieberman, M. (1976). *Last home for the aged—critical implications of institutionalization*. San Francisco: Jossey-Bass.

Wertlieb, D., Weigel, C., Springer, T., & Feldstein, M. (1988). Temperament as a moderator of children's stressful experiences. In S. Chess, A. Thomas, & M. E. Hertzig (Eds.), *Annual progress in child psychiatry and child development*. New York: Brunner/Mazel.

Witt, R., & Mitchell, P. (1973). Psychosocial and mental-emotional status. In P. H. Mitchell (Ed.), *Concepts basic to nursing*. New York: McGraw-Hill.

Youmans, E. (1969). Some perspectives on disengagement theory. *Gerontologist, 9*, 254–258.

Ziller, R. C. (1969). The alienation syndrome: A tragic pattern of self-other orientation. *Sociometry, 32*, 287–300.

Concept Clarification: Using the Norris Method in Clinical Research

Nancy R. Lackey

Catherine Norris (1982) stated in the preface of her book that one of her goals "is to foster the development of increasingly meaningful descriptions of nursing phenomena. Out of these descriptions will come critical questions and hypotheses that nurses will need to explore. Out of these descriptions, nurses will ultimately build the base for a substantive body of knowledge for the discipline called nursing" (p. xv). Norris has developed a method of concept clarification that can be used by nurse researchers to clarify phenomena that are germane to the knowledge base of nursing. The components from such clarification, once operationalized, can be used as variables in studies. The results of these studies will ultimately form a solid foundation from which effective nursing interventions can be derived.

Nurses in a variety of settings and roles care for a very diverse clientele: from the homeless to the very affluent, from the newborn to the frail elderly, from the single individual to the extended family. Lindsey (1991) stated that only through research will the quality of care provided by nurses improve. According to Lindsey, there are three critical stages in the development of a scientific base and in the integration of research findings into practice. These stages are: (1) generation of nursing knowledge; (2) utilization of research; and (3) evaluation of the effectiveness of the specific changes in practice (p. 93). Before nursing knowledge can be generated, concepts pertinent to each of these diverse settings and roles must be identified and clarified, and the components of the concept derived from the clarification incorporated into research questions or hypotheses that ultimately will be tested empirically. Norris (1982) has derived a method of concept clarification that can be used to identify the components of a concept that ultimately can be used to generate nursing knowledge to form the basis of more effective care for the diverse clientele that nurses serve.

The overall purpose of this chapter is to review and discuss Norris's method of concept clarification and delineate how nurses can use this method in their research to generate nursing knowledge as a solid foundation for nursing care. Discussed in this chapter are Norris's philosophical underpinnings for her method of concept clarification, the method itself, and an example that will illustrate the utility of her method of concept clarification for research.

PHILOSOPHICAL FOUNDATION OF NORRIS'S METHOD

Norris (1982) wrote that research in nursing has suffered due to the lack of a well-defined body of knowledge and, conversely, the body of knowledge suffered because nurses have not done appropriate descriptive work, particularly concept clarification. She believed that there were some differences between the descriptive research done in medicine and the descriptive research needed in nursing. According to Norris, the research that had been done in medicine utilized the psyche-soma dualistic model. As a result, separate or several theories were developed for each disease studied by medicine. Because these theories were not analyzed or synthesized, medicine tended to view human beings in terms of a mind-body dichotomy and failed to recognize humans as a unique whole. Norris (1982) believed that nursing functioned independently from medicine and was consistent with a "humanistic, holistic approach to individuals and communities" (p. 6).

Important components of the knowledge base of nursing are the concepts used in nursing theory and practice. Norris (1982) stated that a concept is a "basic idea," an "abstraction of concrete events," and the "only means of connecting an empirical science to the 'real world'"; the term *concept* is the "word symbol, not the act itself" (p. 11). Nursing requires two types of concepts: "one that relates to abstract knowledge and knowing (such as the concept *wellness*), and one that is process-oriented and answers questions about how to solve nursing problems" (such as cardiovascular fitness) (p. 13). The concepts of nursing knowledge and practice articulate the essence of nursing science; that science is dependent upon precise language to convey the phenomenon. The effective use of language requires the precision of adequate concept clarification. Norris stated that concepts are "generalizations about particulars, such as cause-effect, duration, dimension, attributes, and continua of phenomena or objects" (p. 11). The process of concept clarification allows nurses to make generalizations and to systematize the particulars. From these generalizations and systematizations, an operational definition of the concept can be derived. Operational definitions allow us to know when the concept under study is in operation, and thus, they can become the basis for research. Operational definitions, because of their preciseness, articulate the essence of nursing science.

In Norris's (1982) review of the history of concept clarification, it was apparent that very few researchers actually attempted an empirical approach to concept clarification. Norris believed that the only way to build nursing knowledge was by a systematic empirical process that should be applied without exception. Historically, the method of concept clarification used by nurses was focused on a review of the literature regarding a specific concept and then presented as a summary of that literature review. Norris concluded that the existing methods of concept clarification were inadequate and new methods were needed to produce operational definitions and conceptual models from which testable hypotheses could be devised. She proposed that (a) concepts explored generally in the past be studied to clarify their components and roles in specific situations; (b) current methodologies for concept clarification be refined and new methodologies be developed; and (c) nurses become familiar with various modes of synthesis. Attention to these three issues would expedite nursing research and, consequently, enhance the development of a body of knowledge for the profession.

Norris (1982) further believed that concept clarification without experimental research was ineffective because the method by itself could not fulfill the requirements of knowing. Similarly, she argued that "experimental research without concept clarification is meaningless" (p. 11). Consequently, Norris believed that concept clarification should culminate in an operational definition for use in further research. She advocated the development of a model of the concept that specified its components and the relationships among these components as a product of the inquiry. Such a model puts the concept into proper perspective with existing theories. Then, after the independent and dependent variables were identified, hypotheses could be derived that could be tested empirically. Based on these beliefs, Norris developed the following method of concept clarification.

NORRIS'S METHOD OF CONCEPT CLARIFICATION

Nursing theory can be developed inductively, deductively, or through a combination of the two forms of inquiry. Norris (1982) stated that the inductive approach to theory development was based on empirical evidence and from clinical practice. She further stated that the inductive collection of data from practice identified behavioral phenomena that relate to human health, illness, and comfort, phenomena with which nurses were confronted in their interactions with clients. Using the inductive approach, a nursing phenomenon would be observed and analyzed. From the analysis, concepts could be constructed that explained the observed phenomenon. Models would be derived that would help to further explain the observed phenomenon.

The goal of Norris's (1982) method is to collect empirical data and analyze it in ways that increasingly build to higher levels of abstraction. As a result, theories of human behavior in health and illness could be constructed. Ultimately, nurses could understand, predict, and control phenomena. Inductive inference should begin with a specific case and move toward generalities until an inductively derived model would fit into one or more of the deductively constructed theories. In her discussion of concept clarification, Norris never discussed how her method could be used to develop nursing theory deductively or through a combination of the two forms of inquiry.

There are five steps in Norris's (1982) method of concept clarification:

1. After identifying the concept of interest, observe and describe the phenomena repeatedly and, if possible, describe the phenomena from the point of view of other disciplines.
2. Systematize the observations and descriptions.
3. Derive an operational definition of the concept under study.
4. Produce a model of the concept that includes all its component parts.
5. Formulate hypotheses.

The following is a description and discussion of each of the five steps of Norris's method of concept clarification.

Observing and Describing Phenomena

The purpose of the first step is to "describe, explain and give meaning to human behavior" (Norris, 1982, p. 16). This step begins with identification of the concept or phenomenon of interest. When the researcher has determined this focus of the inquiry, he or she then identifies and observes the phenomenon in a variety of clinical settings and describes, in detail, the sequence and context of events and the antecedents and consequences involved in the phenomenon. This description can either be written or tape-recorded for later transcription.

In this step, the researcher also tries to identify examples of the phenomenon as it occurs in other disciplines. After speculating in what other disciplines the phenomenon might occur, the researcher consults representatives of those disciplines to determine if they have observed the phenomenon. For example, if the nurse researcher is studying the concept of abandonment, he or she may wish to consult with individuals in a department of social work. Social workers would be asked if they have seen the occurrence of this phenomenon and, if so, to give as complete a description as possible. This process enables the researcher to describe the phenomenon as completely as possible from a variety of perspectives. The researcher then records those varied descriptions of the phenomenon. After observing the phenomenon in as many situations and from as many relevant viewpoints as possible, the researcher conducts a thorough review of nursing and other literature to examine published reports and descriptions of the occurrence of the phenomenon. The researcher thinks carefully about and reflects on all the possible meanings, relationships, sequences or orders, and causes and effects of the phenomenon in preparation for the second step, systematizing the observations.

Systematizing the Observations

After the researcher has pondered all the possible meanings, relationships, sequences, and causes and effects of the phenomenon, he or she begins to systematize the observations and descriptions. Norris (1982) defined systematization as "establishing categories, continua, hierarchies, and the like" (p. 16). She also stated that systematization activities include "observing, discovering, commonsense thinking, engaging in logical deduction and induction, searching for meaning, developing insights, testing out ways to organize, and speculating about types of relationships" (p. 19) that would help to further describe the concept under study. In this step the researcher is also looking for a sequence of events and for relationships to other events in the environment. Systematizing the observations involves classifying various aspects, components, or elements of the concept based on similarities and differences The categories usually are based on properties of the concept, such as size, width, mass, bulk, color, capacity, location, temperature, time, frequency, duration, type, form, intensity, seriousness, and context in which the concept under study occurs. Categories are more valuable to researchers because they provide more information by indicating possible associational relationships. The following are some of the questions that might be asked during this step: In what type of situation did this phenomenon occur? What events triggered the phenomenon? Are there events that were triggered by the phenomenon itself? Are there certain patterns, categories, or a process that evolve as the phenomenon occurs? What happened as a result of the occurrence of this phenomenon? Upon completion of this step, the researcher should have an understanding of the scope and depth of the concept under study.

Developing an Operational Definition

In the third step, an operational definition of the concept is formulated. Norris (1982) stated that an operational definition answers at least one question, "How will I know the concept when (in the broadest sense) I see it in operation?" (p. 16). Other views concerning operational definitions emphasize *measurement,* however. Chinn and Kramer (1991), for example, indicated specifically that an operational definition explicates ways to "measure" the behaviors observed in a phenomenon (p. 99). Similarly, Walker and Avant (1988) pointed out that an operational definition is the "means by which we can classify a phenomenon as an example of the concept . . . and . . . a means by which to measure the concept in question" (p. 138). Also emphasizing measurement, Waltz, Strickland, and Lenz (1991) indicated that "an operational definition provides meaning by defining a concept in terms of the observations and/or activities that measure it" (p. 34). The emphasis on measurement in operationalizing a concept is a significant outcome of concept clarification because it provides a basis for future research through the quantification of variables.

In her own study of nausea and vomiting, Norris (1982) identified three distinct stages of nausea and, consequently, created three operational definitions of the concept. Because she thought that there were no observable indicators of nausea in its early stage and that the experience was subjective, "early nausea" was operationally defined in regard to the verbal statements of individuals. Statements included the clients' expressed sensations:

- queasiness, uneasiness over the area of stomach, esophagus, and pharynx associated with the subject naming it "nausea"
- verbal statement by subject of heaviness, pressure, or sinking feeling over area of stomach or sternum associated with the subject naming it "nausea"
- verbal statement by subject of inclination to vomit (p. 99)

A second operational definition was proposed for the "late phase" of nausea (Norris, 1982). This definition combined signs and symptoms with the parasympathetic stimulation and indicated all of the manifestations of early nausea. In addition, the late phase of nausea also included:

- vasomotor changes, that is, diaphoresis, feeling of being hot or cold
- increased salivation (p. 101)

The last definition of nausea included:

- forced inspiration
- retching, that is, labored, rhythmic respiratory activity

- rhythmic contraction of abdominal muscles
- vomiting posture, that is, head and neck extended, mouth open (p. 101)

Finally, an operational definition of vomiting was provided:

- liquid and/or semisolid matter that represents the stomach contents is ejected through the mouth
- simultaneously with this ejection, the diaphragm and abdominal muscles contract in unison (p. 103)

Nevertheless, as Norris (1982) noted, the formulation of operational definitions may be difficult because of the imprecise use of terms, lack of clarification of nursing phenomena, and the lack of discriminatory skills needed to identify relevant aspects of the concept of interest. Norris did not provide any insights as to how to rectify this issue.

Constructing a Model

The fourth step is the construction of a model. The model gives meaning to the data by increasing the generalization about the concept and distinguishing the relationships among the various kinds of categories in some communicable way. Norris identified two functions of the model. First, it enables the researcher to reexamine the previously defined categories, continua, hierarchies, and so forth, that were developed in step 2 in order to move the concrete data to a higher level of abstraction or to increase the generalization of the data. The model also facilitates the recognition of relationships among the previously established categories of data (Norris, 1982). Although higher levels of abstraction require causal relationships, other types of relationships can be determined at this time, including independence-dependence, concomitance, concurrence, sequence, temporal rate of relationships, and outcomes.

Models generally are not precise but serve as a medium to convey the phenomenon to others. Models are not the "real thing" but are depictions of the concepts or phenomena that they represent. Models can be constructed in many forms, including the use of mathematical symbols or physical materials, such as a model of human anatomy. In some instances, a combination of forms may be used to construct the model (Chinn & Kramer, 1991). Often, the more abstract the phenomenon, the more difficult it is to develop a model.

Developing Hypotheses

The last step of concept clarification according to Norris (1982) is hypothesis formation. A hypothesis is a statement that predicts a relationship between two or more variables and is derived directly from the model. Hypotheses are formed by the questions that the model creates, the inconsistencies observed, and the inadequacies or "holes" in the schematic representation. The researcher does an in-depth analysis of the relationships within the model to determine which ones, if any, are already supported by empirical research and which of the relationships need further study. Hypotheses based on these relationships and observations can then be tested using experimental research methods. Norris (1982) stressed that the "role of research is paramount in confirming or refuting whether categories assigned and whether causal, coexistence, or sequential relationships exist" (p. 35).

AN EXAMPLE OF CONCEPT CLARIFICATION USING NORRIS'S METHOD

While a graduate student in 1989, Marilyn Stockdale wanted to learn more about Norris's method of concept clarification and to be a part of a research program. Because Norris's research program revolved around identifying the needs of various groups of clinical patients, Stockdale used this method to clarify the concept *human needs.* Nurses in all clinical areas deal with human needs, and this concept is fundamental to the nature and scope of nursing. Yet this concept had not been clarified for use in the profession. What is a human need? How does one distinguish between the individual concepts of need, problem, goal, want, wish, or desire? Are there levels of human needs and, if so, which levels should nurses be dealing with? The following describes the process used by Stockdale (1989) and her findings.

Step 1: Observing and Describing the Phenomenon

The first step is to observe and describe the phenomenon repeatedly and if possible describe it as it occurs in other disciplines (Norris, 1982). Stockdale had observed patients in her clinical practice with various needs that she classified as "human needs," and she described in detail several of these situations. She also knew that this phenomenon existed in other disciplines. Instead of approaching individuals in these varied disciplines and asking them to describe the phenomenon, she conducted an integrative review of the literature. A cursory review of the literature indicated that the concept occurred and had been the focus of literature in nursing and many other disciplines over the years but that there had not been any agreement on a specific taxonomy or classification or on an operational definition of the concept.

Stockdale (1989) made the following assumptions about the concept of human needs:

- All human beings have needs.
- Humans experience needs which have subjective meaning and importance.
- Needs change and have varying degrees of urgency and strength.
- Needs are not always recognized or acknowledged by the individual.
- Significant deprivation of needs will result in physiological and/or psychosocial harm.
- Nursing intervention has the potential to improve the well being of the human condition.
- Need theory is applicable to all aspects of nursing practice. (p. 7)

Stockdale (1989) also found writings from several disciplines that addressed the concept of human needs. As Lederer (1980) noted, the fields of psychology, sociology, philosophy, biology, anthropology, economics, as well as other disciplines, all have contributed to the study of human needs. Similarly, Stockdale found the range of theoretical approaches to the concept of human needs to be very diverse. She found that *need* and *problem* were two different concepts but that they were frequently used interchangeably in the literature. Stockdale cited Block (1974) as stating that because these concepts are used in the nursing process and because many states use these two terms in their nurse practice acts, it was important for nurses to agree on their meanings and use the concepts consistently.

In her review of literature, Stockdale reported that there were four established theories of needs. The earliest of these was proposed by Murray (1938), who postulated that human behavior is attributed to the force of need from within as:

> a construct (a convenient fiction or hypothetical concept) which stands for a force (the physio-chemical nature of which is known) in the brain region, a force which organizes perception, apperception, intellection, connotation, and action in such a way as to transform in a certain direction an existing unsatisfying situation. (pp. 123–124)

Murray thought the concept of need was closely related to the concept of drive, and subsequently identified two types of needs. Primary or viscerogenic needs were described as basic in nature and included needs for air, water, food, sex, lactation, urination, defecation, harm-avoidance, heat-avoidance, cold-avoidance, and sentience. Secondary needs were described as dependent on primary needs and included common reaction systems and wishes, such as nurturance.

Maslow's (1954) theory of the hierarchy of needs is perhaps one of the best known of all the need theories. Maslow's theory of motivation included a five-level hierarchical structure of basic needs that included physiological needs as the most fundamental, followed by safety, belongingness and love, esteem, and self-actualization. The gratification of each stage of needs submerged it and allowed the next higher set of needs to emerge. Unsatisfied physiological needs dominate an individual, whereas higher levels of needs are less imperative for survival and produce more desirable subjective results within the human being.

A theory of existence, relatedness, and growth needs was developed by Alderfer (1972). Alderfer thought there was no reason to distinguish among the concepts of *desire*, *satisfaction*, and *need* and defined *need* as "a concept subsuming both desires and satisfactions (frustrations)" (p. 8). In his theory, existence needs were a person's requirement for the exchange of material and energy to reach and maintain equilibrium with regard to material substances. Relatedness needs acknowledged that a person must engage in an interaction with the environment. Growth needs originated from the tendency of open systems to increase in internal order and differentiation over time as a result of interacting with the environment.

The last theory of needs reviewed by Stockdale was a nursing human need theory developed by Yura and Walsh (1988). These authors applied the concept of human needs to the nursing process and subsequently constructed a theory for use with what they proposed to be basic concepts in nursing: person, family, and community. In their theory, 35 human needs were identified and categorized into survival, closeness, or freedom needs. Human need was defined as a fulfillment of a state in which a person experiences satisfaction of the need with the approximate or target satisfier in an amount sufficient to create a wellness state for the person.

Several other works that specifically addressed the concept of need were discovered by Stockdale as well. Etionzini (1984), for example, suggested there is a universal set of human needs that have attributes of their own and that are not determined by social structure, cultural patterns, or socialization processes. He differentiated between those needs that were shared with the animal kingdom and those that he thought were uniquely human such as affection and recognition. Montagu (1951), however, viewed humans as animals that must breathe, eat, drink, excrete, sleep, maintain adequate health, and procreate. Basic needs were defined by Montagu as "any urge or need with which must be satisfied if the organism or the group is to survive" (p. 51). However, Montagu also pointed out that humans have other needs, such as emotions or biological urges, that are not necessary for physical survival but that must be satisfied if the person is to develop and maintain adequate mental health. According to Stockdale (1989), the needs identified by Montagu dealt with acquired needs that grow out of the person's relation to derived or socially emergent needs. Although these needs are not necessary for survival, they are necessary for maintaining mental health. Galtung (1980) similarly defined needs as "a necessary condition, as something that has to be satisfied at least to some extent in order for the need-subject to function as a human being" (p. 3). Nevertheless, this author categorized needs into four broad categories: security, welfare, identity, and freedom.

In nursing, the works of Peplau (1952) and Roy and Andrus (1996) were found to have made a substantial contribution to the understanding of human needs (Stockdale, 1989). Peplau (1952), a nurse theorist, developed a framework for psychodynamic nursing based on the psychology of personality. Peplau saw nurses as helpers who assisted clientele to meet their needs by providing certain specific conditions. For example, Peplau identified primary needs such as food, drink, rest, and sleep and also noted that secondary needs existed, including human needs for prestige, power, or participation with others. She believed that individuals alone know what their needs are, yet they may not be able to recognize or articulate them.

Roy and Andrus (1996) defined need as a "requirement within the individual which stimulates a response to maintain integrity" (p. 22). Stockdale listed the needs that Roy identified as the basis for physiological integrity. These were exercise and rest, nutrition, elimination, fluid and electrolytes, oxygen, circulation and regulation, temperature, the senses, and the endocrine system. According to Stockdale (1989), Roy and Andrus stated that as internal and external environments change, so does the degree of satiety.

Norris (1982) stated that in this first step the phenomenon under study should not be observed and described only from nursing's point of view but that it should be studied from the viewpoints of various disciplines. Stockdale, realizing that the concept of *human needs* was a pertinent concept for many disciplines, decided to do an extensive review of the literature to determine how the concept was described in other disciplines. This adaptation of Norris's method is very useful, appropriate, and economical of time for highly abstract concepts that are widely used in other disciplines, especially if there have been attempts by individuals in other disciplines to clarify the particular concept.

Step 2: Systematization and Description

The second step in Norris's (1982) method, systematizing the observations and descriptions, is a cognitive process, thus difficult to demonstrate on paper. It involves rereading both the descriptions of the phenomenon given by workers in various clinical settings and the selected literature several times. As the researcher becomes immersed in the descriptions and literature, he or she begins to see patterns, categories, or hierarchies emerge. As the researcher looks for the categories, a definition tends to form.

As Stockdale carried out this step, she was able to identify two categories of needs: universal, or basic human needs, and needs that are unique to the individual. It was during this step of clarification that Stockdale identified a pattern: The fulfillment of needs is a process that is in continuous operation within the individual. As she continued with Norris's method of concept clarification, she developed further insights regarding the concept and repeatedly returned to this step, reexamining her categories, and refining the derived patterns. During this process, Stockdale realized that the steps were not mutually exclusive but often needed to be carried on concurrently.

Step 3: Operational Definition

According to Norris (1982), "the goal of concept clarification was to derive an operational definition" (p. 16). Because of the imprecision in the use of terms, lack of clarification of the phenomenon, and lack of discriminatory skills, it may be difficult for the researcher to construct an operational definition. Stockdale (1989) found this to be true as she reviewed the vast amount of literature about the concept of human needs. She did not find an operational definition of the concept in the literature review. Stockdale proposed the following definition of human needs applicable to nurses for clinical practice:

> Human need is defined as a process of regulating survival, closeness, and freedom requirements. These may be partially fulfilled by the individual or a provider to prevent disequilibrium which is manifested in illness or maladjustment states. The extent that significant needs are restored is dependent on available resources and functional ability of the individual or society to receive the appropriate intervention. Satisfaction of human needs is based on subjective evaluation by the individual. (p. 43)

Forming an operational definition is a cognitive process. This definition was formed based on the results of step 2, systematization and description. The categories and patterns derived were reviewed, and statements were formed that began to link these together. The definition was rewritten several times until the researcher thought it reflected the categories, patterns, and hierarchies derived from the observations made and the review of the literature.

Step 4: Model

The fourth step in Norris's (1982) method is the production of a model. As previously stated, models help give meaning to the data by increasing the generalization about the concept and distinguishing the relationships among the categories, patterns, and hierarchies that have been derived. A well-constructed model should enhance communication of the results of concept clarification. Stockdale (1989) proposed a model that depicted the impact that nursing has on meeting the needs of individuals within society. In Stockdale's model of human needs, nursing is seen as a force that diagnoses and treats human needs. In Figure 11-1, nursing is encased within a rectangle and the bold arrow depicts the force. The human being is seen as complex and holistic and is represented by the large circle at the center of this figure. Central to the internal structure of the human being are human needs. The pyramidal shape, outlined by arrows, illustrates the changing priority and urgency of the needs. These needs are interrelated with changing survival, closeness, and freedom needs. Stockdale further explained that external to a human are forces within society that also change and affect human needs. These forces are represented by a series of interrupted arrows surrounding the circle designated as man. The long

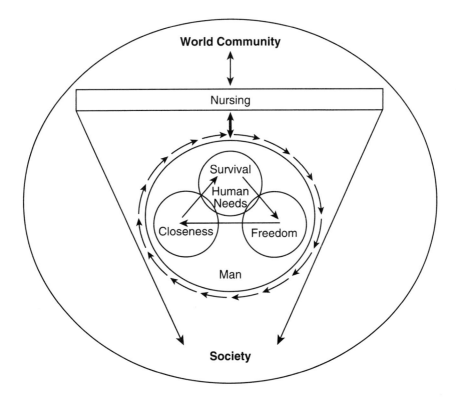

Figure 11–1   Stockdale's proposed model of human needs.

Reprinted with permission from Stockdale, M. (1989). *Human needs: Toward theory, conceptual clarification, and application to nursing.* Unpublished master's project, University of Kansas, Kansas City, Mo., p. 45.

arrows on the sides, showing a connection between the box labeled nursing and society, represent the direct impact nursing has on society through its relationships with people. The outermost oval shape represents the world community; the bidirectional arrow between nursing and this world community reflects the global orientation of nursing in its interaction with people, an interaction that ultimately reaches the whole community of human beings.

Step 5: Hypothesis Formation

Norris (1982) stated that "testing the hypothesis moves the work into the experimental mode, where conclusions are stated with more certainty—that is, one learns whether the hypothesis was or was not supported by the results" (p. 18). Hypotheses are derived from the operational definition and the model. Following are some of the hypotheses that could be developed based on Stockdale's (1989) operational definition and model: the diagnosis of cancer does not change the number of human needs that an individual has; the extent to which some of the significant needs of patients with cancer can be met is dependent on their knowledge of available resources; the greater the decrease in functional ability of the patient with cancer, the greater the survival needs; closeness needs of patients with cancer who attend a cancer support group are not as great as those of patients who do not attend a cancer support group; and patients with cancer who are scheduled to see a clinical nurse specialist each time they come for their clinic appointments have more of their needs met than do those patients with cancer who do not see a clinical nurse specialist every time they come for their clinic appointments.

After the hypotheses are derived from the operational definition or model, they are subjected to empirical testing. Such testing will either accept or reject the hypotheses. The operational definition and model derived from the process of concept clarification can then be revised to reflect the outcomes of such testing and, then, more hypotheses can be developed for empirical testing. This process continues until the researcher is satisfied that the operational definition and model really do describe the phenomenon under study.

SUMMARY

Norris (1982) has stated:

> In that nursing seeks to describe, clarify, predict, and control certain aspects of the world in which nurses work, it can be classified as an empirical, rather than a nonempirical, science. All advances in science require clarifying and relating the basic ideas involved. Specifically, advances in nursing science require clarifying the basic ideas in nursing

and relating them to nursing's unique purposes, perspective, and universe of discourse (p. 12).

In this chapter, Norris's five steps of concept clarification—(1) observing and describing phenomena, (2) systematizing and description, (3) developing an operational definition, (4) constructing a model, and (5) developing hypotheses—have been defined and described. An example using this method has been presented.

There are some strengths and weaknesses inherent in Norris's method. One of the strengths of her method is that it is described in five succinct steps. However, while using her method to clarify a very abstract concept, this author frequently wanted more detail as to how one carried out some of the steps. For example, exactly how is an operational definition constructed from the systematization of the observations and descriptions identified in step 2? Her description of the five steps gives the reader the impression that each step is completed before the next is begun. In actuality, as the investigator goes through the process, he or she finds that the tentative conclusions developed in a step need to be substantiated by the previous step. For example, while trying to derive categories of needs in step 2, Stockdale (1989) had to return to step 1 and reexamine certain relationships and even review her original observations and literature. She repeated this process several times before she was able to complete step 2. This author found the method difficult to use while trying to clarify more abstract phenomena and believes that it can be used more effectively with those phenomena that are more observable (Chinn & Kramer, 1991), such as hemoglobin or nausea and vomiting.

I believe that Norris's (1982) method of concept clarification is relevant and can be used by nurse researchers to define and describe those phenomena that are an important part of nursing's diverse practice. When this occurs, gaps in nursing's scientific body of knowledge will be eliminated.

REFERENCES

Alderfer, C. P. (1972). *Existence, relatedness, and growth: Human needs in organizational settings.* New York: Free Press.
Block, D. (1974). Some crucial terms in nursing: What do they really mean? *Nursing Outlook, 22*, 689-694.
Chinn, P. L., & Kramer, M. K (1991). *Theory and nursing. A systematic approach* (4th ed.). St. Louis: Mosby-Year Book.
Etionzini, A. (1984). Basic human needs, alienation, and inauthenticity. *American Sociological Review, 49*, 870-884.
Galtung, J. (1980). The basic needs approach. In K. Lederer (Ed.), *Human needs* (pp. 55-125). Cambridge, MA: Oelgeschlager, Gunn, & Hain.
Lederer, K. (Ed.). (1980). *Human needs.* Cambridge, MA: Oelgeschlager, Gunn, & Hain.

Lindsey, A. M. (1991). Integrating research and practice. In M. A. Mateo & K. T. Kirchoff (Eds.), *Conducting and using nursing research in the clinical setting* (pp. 93–107). Baltimore: Williams & Wilkins.

Maslow, A. H. (1954). *Motivation and personality.* New York: Harper & Brothers.

Montagu, A. (1951). *On being human.* New York: Henry Schuman.

Murray, H. A. (1938). *Explorations in personality.* New York: Oxford University Press.

Norris, C. M. (1982). *Concept clarification in nursing.* Rockville, MD: Aspen.

Peplau, H. (1952). *Interpersonal relations in nursing. A conceptual framework of reference for psychodynamic nursing.* New York: Putnam.

Roy, S. C., & Andrus, H. (1996). *Introduction to nursing. An adaptation model* (2nd ed.). Norwalk, CT: Appleton & Lange.

Stockdale, M. (1989). *Human needs. Toward theory, conceptual clarification, and application to nursing.* Unpublished masters project, University of Kansas, Kansas City, MO.

Walker, L. O., & Avant, K. C. (1988). *Strategies for theory construction in nursing.* Norwich, CT: Appleton & Lange.

Waltz, C. F., Strickland, O. L., & Lenz, E. R. (1991). *Measurement in nursing research.* Philadelphia: Davis.

Yura, H., & Walsh, M. B. (1988). *The nursing process: Assessing, planning, implementing, evaluating.* Norwalk, CT: Appleton & Lange.

Simultaneous Concept Analysis: A Strategy for Developing Multiple Interrelated Concepts

Joan E. Haase, Nancy Kline Leidy,
Doris D. Coward, Teresa Britt, and
Patricia E. Penn

Systematic concept clarification and differentiation are critical to the advancement of knowledge and the development of scientific disciplines. The clear delineation of concepts is prerequisite to the evolution of theory, the development of measurement techniques, and the generation and testing of hypotheses. It is also necessary for clear, precise communication among members of the discipline.

Unfortunately, many concepts of concern to nurses are difficult to define and operationalize. Compounding these problems are issues of multidimensionality within single concepts and interrelatedness among multiple concepts. As a result, there are troublesome overlaps in definition and meaning, difficulties distinguishing between concepts, and, frequently, the inconsistent and inappropriate use of terminology. Coherent language, a uniform system of symbols that enables people to communicate intelligibly with one another, is critical to the development of any discipline. Thus, problems in terminology and concept clarification are obstacles to the development of the profession and science of nursing. Methods must be developed for the articulation of nursing concepts, removing as much ambiguity as possible and enabling clear communication among theorists, scientists, practitioners, and clients.

The purpose of this chapter is to describe a strategy of simultaneous concept analysis (SCA) designed to extend the clarification process originally proposed by Wilson (1969) and introduced to nursing by Walker and Avant (1988). The strategy employs consensus group process and validity matrices to develop multiple interrelated concepts simultaneously. The purpose of SCA is to achieve clearer conceptual definitions, greater understanding of the meaning of individual concepts and the processes that may underlie their antecedents and outcomes, and insight into the interrelationships that exist among phenomena.

THOUGHTS ON INDEPENDENT CONCEPT ANALYSIS

Strategies have been developed for the systematic analysis of independent concepts. Wilson (1969) provided much of the groundwork for Walker and Avant's (1988) discussion of concept analysis for the construction of nursing theory. Their procedure includes such useful steps as determining the defining attributes of a selected concept, identifying antecedents and consequences, and defining empirical referents, among others. The limiting factor in this process, however, is its failure to suggest a method for considering, simultaneously, other similar or related concepts.

For example, in an analysis of the concept of spirituality, such as that proposed by Burkhardt (1989), questions are raised as to the extent to which defining attributes and outcomes of spirituality are adequately defined, in and of themselves. Burkhardt's description of harmonious interconnectedness as a defining characteristic is compelling, and intuitively meaningful for nursing. It is a critical component of her concept of spirituality, assuming roles as both a descriptive characteristic and a consequence. However, harmonious interconnectedness remains undeveloped in a single concept analysis. By analyzing this concept simultaneously with spirituality, a greater understanding of the characteristics of the concept as well as the interrelationships of the processes of spirituality and harmonious interconnectedness can be attained.

The linkages between relevant concepts are as important to nursing as the static definitions of the concepts themselves. Is it not the dynamic, ever changing nature of human beings that is the focus of nursing intervention? Individual concept analysis is an excellent initiation into the identification and clarification of concepts relevant to nursing. However, additional strategies are needed to capture the breadth of individual concepts, to clarify the interrelationships with other concepts, and to begin to tap the dynamic nature of the processes that underlie nursing-relevant phenomena.

SIMULTANEOUS CONCEPT ANALYSIS

Through the strategy of SCA, concepts relevant to nursing can be more fully developed. In SCA, individual analyses of two or more concepts are accompanied by a critical examination of interrelated antecedents, defining characteristics, and outcomes. This examination leads to the development of definitions that are, by design, unique for each concept. At the same time, interrelationships and distinguishing elements across the concepts' antecedents, critical attributes, and outcomes are highlighted. The goal of this strategy is to gain insight into the potential sources of theoretical, empirical, and practical confusion among concepts, as well as offer greater understanding of the processes that might underlie each phenomenon.

In the remainder of this chapter, the procedures, peculiarities, and precautions of SCA are described. Examples from the authors' experiences in developing and using this strategy will be employed. Specifically, the simultaneous analysis of the following four concepts will be discussed: spiritual perspective, hope, acceptance, and self-transcendence. A more detailed description of these concepts and the results of the SCA have been reported elsewhere (Haase et al, 1992).

The SCA Strategy

Development of the SCA strategy was a group project that evolved over time. The following steps, perhaps more aptly called "sequence of events," became clear in retrospect. Because the evolution of ideas and group processes cannot be condensed to simple steps or a cookbook recipe, these steps are presented as guidelines to be used iteratively and flexibly. Readers may find them most useful when adjusted to the level, goals, and personality of the group involved. In general the steps used in SCA are as follows:

1. Development of the consensus group.
2. Selection of concepts to be analyzed.
3. Refinement of the concept clarification approach.
4. Clarification of individual concepts.
5. Development of validity matrices.
6. Revision of individual concept clarification.
7. Reexamination of validity matrices.
8. Development of a process model.
9. Submission of the SCA results to peers for critique.

Each of these steps will be discussed below. For clarification, we have included descriptions of some of our experiences with the development and use of the SCA strategy.

Development of the Consensus Group

The initial step in SCA is the formation of a consensus group, a set of individuals who are not only interested in several interrelated concepts but also capable of working independently and as a group, and who are able to continue working together for an extended period of time to achieve the desired outcome. Perhaps the greatest advantage of using a consensus group process in SCA is the diversity of perspectives contributing to the final product. Each individual brings certain expertise to the group—a familiarity with use of the concept, knowledge of relevant literature, and representations of the concept in clinical practice. As will be discussed below, each individual uses this expertise to clarify a single concept, bringing ideas back to the group for discussion. Then, group members contribute their own perspectives and expertise to yield a product that reflects a consensus.

Individual expertise, together with a willingness to compromise and contribute, forms the foundation of the group. It is also helpful, although perhaps not necessary, to include a member who is interested in all concepts and the nature of their interrelationships, but is not necessarily committed to or invested in any single concept. This individual can serve as a group moderator, an unbiased participant who attempts to see both forest and trees and facilitates the group's journey along the most productive path.

A healthy alliance of qualitative and quantitative orientations within the group seems to broaden perspective and promote creativity. Members with expertise in qualitative research guide the group toward meaning by encouraging depth, offering case studies, and considering philosophical implications. Complementing this orientation, the quantitatively focused members encourage the group to consider concrete issues, questioning the implications of SCA findings for operationalizing and testing relationships among concepts. Myers and Haase (1989) refer to this approach as seeking maximally conflicting points of view with provision for systematic confrontation by individuals who recognize that both approaches are equally valuable and vulnerable. A pleasant outcome is the understanding group members derive from understanding of the two perspectives, and the tendency to integrate this understanding into individual theory development and research practices.

In our experience with SCA, several factors motivated the formation of a group to study the four concepts of spirituality, hope, acceptance, and self-transcendence. First, overlapping research interests led to frequent informal discussion on the definitions and meanings of various concepts we felt were important to nursing, yet elusive to empirical understanding. Similarly, we were all experiencing difficulty identifying and/or developing adequate measures for these complex, multidimensional concepts and generating adequately refined hypotheses for our individual foci. Finally, we each felt that methods to operationalize these concepts for nursing must be devised. In order to develop these methods, however, clear and accurate theoretical descriptions of the concepts had to be developed.

We began meeting on a biweekly basis to help one another develop individual concept analyses and compare and contrast the results. The group met regularly for over one year, with the membership remaining unchanged throughout this period. The products of those meetings were refined definitions for each concept, identification of the specific elements of each concept and their sequence of occurrence, clarification of interrelationships, and development of the SCA strategy. With communication ability improved with the Internet, we have found a continuing dialogue possible, even as we have moved on to other positions and places.

Selection of Concepts To Be Analyzed

The second step in simultaneous concept analysis is to select the concepts to be analyzed. In reality, Steps 1 and 2 are interrelated. Group formation arises out of common interests, and those interests drive concept selection. What must be realized, however, is the extent to which interests can vary, and be spirited on by group discussion and mutual intrigue.

To this point, we have presented the examples of spiritual perspective, hope, acceptance, and self-transcendence as though they were easily and decisively chosen. In reality, they represent four of many concepts we discussed, including courage, self-actualization, resilience, spirituality, and other, similar concepts that lie at the heart of our common research interests: health and adaptation in chronic illness. Through discussion and group consensus, the four concepts were chosen to best represent the most important, interrelated, and elusive of our research interest areas. With time, it was discovered that some of the other concepts of interest seemed to be subsumed in these four. (Whether this "discovery" reflected a bias of the group members inadvertently introduced into the SCA, and therefore represents a limitation of the method, is an interesting discussion question.)

Subsequent to completing the process, several of us have continued to focus on our selected concepts. However, we have also used the results to further explore related concepts. For example, Haase and Leidy (1996) have further explored the concept of connectedness within the context of chronic illness.

Refinement of the Concept Clarification

After selecting the concepts to be analyzed, the next step in SCA is to determine the specific concept clarification techniques to be used.

Factors to be considered include the extent to which (1) group members are familiar with specific techniques; (2) one technique is expressly preferred over another; (3) certain techniques are believed to be most effective in a group setting, or most effectively modified to meet group needs; and (4) efficiency is a priority inasmuch as group process can be more protracted than independent work and, in some cases, certain deadlines (manuscripts, grants, and graduation, for example) must be met.

The group must reach consensus and a sound understanding of the technique and terminology to be employed in the individual concept clarification process (Step 4). It may, in fact, take several sessions to reach this understanding. However, it is imperative that each group member understand and use the same approach in order to permit later cross-concept comparisons.

In our analyses, we primarily used Wilson's (1969) concept clarification method. Several group meetings were spent discussing the basics of the method so that each member had a good understanding of the meaning of antecedent, critical attribute, and outcome. As we became immersed in the process, we found the need to devote time during later sessions to reclarification and redefinition of the approach selected. We also made the decision that it would be more efficient and effective to conduct case identification (i.e., model, related and contrary cases as described by Wilson) informally during group discussion, rather than by the individual responsible for a given concept analysis. This permitted all group members to contribute examples of cases derived from clinical, research, and personal experiences during group discussion. It also proved to be one of the more insightful and interesting aspects of the discussions.

Clarification of Individual Concepts

The fourth step in simultaneous concept clarification is the clarification of individual concepts. Each concept is initially analyzed by the respective expert. Working independently, the expert drafts preliminary definitions, critical attributes, antecedents, and outcomes based on a thorough review of existing theoretical and empirical literature, clinical experience, empirical data, and, when appropriate and useful, lay literature. Individuals may also employ expert consultants to assist in concept clarification.

The written "drafts" are discussed and critiqued in a group setting. Group members attempt to apply the concept in the context of their own knowledge base and clinical experiences. Any missing or unnecessary elements and any discrepancies or disagreements about what elements should be included in the concept are discussed and debated. Based on group feedback, each draft is rewritten by the individual expert and discussed in subsequent group sessions until all group members feel the definitions, antecedents, critical attributes, and outcomes contain the critical and the essential elements. That is, this process continues until the group reaches consensus on each concept analysis.

In our own experience, it took several months to accomplish the individual analyses of the four concepts. Each meeting was devoted to one concept, considered as "le concept du jour." Adequate time (one to two hours) was necessary to allow the discussion to build momentum and decrease the time spent reviewing or "rehashing" previously addressed issues. We found that fewer meetings of longer duration, though more difficult to schedule, was the most effective and efficient strategy. Following the meeting, the draft was reworked independently by the respective expert, while the group rotated to another concept for the subsequent discussion.

In retrospect, it became apparent that we were becoming involved in a simultaneous concept analysis. In any given discussion, concepts were considered in light of the others. For example, while discussing self-transcendence as an outcome of hope, consideration was given to the critical attributes of self-transcendence discussed in an earlier meeting. Similarly, when energy was identified as a critical attribute of acceptance, consideration was given to this attribute in hope and spiritual perspective. This is a strength of SCA and the rationale behind using group process during the individual concept clarification step of this strategy.

During the individual clarification stage, we made several observations about group process that may be helpful to others using SCA or other similar approaches. First, challenges to assertions were done in respectful and valuing ways. Second, the individual doing the initial work on the concept was considered the expert. The group would push that person hard for clarification or justification of their work. We expected challenges to be met through specific theoretical writings, research, case examples, and/or other acceptable references.

Third, debate was not concluded until all group members felt the essence of the idea was complete and accurate based on the available theoretical, empirical, and experiential knowledge base. The massive amounts of information we were juggling forced us to deal with only essential elements. There were times, however, when the expert was heavily invested in the concept during this phase and the group had to work diligently to eliminate all but the essential elements. We often felt that, to achieve theoretical parsimony, some of the interesting and rich subtleties of a concept were necessarily put aside. In the interest of breadth, understanding, and a glimpse at the processes underlying multiple concepts simultaneously, individuals learned to let go of certain aspects of "their" concept, for the time being, and continue the analysis process.

Fourth, although several content experts were consulted about specific concepts during this phase of the process, consultants were not included in group discussion. Again in retrospect, limiting meetings to the work group contributed to its cohesiveness and enhanced group process. The use of consultants, however, strengthened the group's knowledge base and enhanced its image as scholarly, open, and task oriented.

Finally, all group members contributed to the background information necessary for individual concept analysis. Individuals shared their knowledge of the literature, philosophical bases, and clinical and/or personal experiences. Each source was considered legitimate and highly valued by the group. However, all sources of knowledge were critically evaluated before being accepted as valid.

Results of Individual Concept Clarification. The results for this step in the SCA strategy are, simply stated, definitions, critical attributes, antecedents, and outcomes with supporting references for each concept. Figure 12-1 displays the antecedents, critical attributes, and outcomes we identified for one of the concepts analyzed in our group, spiritual perspective. At this point, disregard the boxes, arrows, and bold print. The realization of these elements came much later in the SCA process.

For illustrative purposes, let us examine this concept in more detail. The few words in Figure 12-1 do not convey the depth of discussion that preceded this version of the concept analysis. For example, notice that spirituality is considered an antecedent. Although spirituality is the term most frequently found in the literature, and the term we were using at the beginning of the SCA process, group discussion yielded a

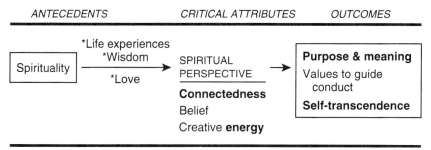

* Enablers
→ Indicates the direction of the process
Bold Indicates that the element occurs more than once

Figure 12-1 Process model for spiritual perspective.

consensus that spirituality was a basic or inherent quality of all humans. We concluded that the phenomenon that varies between individuals is spiritual perspective, a highly individualized awareness of one's spirituality and its qualities. Notice, too, that love, knowledge (understanding and wisdom), and life experiences have been placed between antecedents and critical attributes. It was the group's decision that these elements were not antecedents, per se, but rather potential enablers, each serving as an impetus for the development of spiritual perspective.

The following conceptual definitions were derived for each concept from the discussions leading to identification of the critical attributes: Spiritual Perspective—an integrating and creative energy based on belief in, and a feeling of interconnectedness with, a power greater than self; Hope—an energized mental state involving feelings of uneasiness or uncertainty and characterized by a cognitive, action-oriented expectation that a positive future goal or outcome is possible; Acceptance—a present-oriented activity requiring energy and characterized by receptivity toward and satisfaction with someone or something, including past circumstances, present situations, others, and ultimately, the self; Self-Transcendence—the experience of extending oneself inwardly in introspective activities, outwardly through concerns about the welfare of others, and temporally, such that the perceptions of one's past and anticipated future enhance the present (Reed, 1991). It is interesting to note that, after a great deal of discussion and analysis, the group adopted Reed's (1991) definition of self-transcendence, providing theoretical validation for her work with this concept. The results of the clarification of individual concepts, including antecedents, critical attributes, and outcomes, can be discerned by each concept horizontally across Figure 12-2. Again, do not pay too much attention to the arrows, boxes, and bold type yet.

Group Process Outcomes. Several group process outcomes also resulted from this phase. After several months of meeting, group members felt more comfortable implementing concept clarification techniques in a group setting. In addition, mutual understanding of the four concepts increased. That is, group members felt they had a basic understanding of the structure of all concepts and the theoretical and empirical work that had been done in the area. Eventually, we found that all members were so familiar with each concept that when one member questioned the "identified expert," a third member was able to provide case examples or literature references to answer the question.

Development of Validity Matrices

The next major step in simultaneous concept analysis is the identification of similarities and differences across concepts. In reality, Steps 4

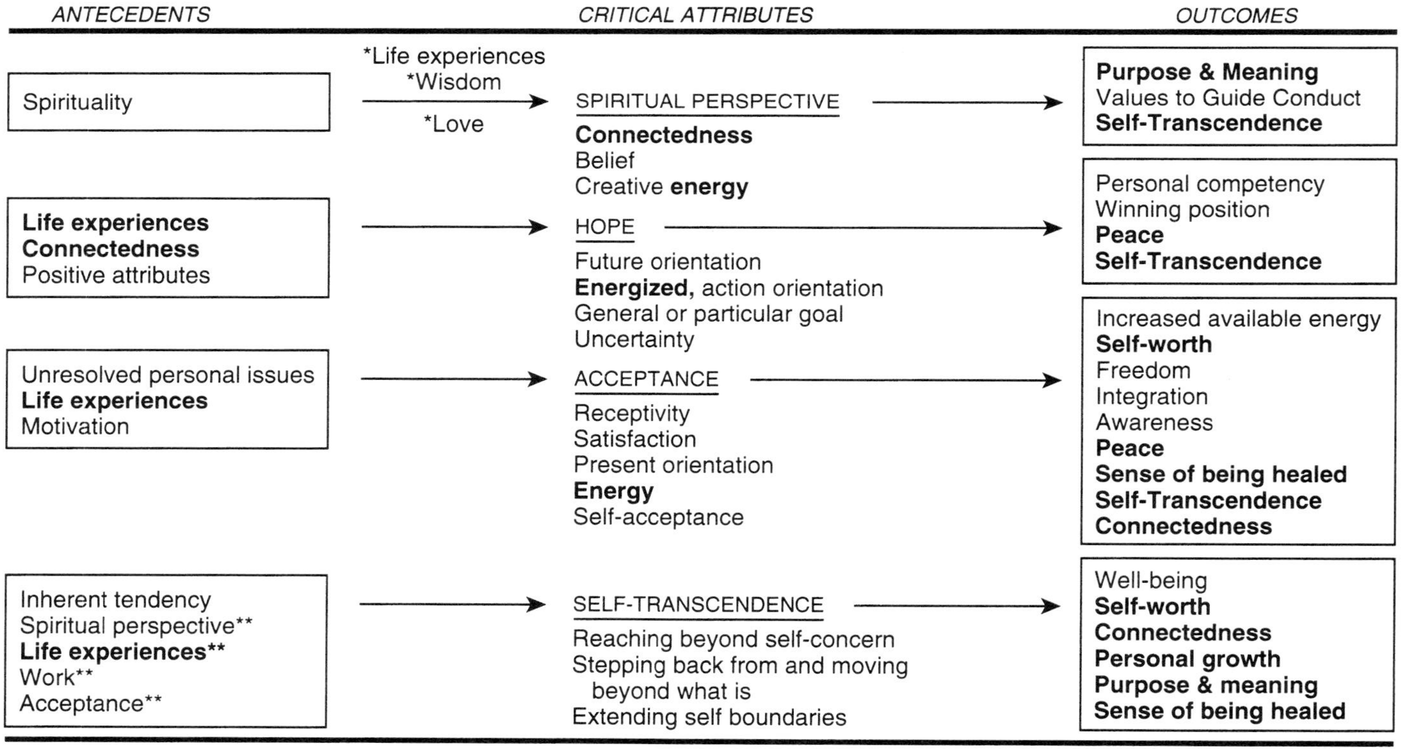

Figure 12–2 Four-concept process model.

ANTECEDENTS	CRITICAL ATTRIBUTES	OUTCOMES
Spirituality	SPIRITUAL PERSPECTIVE **Connectedness** Belief Creative **energy**	**Purpose & Meaning** Values to Guide Conduct **Self-Transcendence**
Life experiences **Connectedness** Positive attributes	HOPE Future orientation **Energized,** action orientation General or particular goal Uncertainty	Personal competency Winning position **Peace** **Self-Transcendence**
Unresolved personal issues **Life experiences** Motivation	ACCEPTANCE Receptivity Satisfaction Present orientation **Energy** Self-acceptance	Increased available energy **Self-worth** Freedom Integration Awareness **Peace** **Sense of being healed** **Self-Transcendence** **Connectedness**
Inherent tendency Spiritual perspective** **Life experiences**** Work** Acceptance**	SELF-TRANSCENDENCE Reaching beyond self-concern Stepping back from and moving beyond what is Extending self boundaries	Well-being **Self-worth** **Connectedness** **Personal growth** **Purpose & meaning** **Sense of being healed**

*Life experiences
*Wisdom
*Love

*   Enablers
**   Potential antecedents
↑   Indicates the direction of the process
Bold Indicates that the element occurs more than once

and 5 begin to intertwine with time. As individual concepts develop, comparing and contrasting should enter the discussion, as indicated earlier. This is an essential component of SCA, and is, in fact, one of its unique characteristics. Unlike individual concept analysis, where a concept can be developed in isolation, each concept in SCA is developed in light of all others. The comparing and contrasting process helps to refine definitions and clarify antecedents, outcomes, and critical attributes. As these elements are developed, however, a more formal means of cross-concept comparison is needed. We labeled this formal mechanism a *validity matrix*.

Description of Validity Matrices. To explore the interrelationships between concepts and achieve theoretical cogency, validity matrices are developed for antecedents, critical attributes, and outcomes. A validity matrix is a tool developed by the authors to identify and display commonalities across concepts; in factor analytic terms, the matrix is used to "extract common factors." An example of a validity matrix for critical attributes is given in Table 12-1. To develop the matrix, concept labels are placed along the horizontal axis and elements assigned to the concepts are listed below their respective labels. Elements that seem to be common across concepts are grouped together. These common elements are given a "common factor" label that is placed along the vertical axis of the matrix. This process is iterative until all the elements are identified within the context of a common factor. The formation of validity matrices forces the group to consider each element in light of all others, comparing and contrasting to identify inconsistencies and gaps and making revisions when appropriate.

In developing the validity matrix for critical attributes (see Table 12-1), five factors were identified that were common across the four

Table 12–1 Validity Matrix for Critical Attributes

Factor	Spiritual Perspective	Hope	Acceptance	Self-Transcendence
Time orientation	—	Future	Present	Across time
Energy	Creative	Action	Nonspecific	Derived
Feeling	Connectedness	Uncertainty	Satisfaction	—
Extrapersonal orientation	Belief Connectedness With others/ universe	Goal toward others	Receptivity to others	Reaching out
Intrapersonal orientation	Connectedness with self	Goal toward self	Receptivity to self	Extends self-boundaries inwardly

concepts: time orientation, energy, feeling, and extrapersonal and intrapersonal orientation. Interestingly, these "common factors" were also used as a means of differentiating the four concepts. For example, three of the concepts were found to be characterized by some form of time orientation, a commonality. However, the concepts could be differentiated from one another by the nature of this time orientation, i.e., future, present, or across time, respectively. Similarly, although energy was a common theme across all concepts, the four could be differentiated by the type of energy involved: creative, action, nonspecific, and derived from other sources (perhaps from hope or acceptance).

Although we found that some factors assisted us in identifying distinguishing characteristics across concepts, other factors helped us to identify commonalities, and potential sources of confusion across concepts. For example, in the validity matrix for outcomes, we found that all four concepts had either connectedness, purpose, and meaning, or self-transcendence as common outcome elements. There were no higher order factor labels for them. That is, we were unable to reduce these characteristics to a common denominator; they were irreducible and contributed in this manner to the meaning of each concept. In addition, self-transcendence was itself an outcome element of all other concepts. Thus, research exploring the outcomes of spiritual perspective, hope, and acceptance may reveal repeating themes that may be, and very likely are, characteristics of self-transcendence. (In the interest of available space, all validity matrices are not reproduced here. The reader is referred to Haase et al. [1992] for a more detailed presentation of these SCA findings.)

The validity matrix also allowed us to examine elements within concepts across factors. For example, in Table 12-1, the goal directed behavior that characterized hope "loaded" on two factors, extrapersonal and intrapersonal orientation. This highlights the proposition that hope-oriented goals can have different referents, either self or others, but not necessarily both.

Revision of Individual Concepts

The construction of validity matrices is designed to help the group critically evaluate the clarity of the identified antecedents, attributes, and outcomes, and the interrelationships and differences that exist across concepts. It is also intended to point out any glaring omissions or inconsistencies in the work accomplished to this point. Logically, the next step in the SCA process is to reexamine the previous concept clarifications and make any necessary revisions. Steps 5 and 6 are clearly interrelated and iterative processes.

For example, our original work on the concept of acceptance did not include receptivity as a critical attribute. When we constructed the matrix and initially found no element for acceptance that fit extra- or intrapersonal orientation, we began to question whether we had overlooked a critical attribute of acceptance. We identified receptivity to self and others as a critical attribute. Although receptivity seems an obvious component of acceptance now, it may not have been realized had it not been for the use of SCA and validity matrices.

Reexamination of Validity Matrices

Once again, the iterative nature of the SCA process is apparent. Group discussion, examination, and reexamination of the concept analyses and validity matrices are essential to the development of multiple concepts. Our experiences with the development of the validity matrix method and its subsequent use have led to several precautions: First, as indi- cated, there is a danger of trying to force-fit elements into a common factor. In re-examination and review it is imperative that the group avoid the temptation to overwork the concept, to the point that insignificant characteristics are included that contribute little to our understanding of the concepts or their underlying processes. In analyzing the four concepts discussed here, some commonalities among elements were relatively easy to identify and label. Others were more difficult to reconcile. Perhaps the best words of advice: "if it ain't broke, don't fix it"—change only that which really needs to be changed.

Second, careful consideration should be given to semantics and termi- nology. This is particularly important in exercises such as this, where language, i.e., communication, is the central issue. For example, in the validity matrix for outcomes we held lengthy discussions about the difference in meaning between the common factor label, serenity, and an outcome, peace. Through this discussion and a timely meeting with Kay Roberts concerning her qualitative studies of serenity (Roberts & Fitzgerald, 1991), we were able to come to some agreement.

Development of a Process Model

As the definitions, antecedents, outcomes, and attributes become more clearly delineated, the need for a process model evolves. A process model is a structure to further examine the consistency and pattern among concepts under analysis. In many respects it is a reflection of Kaplan's (1964) description of models as "devices by which a system can be shown to be consistent" (p. 267) and that offer "meaningful contexts within which specific findings can be located as significant details" (p. 268). It is a grand overview, a single image of the elements and processes of the concepts in juxtaposition. In one apparently complex but meaningful picture, the group is able to examine each concept, the similarities and differences across concepts, the interrela- tionships across both concepts and processes, and new concepts that appear in strategic locations throughout the model. A process model is not intended, in any way, to represent theory. Rather, it should be seen as an analytic tool and a predecessor of theory.

Figure 12–2 is a process model of the four concepts we analyzed using the SCA strategy. Examples of a few of the insights gained through this model are as follow. Note that spiritual perspective, characterized by connectedness, belief, and creative energy, was found to be an antecedent of self-transcendence. This implies that life experiences, wisdom, and love as enablers of spiritual perspective might contribute to self-transcendence indirectly, through their impact on the development of self-transcendence. Purpose and meaning are outcomes of spiritual perspective and self-transcendence, indicating there are several paths to the evolution of these two outcomes. Note, too, that life experiences are antecedents of all concepts. This is consistent with the notion that personal growth and the development of personal resources of spiritual perspective, hope, acceptance, and self-transcendence arise out of life experiences.

Another theme that became apparent through Figure 12–1 is the central role of intrapersonal characteristics for each of these concepts. That is, wisdom and love are enablers of spiritual perspective, positive attributes such as optimism are antecedents of hope, motivation is an antecedent of acceptance, and spiritual perspective and acceptance are antecedents of self-transcendence. Intrapersonal characteristics appear as critical attributes as well, and include, for example, connectedness with self, receptivity, and extended self boundaries. Many outcomes also reflected the intrapersonal characteristics theme, including such personal growth characteristics as the development of personal values, competency, self-worth, and well-being.

Finally, a very important "new" concept emerged as a central theme: connectedness. Connectedness with others is an antecedent of hope, a critical attribute of spiritual perspective, and a consequence of acceptance and self-transcendence. This suggests that the apparent theoretical overlap among the four concepts may also be due, in part, to a connectedness that crosses all four psychosocial phenomena. In some sense, this finding was not surprising, nor, of course, is the concept really new. Burkhardt's (1989) concept analysis proposed harmonious interconnectedness as the central characteristic of spirituality, and, intuitively, a sense of connectedness with others should be an important part of each of these concepts. Yet, the centrality of connectedness to all four concepts was made apparent to us through the SCA strategy. Furthermore, because the four concepts were selected because of their perceived importance to nursing, the implications of connectedness for the nursing profession seem even more meaningful and dynamic. Connectedness has received increasing attention in recent literature (e.g., Conco, 1995; Schubert & Lionberger, 1995; Weeks & O'Connor, 1994).

Submission of the SCA Results to Peers for Critique

The final step in the SCA process is to submit the findings to one or more peers for review. After working closely with multiple, complex concepts, it is easy for the researchers to lose perspective. Thus, it is helpful to seek objective evaluation of the results. Do they seem logical? Are the terms consistent across concepts? What are the implications of the findings for theory development and research? Do the findings have potential meaning for nursing practice?

By presenting the results informally to peers, to colleagues in seminar, or to refereed journals for broader review, the SCA process can come full circle, presenting opportunities for reworking the same concepts, or moving on to new ones.

IMPLICATIONS

What Can SCA Tell Us About Empirical Methods?

It is interesting that implications concerning qualitative and quantitative empirical methods arise from the simultaneous clarification process. Qualitative implications include the need for field studies to further clarify the concepts of interest, as well as those emerging from the SCA strategy. Among the quantitative implications are issues related to measurement, model specification, the use of latent variables, and assumptions underlying commonly used statistical methods. In addition, SCA can provide guidance for programs of research, suggesting empirical work to explore, verify, or test SCA findings.

Schwartz-Barcott and Kim (1986), in their hybrid model, obtain an understanding of the structure of the concept, whereas ethnographic or grounded theory approaches could contribute to clarifying the social and cultural processes associated with the model (Morse, 1995).

In terms of quantitative measurement issues, confirmatory factor analyses of instruments designed to measure multidimensional concepts should be performed in order to evaluate factor structures in light of the definitions, interrelationships, and validity matrices proposed through SCA. Because multidimensional concepts, such as those presented in this chapter, often represent changing processes, investigators should anticipate low to moderate test-retest reliability in their instruments, particularly during times of pivotal life events or experiences. In selecting or developing instruments to measure multidimensional and interrelated concepts, consideration must be given to the nature of their interrelationships and the goal of the study or program of research. If a critical goal is to differentiate among any combination of the variables, for example, the instruments should be restricted to critical attributes, the area least likely to contain overlap. On the other hand, if the goal is to measure outcomes, the investigator must remain aware of the similarities and differences obtained in SCA, and how these are reflected in the various instruments. High correlations among the outcomes of spiritual perspective, hope, acceptance, and self-transcendence would be expected due to their similarities along this dimension. To gain more accurate insight into the interrelationships among outcomes of these four variables, the researcher might consider restricting measurement to one unique outcome for each concept, rather than attempting to tap all dimensions.

Concepts amenable to SCA often involve dynamic and interrelated processes. Hence, they are likely to be excellent candidates for latent variable and nonrecursive models. Latent variable modeling, a statistical procedure that uses multiple indicators to measure a single factor, would enable the investigator to account for the shared and unique variances of both instruments and latent factors. Nonrecursive modeling, a statistical procedure that can accomodate feedback loops, is the appropriate technique for examining the various recurring processes that may be suggested by simultaneous concept analysis. Process models may be used as an initial step in the development of theoretical models to be subjected to empirical testing.

Clearly, the study of interrelated concepts can create numerous analytical problems. SCA may assist the investigator in anticipating and visualizing some of these. For example, simple regression analysis is designed to handle a certain degree of multicollinearity, the intercorrelation among the independent variables. However, when multicollinearity is extreme, problems arise, specifically large standard errors of estimation and failure to achieve statistical significance. This, of course, makes it difficult to obtain a unique solution for the parameter estimates, i.e., it becomes difficult to separate out the effects of the interrelated variables, often the task of greatest interest (see Berry & Feldman, 1985; Lewis-Beck, 1980; or Pedhazur, 1982, for more complete discussions of multicollinearity). SCA should provide the investigator with some insight into the potential for multicollinearity, especially its source and potential solutions. For example, the degree of overlap among outcomes of the four concepts considered here suggests that unless special precautions are taken, a high degree of multicollinearity would be inevitable. Hence, these four concepts do not appear to be good candidates for the role of independent variables in a simple regression model.

Finally, implications for specific empirical work should arise from the SCA process. For example, life experiences, connectedness, and positive attributes were found to be antecedents of hope in our SCA. The qualitative and quantitative research implications of this statement are important. What is connectedness? How is it experienced? What are positive attributes? How do these characteristics differ for people experiencing hope (according to the critical attributes identified) and those who are not? Is self-transcendence an outcome of hope? In what way are hope and self-transcendence helpful to clients of nursing? In what way can (do) nurses facilitate hope through connectedness? Are there specific interventions that can be tested? The ideas that arise from SCA can be endless.

What Does SCA Tell Us About the Philosophical Aspects of Concept Development in Nursing?

It is difficult to say whether the SCA has inherent philosophical implications, or if the method reflects the philosophical bases of the group developing the strategy. In any event, there are philosophical underpinnings to the SCA approach, and it is to these that we must now turn before discussion of this strategy can be considered complete.

Several philosophical assumptions clearly underlie the SCA strategy. First and foremost, concepts relevant to nursing are viewed as complex, interrelated, dynamic processes. Thus, to consider or analyze them as static terms provides a false understanding of their underlying structure or processes. Second, because such interrelationships exist, many concepts cannot, and should not, be analyzed in isolation. The influence of related concepts can significantly alter the dynamic processes that occur, hence the development of the SCA strategy. Third, to obtain a holistic product, concept analyses should reflect diverse perspectives. And, to the extent possible, results should be useful to theorists, investigators, and practitioners in a variety of settings. This is the most useful contribution concept analysis can make to the language of nursing and its development as a discipline. Finally, qualitative and quantitative research have important, complementary, noncompeting roles in nursing science. Together, these methodologies can provide a scientific data base for nursing practice and further the development of nursing theory.

SOMEWHAT ANSWERED QUESTIONS

In the first edition of this book, we included a section called Unanswered Questions. Some of these questions have at least partial answers now. In the first edition we stated that although we found the SCA strategy to be very effective in deriving greater understanding and insight concerning concepts of interest to us, others must use and evaluate the method in order to prove its utility. Since that time, SCA has been referenced as a useful strategy for concept development and clarification (Meleis, 1997; Morse, 1995). Meleis (1997) evaluates the process as an "innovative and discipline-congruent strategy." She further evaluates the strategy as based on "collaboration, critical thinking, expertise of participants, complementarity, mutual trust building and mutual consensus building. These are attributes congruent with the nature of nursing as a human science and caring discipline" (p. 211).

SCA has been used in an academic setting with doctoral level students to clarify a nursing concept. Class members formed small groups based on their identification of similar concepts with which they wanted to work over the course of the semester. For example, one group included students interested in the concepts of recovery, healing, transcendence, and dying. Another group of students worked with the concepts of well-being, quality of life, faith, and ethical dilemma.

After sessions to familiarize the students with the SCA process, students met in their small groups over several class sessions to assist each other in developing the analysis of their individual concepts. Each week a student took a turn leading discussion about one concept, based on a review of the literature. The group members assisted with concept clarification in light of knowledge of their own concepts of interest. For example, both recovery and healing were identified as similar processes by students. Questions were raised about whether healing was an attribute of recovery or whether recovery was an outcome of healing. A return to the literature on both recovery and healing led to the group decision that both recovery and healing were processes—but recovery had a finite end point and could be an outcome of healing whereas healing might require a lifetime.

Although the students did not develop validity matrix models, they did use a group consensus approach to examine the interrelationships and theoretical overlaps among their chosen concepts and to develop a process model for each group of concepts. As such, they used two of the three critical components of SCA. This variation of the SCA process greatly facilitated the students' development of their own concepts. Students commented that the group process was far more beneficial than their previous attempts to clarify concepts while working independently. Students also said that they thoroughly enjoyed the interactions with each other during the scholarly group consensus process.

Another unanswered question was whether SCA is feasible without a consensus group? That is, is it possible for one individual to "objectively" conduct an SCA? To "master" more than one concept without group challenge? We continue to think it is not. The group consensus process is an integral part, and strength, of SCA. To attempt simultaneous analyses alone would yield different, and perhaps less interesting, results due to the loss of varied perspective offered by the group approach. However, the opportunities for individuals to join together for SCA requires planning, time, and commitment that is not always available.

Another question we raised in the first edition of this book concerned the laying aside of interesting and rich subtleties of individual concepts in an attempt to handle large quantities of information more efficiently and gain breadth of understanding across concepts. This problem was introduced in the discussion of Step 4. We raised the question of what to do with these rich subtleties. What, if anything, was lost? Did the gain in breadth offset any loss in depth? Should the group return to earlier steps in the SCA process and reevaluate each concept, integrating the information that was set aside? Or should this task be left to individuals during their research pursuits? Could further individual analyses be done without threatening the validity of findings from SCAs? We mentioned that groups using the SCA might "revisit" some of their earlier work and evaluate the extent to which information that was lost might be reintegrated into the SCA results. Not all groups have this opportunity, however. Our group as a whole did not revisit the SCA results. However, we have used the results in subsequent projects with much greater insight (Coward, 1990, 1991, 1994, 1995, 1996a; 1996b; 1998; Coward & Reed, 1996; Coward & Lewis, 1993; Haase et al., in press; Haase & Braden, in press; Haase & Rostad, 1994; Hinds & Haase, in press; Leidy, 1994a, 1994b). For example, Leidy and Haase examined the embedded concept of connectedness in work on functional performance in persons with COPD. The concept has been incorporated into the beginning of a model of the process of preserving integrity in the face of chronic illness (Leidy & Haase, 1996, 1999).

SCA is designed to be one of many strategies used to clarify concepts and strengthen professional language. It should complement other approaches and withstand the test offered by subjecting the results to further concept clarification.

SUMMARY

Simultaneous concept analysis (SCA) is a strategy designed to generate and refine conceptual definitions, critical attributes, theoretical definitions, antecedents, and outcomes of multiple interrelated concepts. Critical components of this strategy are consensus group process, the application of validity matrices, and the development of a process model. Unlike the individual concept analysis approach proposed by Wilson (1969), and Walker and Avant (1988), the SCA strategy is designed to analyze interrelationships and identify theoretical overlap, common themes, and distinguishing characteristics among similar or complementary concepts. It is still a relatively new strategy that must be subjected to further scrutiny and evaluation. However, the method proved very useful to us in clarifying four complex, interrelated, and empirically elusive concepts. We have subsequently found usefulness in the approach in educational settings and as we continue our own projects. We hope that it will prove useful for others as well.

REFERENCES

Berry, W., & Feldman, S. (1985). *Multiple regression in practice.* Beverly Hills: Sage.

Burkhardt, M. (1989). Spirituality: An analysis of the concept. *Holistic Nursing Practice, 3*(3), 9–77.

Conco, D. (1995). Christian patients' views of spiritual care. *Western Journal of Nursing Research, 17*(3), 266–276.

Coward, D. D. (1990). The lived experience of self-transcendence in women with advanced breast cancer. *Nursing Science Quarterly, 3,* 162–169.

Coward, D. D. (1991). Self-transcendence and emotional well-being in women with advanced breast cancer. *Oncology Nursing Forum, 18,* 857–863.

Coward, D. D. (1994). Meaning and purpose in the lives of persons with AIDS. *Public Health Nursing, 11,* 331–336.

Coward, D. D. (1995). The lived experience of self-transcendence in women with AIDS. *Journal of Obstetric, Gynecologic and Neonatal Nursing, 24,* 314–318.

Coward, D. D. (1996a). Self-transcendence and correlates in a healthy population. *Nursing Research, 45*(2), 116–121.

Coward, D. D. (1996b). Self-transcendence: Making meaning from the cancer experience. *Quality of Life: A Nursing Challenge, 4*(2), 53–58.

Coward, D. D. (1998). Facilitation of self-transcendence in a breast cancer support group. *Oncology Nursing Forum, 25*(1), 75–84.

Coward, D. D., & Lewis, F. L. (1993). The lived experience of self-transcendence in gay men with AIDS. *Oncology Nursing Forum, 20,* 1363–1368.

Coward, D. D., & Reed, P. G. (1996). Self-Transcendence: A resource for healing at the end of life. *Issues in Mental Health Nursing, 17,* 275–288.

Haase, J., Berry, C., Heiney, S., Kuperberg, A., Leidy, N., Myers, S., Rostad, M., Ruccione, K., & Stutzer, C. (in press). Resilience and quality of life in adolescents with cancer: Instrument and Model Development. *International Journal of Cancer.*

Haase, J. & Braden, C. (in press). Concepts related to quality of life. In C. King & P. Hinds (Eds.), *Quality of life: Theory, research, and practice.* Boston: Jones & Bartlett.

Haase, J., Britt, T., Coward, D., Leidy, N. K., & Penn, P. (1992). Simultaneous concept analysis of spiritual perspective, hope, acceptance, and self-transcendence. *Image, 24,* 141–147.

Haase, J., & Leidy, N. K. (1996, June). Connectedness: Concept development through empirical analysis. American Nurses Association Council for Nursing Research: 1996 Scientific Session, Washington, DC.

Haase, J., & Rostad, M. (1994). Experiences of completing cancer therapy: Children's perspectives. *Oncology Nursing Forum, 21,* 1483–1492.

Hinds, P. & Haase, J. (in press). Quality of life in children and adolescents with cancer. In C. King & P. Hinds (Eds.), *Quality of life: Theory, research, and practice.* Boston: Jones & Bartlett.

Kaplan, A. (1964). *The conduct of inquiry.* Philadelphia: Chandler.

Lewis-Beck, M. S. (1980). *Applied regression: An introduction.* Beverly Hills: Sage.

Leidy, N. K. (1994a). Functional status and the forward progress of merry-go-rounds: Toward a coherent analytical framework. *Nursing Research, 43,* (4), 196–202.

Leidy, N. K. (1994b). Operationalizing Maslow's theory: Development and testing of the Basic Need Satisfaction Inventory. *Issues in Mental Health Nursing, 15*(3), 227–295.

Leidy, N. K., & Haase, J. (1996). Functional performance in people with chronic obstructive pulmonary disease: A qualitative analysis. *Advances in Nursing Science, 18*, 77–89.

Leidy, N. K., & Haase, J. (1999). Functional status from the patient's perspective: The challenge of preserving personal integrity. *Research in Nursing and Health, 22*, 67–77.

Meleis, A. (1997). *Theoretical nursing: Development and progress.* Philadelphia: Lippincott.

Morse, J. (1995). Exploring the theoretical basis of nursing using advanced techniques of concept analysis. *Advances in Nursing Science, 17*(3), 31–46.

Myers, S., & Haase, J. (1989). Guidelines for integration of quantitative and qualitative approaches. *Nursing Research, 38*, 299–301.

Pedhazur, E. (1982). *Multiple regression in behavioral research: Explanation and prediction.* (2nd ed.). New York: Holt, Rinehart, & Winston.

Reed, P. (1991). Self-transcendence and mental health in oldest-old adults. *Nursing Research, 40*, 5–11.

Roberts, K., & Fitzgerald, L. (1991). Serenity: Caring with perspective. *Scholarly Inquiry for Nursing Practice, 5*(2), 127–142.

Schubert, P. E., & Lionberger, H. J. (1995). Mutual connectedness: A study of client-nurse interaction using the grounded theory method. *Journal of Holistic Nursing, 13*(2), 102–116.

Schwartz-Barcott, D., & Kim, H. S. (1986). A hybrid model for concept development. In P. Chinn (Ed.), *Nursing research: Methodology issues and instrumentation.* Rockville, MD: Aspen.

Walker, L., & Avant, K. (1988). *Strategies for theory construction in nursing.* (2nd ed.). Norwalk, CT: Appleton-Lange.

Weeks, S. K., & O'Connor, P. C. (1994). Concept analysis of family + health: A new definition of family health. *Rehabilitation Nursing, 19*(4), 207–210.

Wilson, J. (1969). *Thinking with concepts.* New York: Cambridge University.

CHAPTER

13

Integrative Literature Reviews for the Development of Concepts

Marion E. Broome

Any individual who chooses to systematically build a base of knowledge about a selected concept will be involved in searching, reading, analyzing, synthesizing, and eventually reconceptualizing existing literature on the concept. Interestingly, searching the literature is one of the earliest skills required in education, yet one most often taken for granted. Often little attention is given to teaching the students the skills required to conduct a thorough literature search, critique the research, and report their findings. Instead, most students develop a routine approach to selecting and reviewing the literature and consistently follow this routine without regard to its effectiveness.

The volumes of information published daily on any given topic have become overwhelming (Cooper, 1989). The average university library has the capability of searching over 700 data bases for retrieval of articles from journals in a variety of disciplines (University of Wisconsin-Milwaukee, 1997). In recent years the search for information has expanded to the Internet and web sites. Hence, anyone beginning the study of a concept must use systematic, thorough, and time-efficient methods to search and analyze the literature in order to minimize effort and maximize knowledge gained.

The primary purpose of a review of existing knowledge, usually in large part the literature, is to gain an in-depth understanding of a phenomenon by building on the work of others. This process is especially important in concept development. Concept building requires a working knowledge of what previous work has been done in the area, what limitations in conceptualization and methods have influenced the development of the concept, as well as what questions remain unanswered. Such a review can assist the individual to understand how others have defined the concept, develop a personal definition of the concept, and to understand how others have measured related phenomena.

It is essential that the sources chosen are as representative of the entire body of knowledge as possible and that the knowledge that is used to gain understanding is valid. This is especially important when the reader is interested in broadening knowledge about a concept. How the investigator organizes the search, how the content of the literature is documented, what methods are used to critically analyze each piece of the literature, and finally, how the content is organized, synthesized, and presented is very important. This work can become frustrating and unproductive if the entire process lacks organization and direction.

Rigorous, systematic reviews of the literature are critical to developing a substantial knowledge base about a concept. Approaches to learning and, eventually, to contributing knowledge about a concept should be as uncompromising as any other step in the knowledge building and testing process. The purpose of this chapter is to discuss methods that are used by researchers to systematically search and analyze the literature as well as strategies that investigators use to critically evaluate sources and organize and synthesize their findings.

TYPES OF LITERATURE REVIEWS

There are several types of reviews of knowledge commonly published in journals, books, or manuscripts. These vary in purpose, scope, depth, breadth, and organization of the material. Literature reviews take many forms including: (1) abbreviated synopses of the literature found in most data-based research articles; (2) methodological or theoretical reviews; (3) critical analyses; (4) integrative reviews; and (5) meta-analyses. These various approaches share some commonalties, yet have divergent goals. For instance, the purpose of a theoretical review is broad and inclusive of the literature evaluated and discussed. Theoretical reviews often include a historical analysis of the "state of the science" and recommendations for further theory development and research in the area. The primary purpose of most meta-analyses, on the other hand, is to examine the overall effectiveness of specific experimental effects, and is usually more focused on a review of selected intervention studies.

Abbreviated Reviews. Abbreviated reviews found in journal articles are typically much shorter than other types, due to space limitations in journals. These reviews are narrowly focused around a discussion of the variables and empirical data in that specific study. A limitation of such reviews is the limited scope and selective nature of what is presented; usually only research that is supportive of the argument for the present research is included. The arguments found in these reviews tend to be much more persuasive and selective of what literature is used to present a picture of what is known about the concepts (variables) of interest.

Methodological Reviews. A methodological review is focused on critiquing the designs, methods, and analyses in a series of studies. An example of such a review is "Personality disorders in the chronic pain population: Basic concepts, empirical findings and clinical implications" (Weisberg & Keefe, 1997). These authors reviewed research conducted over the past 15 years and discussed the process, structure, and outcomes of these studies. Limitations of the studies were described and specific suggestions for further research were provided.

Theoretical Reviews. A theoretical review is perhaps the most challenging to write and yet can be very instrumental in moving collective thought ahead in a discipline. These reviews usually propose models that describe the relationships among variables previously studied, and often propose new variables and relationships to investigate. Hence, they tend to be most useful for and relevant to concept development. Occasionally, these reviews result in the identification and description of a new concept or theory or in refining an existing one. An example of such a review is "Wellness motivation theory: An exploration of theoretical relevance" (Fleury, 1996), in which the results of a qualitative study were used to examine the validity and cultural relevance of an existing theoretical framework on the topic of wellness motivation in health behavior change. Many experts argue that theoretical reviews are critical to the development of a substantive knowledge base in a discipline, which cannot be achieved solely through the description of existing research (Cooper, 1989; Kirkevold, 1997).

Critical Reviews. Critical reviews are extensive analyses of literature in a selected area that usually have a specific focus. Such reviews do not include original data but rather are interpretations of findings from different studies. A specific concept (e.g., day care) is defined, and a concise historical perspective on the topic is provided. Critical reviews are comprehensive and include both a theoretical analysis and methodological critique of the research. Most authors use this synthesis of the literature to develop theoretical propositions that generate many fruitful ideas for future research. An excellent example of a comprehensive, critical review article is "Nursing blood pressure research 1980–1990: A bio-psycho-social perspective" (Thomas et al., 1993). The authors reviewed empirical studies in the area, identified key variables in the environment that influenced the measurement of blood pressure, the methods used to measure the phenomenon, and the statistical analyses employed to study blood pressure. They identified several key areas for imposing the conceptualizations about and designs used to study blood pressure that future researchers can apply.

Integrative Reviews. An integrative review is defined as one in which past research is summarized by drawing overall conclusions from many studies. Although this is very similar to the kind of work done and presented in a critical review, there are some distinct differences. Cooper (1989) recommended formulating a research problem that will guide the integrative review. He defined research problem broadly and stressed that definitions of important variables and a description of how the variables relate to each other should be included. This first step of identifying the research problem or question is important in order to delimit the scope of the review. For instance, even in a topic area with a relatively recent research history, such as neonatal pain, there is a large volume of literature. This literature varies a great deal and includes studies of behavioral responses of the neonate to painful procedures as well as comparative studies of both pharmacological and nonpharmacological options for managing pain in neonates.

For instance, a question or hypothesis such as "Is morphine or fentanyl more effective in reducing pain in the neonate?" or a broader question such as "Which analgesics are most effective in reducing pain?" is very effective in delimiting the review. Although this second question broadens the scope of the review, it still restricts the type of literature to that reporting pharmacological interventions and would exclude studies in which the primary purpose was to examine behavioral responses to neonatal pain.

Meta-Analysis. Meta-analysis is a special case of the integrative review. The purpose of meta-analysis is to conduct an integrative review and, in addition, to determine the overall effectiveness of interventions using statistical analyses that combine the results of many independent studies (Anello & Fleiss, 1995). Studies are systematically chosen, critiqued, and coded using protocols in an attempt to reduce bias and subjectivity (Rosenfeld, 1996). In a meta-analysis, selected variables related to research or the phenomenon itself are examined to determine their influence on an intervention's effectiveness.

QUESTIONS THAT GUIDE REVIEW PROCESSES

As any student or scholar knows, there is much to be gained from reading a variety of reviews on a selected topic. For individuals interested in concept development, these reviews are invaluable and facilitate mastery of a broad literature. During the review process answers to the following questions should be sought:

1. How has the concept been defined by authors and what are the various theoretical perspectives that have been used to describe the concept?
2. What work has already been done and what can be expanded?
3. What relationships have been discovered between dimensions of this concept and other related phenomena?
4. What research approaches (e.g., phenomenology, experimental) have been used to understand and study the concept?

INTEGRATIVE REVIEWS AND META-ANALYSES

There have been several attempts by nurse authors to direct attention to the need for a more systematic and rigorous approach to the review of the literature (Ganong, 1987; Kirkevold, 1997). Ganong (1987) critiqued 17 integrative reviews in nursing published from 1978 to 1983 in four major research journals. One meta-analysis was included in this sample. Ganong found that only 9 of the 17 reviews included discussion of methodological problems, while 3 presented a systematic search for effects. All but 1 review provided suggestions for further research, and 6 reviews discussed implications for policy or practice. Ganong concluded that although methods for conducting integrative reviews vary, they should be as uncompromising as methods for conducting primary research, and a systematic, thoughtful process should be used in reviewing the literature. That process is discussed in the rest of this chapter. Meta-analysis, which is a unique, extended form of the integrative review, has received a great deal of attention in most practice disciplines. Nursing is no exception, so a discussion of meta-analysis is included. The processes of conducting integrative reviews and meta-analyses share many commonalties, as shown in Table 13-1. Meta-analysis takes the integrative review one step further, reanalyzes the data reported in each article, and determines the overall effectiveness of a specific research treatment.

Concept Identification and Research Questions

Once the concept is chosen, questions that will guide the review are identified to delimit the search and facilitate identification of the keywords (Smith & Stullenbarger, 1991). Specifically, the questions that guide the review or meta-analysis should be made explicit because they will influence which studies are chosen, what information is extracted from the articles, and which statistical operations, if any, are chosen to

Table 13–1 Process of Integrative Reviews and Meta-Analysis

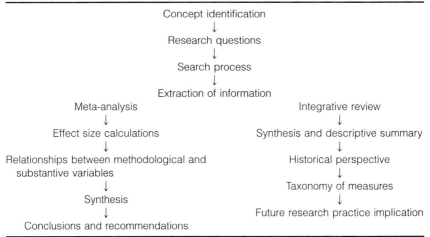

Concept identification
↓
Research questions
↓
Search process
↓
Extraction of information

Meta-analysis	Integrative review
↓	↓
Effect size calculations	Synthesis and descriptive summary
↓	↓
Relationships between methodological and substantive variables	Historical perspective
↓	↓
Synthesis	Taxonomy of measures
↓	↓
Conclusions and recommendations	Future research practice implication

analyze the data. The research questions for reviews can be broad or narrow; however, broad questions will usually require a review that is more labor intensive.

The research questions will be a reflection of the theoretical perspective and underlying assumptions held by the investigator, and can heavily influence the interpretation of the findings. For instance, in two different meta-analyses of the pain literature (Broome et al., 1989; Fernandez & Turk, 1989), different categorizations of cognitive coping strategies were used. Broome et al. restricted their meta-analysis to research interventions with children and reported types of interventions (cognitive, biophysical, affective), whereas Fernandez and Turk restricted their review to cognitive strategies only, using studies with primarily adult subjects. Both groups of researchers reported that cognitive strategies were beneficial in reducing pain and distress ratings. The intervention categories in Fernandez and Turk's paper were more discrete, which reflected the purpose of the paper as well as the background and interests of the authors, who were psychologists.

Once the research questions are specified, decision making related to the sample of studies to be reviewed begins. For instance, the reviewer has to decide if the literature search will be restricted to one or several disciplines, what journals and how many years will be searched. These decisions are heavily influenced by the historical evolution of the concept itself as well as how discipline-specific a concept is. For instance, the concept of maternal confidence is prevalent in the nursing literature, nonexistent in medicine, and often labeled as "self-efficacy" in psychology. Some of these decisions will vary depending on the nature of the concept, purpose of inquiry, etc., with different investigators choosing different options to guide their search.

The Search Process

Most research texts contain a comprehensive list and descriptions of the various computerized literature searches. There is a certain degree of skill and knowledge required to conduct a computerized search, and anyone who is seriously considering conducting one should spend time in the library either with a reference librarian, a tutorial specific to literature searches, or in a library-sponsored class. In the long run, much time will be saved and the outcomes of the search will be maximized.

If the literature to be searched is extensive, the use of questions that can guide the review is critical. These questions will also help the reviewer to later identify keywords to delimit the search. For instance, the concept of pediatric pain is extremely broad and will yield over 1,500 citations on MEDLINE from 1986 to 1997. Some narrowing is necessary in order to conduct a timely, efficient, but thorough search. The following questions are examples of how such a broad topic could be narrowed:

1. When was pain first identified in the pediatric literature?
2. How is pain defined?
3. How is pain measured (operationally defined) in children? How does this differ from adults?
4. What kinds of pain do children have?
5. What are the common modalities used to treat pain in children?
6. What other factors influence the expression of pain and its treatment in children?

Obvious keywords in a search of literature to answer these questions are *child*, *pain*, *measurement*, and *intervention*. However, it is possible that very little would emerge from an initial search using just those keywords especially to answer questions 5 or 6. The reviewer may need to search a broader literature on pain assessment and management using computerized online search procedures such as MEDLINE and CINAHL (Table 13-2). To use these most efficiently, the reviewer must continue to identify *keywords* that will assist the individual conducting the search and narrow the field.

For example, a search that begins with a global concept such as *pain* is narrowed considerably by the descriptor *pediatric pain* and even further with *pediatric pain assessment*. Additional keywords that could be used to narrow the search for articles reporting research in pediatric pain assessment may be *child response*, *pain measurement*, and *procedural pain*.

Table 13–2   Selected Computer Search Services

Health Sciences

AIDSLINE: a dynamic data base with over 48,000 citations from 1980 to the present on acquired immunodeficiency syndrome, covering research and clinical aspects of the disease. Available from the National Library of Medicine.

BIOSIS: contains 11 million citations (50% abstracts) from life sciences, both Biological Abstracts and Biological Abstracts/RRM. Research literature in the life sciences is comprehensively covered through the abstracting of articles from 6,000+ journals, congresses, reviews, reports, and research communication.

CANCERLIT: (sponsored by the National Cancer Institute) contains 1 million citations and abstracts from journals, congresses, conferences, and texts from 1963 to the present. All aspects of cancer are covered including etiology, prevention, diagnosis, treatment, and biology.

MEDLINE: contains more than 6.8 million citations (60% abstracts) in biomedicine including research, clinical practice, administration and policy and corresponds to three printed indexes: Index Medicus, International Nursing Index, and Index to Dental Literature. Indexing articles from 3,900+ journals, published in over 70 countries.

NURSING & ALLIED HEALTH LITERATURE (CINAHL): contains citations to English language journal articles and some pamphlet and other ephemeral materials in the disciplines of nursing, medical technology, physical therapy, and other allied health science professions.

BIOETHICSLINE: indexes and abstracts the world's English language literature related to ethical and public policy aspects of medicine and health care; includes interdisciplinary coverage of bioethical topics such as euthanasia, abortion, biotechnology. Information is compiled from a variety of formats: books, journals, newspapers, court cases, and audio-visuals.

Psych INFO: produced by the American Psychological Association, contains over 1 million citations and abstracts to the literature of psychology and related disciplines. The formats of the indexed literature include periodicals, dissertations, technical reports, and conference proceedings.

SOCIAL SCISEARCH: a multidisciplinary database indexing 3,200 journals in the social sciences and selected articles from 2,000+ additional journals in other fields. The unique feature of this data base is the capability of producing lists of current references that have cited a well-known paper or author.

Developed from Novallo, A., Alampi, M., & Nolan, K. (1997). *Gale directory of databases.* Detroit, MI: Gale Publishing.

In most libraries, anyone can search a number of data bases at no charge using the mini-MEDLINE on a library information system. Other searches that are more comprehensive require the use of personnel and computer time and may be costly. Each data base charges a different fee depending on the number of citations retrieved, the computer time used, and the extent of the entire literature base. Computerized searches of the literature have expanded phenomenally over the past decade. In fact, there are even directories of data bases (Novallo et al., 1997) that provide the reviewer with information on over 5,000 publicly available online data bases.

In addition to the computerized search, the investigator can initially use article bibliographies or reference lists from very recent books on the subject. This is a rather commonly used approach called the "despondency method" (Cooper, 1987). A study of 57 authors of research reviews published in psychology and education revealed the use of references in published review papers to be the most frequently reported strategy for searching the literature (Cooper, 1987). Computer searches of abstract data bases, such as MEDLINE, ERIC, or Psychological Abstracts, also were used. In addition, authors of the review articles that were examined stated they often communicated with others who shared their work or ideas, a concept commonly referred to as "the invisible college" (Crane, 1969). The use of this "invisible college" also will uncover unpublished studies that can be accessed through colleagues and then added to the review. The use of unpublished studies often is recommended for integrative reviews, and especially meta-analyses, because there is a bias toward publishing positive results in the literature (Cook et al., 1993).

Even in searches limited by time, resources, and money, the goal should be to avoid obvious bias in a search within the limits of cost (Cooper, 1989). It is important to not over-represent any one segment of the literature and thereby reduce generalizability of the conclusions. Yet, cost of retrieval, breadth of the literature, specificity of the research questions, and time restrictions all influence how extensive the search will be. When decisions are made about the search process, they should be documented by the investigator, and the search must reflect these decisions. For example, in the meta-analysis by Broome, Lillis, and Smith (1989), a decision was made to begin the search with 1967 and extend over the next 20 years through December, 1987. The beginning date was chosen because it was 10 years before the first systematic studies of pediatric pain emerged. To increase comprehensiveness and include literature from several disciplines, these authors scanned an index of health profession journals that listed 1,000 journals. Journals that were chosen from this index were those thought to include pediatric pain intervention studies. All of these decisions and procedures were documented, and the records were kept in a notebook. This documentation enabled the investigators to record decisions to refer to later when publishing the study.

Searches often proceed in levels that begin broad and increasingly narrow. Searching the literature is never strictly a linear process but rather one in which the author returns many times to the initial questions and decision criteria when choosing what to do next. Initially, as was discussed earlier, keywords are developed to assist in screening the studies. During the meta-analysis discussed earlier, Broome, Lillis, and Smith (1989) identified 32 keywords such as *pain, interventions,* and *child* for a computerized search using MEDLINE and Dissertation Abstracts International. This Level I search yielded 125 articles and dissertations on pain interventions with children. Many of these were descriptive studies or clinical case studies. In a second level of review, it was decided that the research study must report use of an intervention, include more than 10 subjects, and contain the statistical information necessary to calculate effect sizes. These criteria were based on both initial research questions and meta-analysis methodology.

A total of 27 studies were finally included in that meta-analysis. Nonpublished studies and unpublished theses were not included because the investigators decided that using only published material and dissertations would provide assurance of a minimal quality of the study. Their assumption was based on the belief that journal referees and university dissertation committee members provide some consistency in the quality of written research reports. Time limitations and cost constraints on this meta-analysis also influenced this decision. If master's theses and solicitation of unpublished studies are used, the search process is extended considerably. However, some meta-analysts recommend using unpublished studies in order to access the full range of studies, even those likely not to have reported significant findings (Hasselblad et al., 1995; Hedges & Olkin, 1985). This decision is an example of one of the decisions that can differ depending on the reviewer, as others might choose to invest more time and money to include a wider range of sources. Again, decisions were documented and studies that were excluded in the meta-analysis were listed in a bibliography with a notation as to the reason for the exclusion. The authors found this documentation very helpful later when responding to questions about why specific articles were not included.

Extraction of Information

Annotation of articles from the literature involves the extraction of specific information from each article. The purpose of annotation is to summarize and document, in a concise and easily retrievable way, information from each piece of literature. Important content can vary with each reviewer's purposes but generally includes the purpose, methodology, and findings of the study. Annotation can be done in a variety of ways. Traditionally, index cards have been used by reviewers to organize their assessments of each article. With the increasing popularity of personal computers, many reviewers now use charts or tables (Table 13-3) to organize relevant content using word processing software programs. There are also bibliographical software programs avail-

Table 13–3   Interventions for Children in Preparation for Painful Procedures

Source	Sample	Methods	Intervention	Findings

able that allow the reviewer to catalogue references for easy access and retrieval of key information. One advantage to the chart system for annotation is that studies can be viewed and compared easily as a whole. Although categories in the chart are flexible, they should reflect the overall purpose of the review. Organizing the articles chronologically allows the individual to develop an appreciation for the historical evolution of knowledge in the area.

Coding

Coding information taken from the articles is a two-step process. First, the reviewer develops a codebook that guides which information is retrieved from the article. The second step requires an assessment of the quality of the research. Codebooks are used in both integrative reviews and meta-analyses (Cooper, 1989; Smith & Stullenbarger, 1995). Selection of what information to extract varies. Investigators must have a working knowledge of the concept as well as methodologies used in the research in order to develop the codebook (Smith & Stullenbarger, 1991). An example of a section of the codebook can be found in Table 13-4. Relevant methodological and substantive variables are listed and applied to each article. Information in the codebook is very important and will be used in later analyses to determine if overall effect sizes were affected by any methodological or substantive variables. For example, the researcher might want to consider whether the type of intervention used, such as distraction or parental presence, was related to children's responses to pain, or whether sampling methods were reflective of sample size.

Developing the codebook and coding the initial studies is a reciprocal process requiring many revisions as it becomes clear that data are missing or not available in the form required (Cooper, 1989). A draft of the codebook should be developed and used in the review of several research reports. Revisions should be made as needed before the actual coding process begins.

Table 13–4 Selected Examples of Variables in a Codebook

Methodological Characteristics	
Journal type (nursing, medicine, dental)	Nursing (1)
Sample (infants, toddlers, male, female)	Preschoolers (3), both genders (3)
Sampling procedures (random selection, convenience)	Random assignment (2)
Size of experimental group, control group	n = 37, n = 36

Substantive Characteristics	
Type of intervention (cognitive, affective, biophysical)	Cognitive (1)
Time of intervention	Immediately before stimulus (1)
Participants (individual, group)	Group (2)
Medium of intervention (person, videotape, play book, medication)	Person (1), play (3)
Outcome of measure (physiological, behavioral, self-report)	Pulse rate (1), blood pressure (1), behavioral (3)
Type of statistical test used	ANOVA (3)
Critical value	F = 2.53

Numbers in parentheses correspond to the code used to classify variables in codebook.

Critical Evaluation of the Research

A critical analysis of studies included in a review of the literature for an integrative review or meta-analysis requires an organized approach to evaluating the rigor and substance of each study. Some authors recommend excluding certain studies a priori, whereas others have called for inclusion of all studies (Cook et al., 1993). Most experts recommend coding the quality of various dimensions of the study and statistically analyzing whether the quality is related to other variables. For instance, in a meta-analysis, the rigor of the design of a study is reflected in low-quality ratings. Quality rating scores are based on an assessment of all components of a quantitative research study from statement of the problem, sampling techniques, through discussion of findings. These ratings can be used to weigh the overall contribution of the study when calculating effect sizes.

Assessing the quality of studies included has produced a great deal of discussion and controversy in the integrative review and meta-analysis literature. Some authors propose that the use of published literature alone will control for quality, whereas others believe the inclusion of only certain types of designs (e.g., randomized, controlled trials) or use of tightly controlled homogenous criteria for all studies will assure some level of quality (Rosenthal, 1984). Others believe the use of rating instruments that evaluate the various components of the studies is essential (Sachs et al., 1996; Smith & Stullenbarger, 1995). Most recommended instruments require the researchers to rate a variety of research design components (e.g., randomization process, measurement reliability and validity, statistical analyses) for appropriateness (Table 13-5). It is necessary to have more than one individual rate the quality of studies to reduce subjectivity and bias. Two raters are needed to complete the codebook as well as the quality ratings but are especially important for the quality of study ratings because most rating scales require some degree of interpretation (Sachs et al., 1996).

The raters using a quality rating instrument should be trained and should practice until they meet a preset standard determined by the investigator (e.g., 90 percent agreement). Subsequent quality scores must be interpreted carefully because they can be affected by several factors. A quality score is somewhat reflective of the amount of information provided in the study. In published research, space limitations often preclude the inclusion of some information about the study. This is one reason dissertation quality scores are generally higher than published articles. Another factor that influences quality scores is the familiarity of the rater with the area of study. If a rater is familiar with the area, it is easy to read between the lines and unintentionally inflate a score. A third consideration arises when both published and unpublished information are used. Quality scores, as a whole, may be higher in meta-analyses that include only published material than in those that use all sources. More important, they may not be variable, which will make any statistical analysis related to quality scores less meaningful.

The search for and retrieval of articles and documents on the World Wide Web has become an increasingly popular method of locating literature for reviews as well. There are more than 10,000 health-related web sites in existence (Pealer & Dorman, 1997). In fact, there is now an electronic newsletter that features Internet resources for health professionals called *The Internet Healthcare Network* (1997), which provides information on the availability of Internet sites for education, collaboration, and research.

However, searchers must be aware that there can be dramatic variations in the quality of the articles and documents found at various web sites and some evaluation criteria should be applied to those articles and documents taken from web sites. Most sites have no manuscript review mechanism in place as do refereed journals that ensure some minimum level of quality (Bridges & Thede, 1996). The World Wide Web makes no provision for ensuring the accuracy of information provided at each site; therefore it is incumbent on each user to use some valid criteria to determine quality. Several authors have developed some initial guidelines reviewers can use (Bridges & Thede, 1996; Pealer & Dorman, 1997). These guidelines include evaluation of accuracy of content, whether the content is based on current research, review of references provided, and authors' credentials, among other criteria.

Table 13-5 Quality of Study Instrument

Elements and Requirements	1 Low	2 Med	3 High	0 Absent	NA
1.0 Introduction					
1.1 Justification for study					
1.2 Conceptual framework					
1.3 Statement of problem or purpose					
1.4 Critical review of issues					
1.5 Methodological issues					
1.6 Hypotheses or study questions stated					
1.7 Operational definitions					
2.0 Methodology					
2.1 Design described					
2.2 Control of validity threats					
2.3 Sufficient sample size					
2.4 Representative sample					
2.5 Data collection procedures described					
2.6 Instrument validity described					
2.7 Instrument reliability described					
3.0 Data Analysis and Results					
3.1 Statistical treatment					
3.2 Data presentation					
3.3 Results related to problem and/or hypotheses					
3.4 Findings are substantiated by methods used					
4.0 Conclusions/Recommendations					
4.1 Discussion related to background and significance					
4.2 Conclusions logically derived from findings/results					
4.3 Recommendations consistent with findings					
4.4 Alternate explanations advanced					

n =
Sum =
Mean =

From Smith, MC, & Stullenbarger, E. (1991). A prototype for integrative review and meta-analysis of nursing research. *Journal of Advanced Nursing, 16*(11), 1272–1283.

ANALYSIS AND SYNTHESIS IN INTEGRATIVE REVIEWS

The process of conducting integrative reviews and meta-analyses differs somewhat at the point of analysis. Analysis has been defined as "the categorization, ordering, manipulating, and summarizing of data to obtain answers to research questions" (Kerlinger, 1973, p. 134). In most integrative reviews this categorization, ordering, and summarizing of the data are done in a more narrative fashion in which the investigator attempts to group the major findings of studies by variable of interest. Although there are no standard analysis and interpretation techniques for integrative reviews, most reviewers will present summary conclusions and recommendations for further research based on whether the majority of studies support specific relationships among variables (Cooper, 1989). Meta-analysis, on the other hand, is a method that enables reviews to more closely approximate analytic methods of researchers who analyze data from primary (actual) sources.

Meta-analysis is a relatively new addition to the methods used by scientists to examine the body of knowledge in a specific area (Cooper & Hedges, 1994; Hedges & Olkin, 1985; Wolf, 1986). Meta-analysis is the application of measurement and statistical techniques to analyze the combined data from multiple studies and to examine relationships among substantive and methodological characteristics of the studies and their results. The basic question guiding meta-analyses is "Are there patterns that can be observed in a body of studies in a selected area that have produced a variety of divergent results?"

The analysis of findings from qualitative studies is referred to as qualitative meta-synthesis (Sandelowski, 1997). The purpose of this technique is to synthesize the finding across a variety of qualitative studies. This is a relatively new method, but one that holds promise for extending the science of nursing. Qualitative researchers have identified several challenges of meta-synthesis (Sandelowski, 1997). These include the need to develop techniques to establish similarity across topical areas of inquiry and a way to compare different qualitative approaches used across studies, including analysis and integration.

The term *meta-analysis* for quantitative studies was first coined by Glass in 1976. Since that time use of the method has become increasingly widespread, especially in fields such as medicine and nursing, where the effectiveness of interventions must be ascertained yet subject pools remain small and individual studies are very costly. A large number of studies on a particular intervention provide greater statistical power than any individual study can. In addition, a single study often provides inconclusive findings or even no effect. Yet, other studies of the same phenomenon can yield positive results. It is difficult then to decide which study to use as a guide for practice or for further research

(Smith & Stullenbarger, 1991). Meta-analysis enables a more objective look at the domain of studies and includes as much as possible of the relevant research available.

The conceptual basis for the analysis used in a meta-analysis concerns the transforming of research results from multiple and diverse studies into a common metric representing an index of effect magnitude (Glass, 1976). In other words, the meta-analyst is interested in aggregating results from studies that investigated the same phenomenon by pooling data from subjects across studies. There are several types of analyses conducted that enable the investigator to describe (1) the scope of the phenomenon studied; (2) the positive and negative tails of a distribution of studies; (3) any relationships among methodological and substantive variables in the body of studies; and (4) the combined effect of the interventions. Hence, analyses can include descriptive, correlation, analysis of variance, combined probability tests, and effect size estimates.

Scope of the Phenomenon (Domain)

Descriptive statistics are usually used to provide a perspective of what literature comprises the area (i.e., year of publication, authors, and disciplines, etc.). These are also used to describe the positive and negative tails of the distribution (i.e., distribution of effect size estimates). Effect size estimates are calculated to examine the strength of the relationship or treatment and its practical importance and meaningfulness (Wolf, 1986). Correlation procedures are used as well as analysis of variance and regression techniques to determine relationships among selected substantive and methodologic variables. For instance, Broome, Lillis, and Smith (1989), in their meta-analysis of pediatric pain management interventions, found a difference between the quality of study ratings and the type of publication (dissertation or journal). Nevertheless, analysis of variance (ANOVA) procedures revealed no significant differences between the type of intervention (books, play, etc.) and children's responses to pain.

Determining Effect Sizes

Combined probability techniques and effect size estimates have been described in several authoritative texts (Cooper & Hedges, 1994; Hedges & Olkin, 1985; Wolf, 1986). These procedures allow investigators to make conclusions based on a group of studies as opposed to one, or even several, studies. Statistical approaches and techniques have evolved over time and have become more sophisticated. Basically, each technique involves computing an overall effect size for the dependent variable of interest. In some meta-analyses, several effect sizes are computed (e.g., one for physiological measures, one for behavioral observation measures, and one for self reports). Certain types of information are needed to perform the analyses for effect size. Although exactly what information is needed depends on the specific statistical procedure used, there are some commonalties. For instance, important information usually includes the number of subjects in the groups in the study, and the means and standard deviations for each group. In some cases the statistical tests and probability values are also required as when the Fisher combined test is used (Wolf, 1986). An alternative equation, recommended by Rosenthal (1984) and Wolf (1986), uses exact probability values that are converted to standard normal deviations using a table of z values numbers. One effect size is calculated for each study, and all are summed; z_c represents the combined z scores. Another important number to calculate is the Fail Safe N (Rosenthal, 1984). This is defined as the number of studies with null results that have not been published (those finding no significant differences between treatment and control groups) that could potentially counterbalance or nullify the results of published studies. In the Broome, Lillis, and Smith (1989) meta-analysis, this calculation resulted in 649 unpublished studies that reported no significant differences in order to nullify the results.

ISSUES IN META-ANALYSIS

There has been a great deal of controversy in the literature in response to the increasing popularity of meta-analysis. The number of meta-analyses has burgeoned over the past decade, with a search of MEDLINE from 1976 to 1996 documenting over 2,000 (Cook et al., 1992; Sachs et al., 1996). Few authors have questioned the need for a more systematic approach to reviewing and evaluating the literature. However, several issues related to combining results of different studies to reach summative conclusions have been identified and as the method becomes more common, experts have proposed a variety of design controls that should be put in place. These issues center around (1) variable quality of the studies; (2) lack of representation in the research reviewed; and (3) variability of outcome measures and independent variables.

Some authors argue that meta-analysis camouflages badly designed studies (Hasselblad et al., 1995). This concern is related to the varying quality of different studies. Many meta-analysts have attempted to control for the variability in quality by rating each study, as was discussed earlier. Others control for this variability by a priori elimination that can reduce already small sample sizes (Lynn, 1989). Most suggest that the researcher use some method of weighting the studies relative to the strength of the design and the reliability and validity of the research, and factor that weighting into an analysis and discussion of findings.

Another concern is related to the representation of all studies used (Lynn, 1989). This concern results from the difficulty many meta-analysts have in locating all studies in the population. Some studies have not been published or were conducted as master's theses. Accessing these is time consuming and costly. Yet, journal articles are more likely than unpublished works to contain significant findings. This can result in a positive bias in meta-analysis when only published studies are used. As noted previously, it is very important to keep documentation regarding which literature was accessed and why certain decisions were made throughout the analysis.

A third issue is the concern that variability and subjectivity in instrumentation contribute to invalid results (Sachs et al., 1996). Although many authors of meta-analyses do not address this, others use more than one person to code each study and report inter-rater reliability estimates for both codebooks and quality of study ratings. If meta-analysis is to be as rigorous as primary research, then it is essential to measure and report reliability of instrumentation when appropriate and for reviewers of meta-analyses to apply the same rigorous criteria when reviewing.

Other criticisms of meta-analysis include the use of studies with different outcome measures in which more than one outcome measure from each study is used to compute an effect size or different, but similar, outcome measures are compared across studies (Hasselblad et al., 1995). These practices, if not handled appropriately and with adequate statistical and design consultation, can violate statistical assumptions related to independence and can inflate effect sizes. For instance, if more than one finding is used from each study, this gives those particular studies more weight in the overall combined summative statistical conclusion. In studies with more than one outcome, the outcomes cannot be assumed to be independent because they are all taken from the same sample. The meta-analyst must decide whether to use only one outcome per study or to calculate different effect sizes for categories of similar outcomes. Each meta-analyst needs to consider all of these criticisms and plan to control for any threats to the validity of their conclusions.

Integrative reviews and meta-analyses are becoming increasingly common in the nursing literature. Both of these methods use a rigorous, systematic approach that parallels the primary research process in searching, selecting, evaluating, and reporting the literature. Research reviews begin with a problem statement and questions that guide the selection of the literature to be evaluated and extraction of information needed to describe the studies and their findings. Whether to conduct an integrative review or a meta-analysis depends on several factors. The first is the questions one wants to answer. If a reviewer wants to know how effective certain interventions are or the overall strength of the relationship between variables, then a meta-analysis will be necessary. But meta-analysis does take some additional knowledge and skill using certain statistical procedures.

It is clear that meta-analysis is a time-consuming, expensive, and somewhat controversial technique. Nevertheless, many of the necessary approaches used in meta-analysis, such as reporting the statistical test and values used to support conclusions, can only improve the traditional approach to reviewing the literature and reporting research. Meta-analytic techniques promote closer examination of how concepts are defined and measured across studies and can increase clarity about the variable dimensions of a concept and extend knowledge.

SUMMARY

Integrative reviews are useful when an individual is beginning to build knowledge about a concept. A meta-analysis will be necessary if a reviewer plans to build a research program around a specific concept. Meta-analysis extends the integrative review process to determine cumulative effects of combined results of the studies. These methods will provide nurse scientists with evidence on which to develop future studies to contribute to nursing science and to plan changes in nursing practice.

REFERENCES

Anello, C., & Fleiss, J. (1995). Exploratory or analytic meta-analysis: Should we distinguish between them? *Journal of Clinical Epidemiology, 48*(1), 109–116.

Bridges, A., & Thede, L. (1996) Electronic education. Nursing education resources. *Nurse Educator, 21*(5), 11–15, Sept.–Oct.

Broome, M., Lillis, P., & Smith, M. (1989). Pain interventions with children: A meta-analysis. *Nursing Research, 38*(3), 154–158.

Cook, D., Guyatt, G., & Tyan, G. (1993). Should unpublished data be included in meta-analyses? Current convictions and controversies. *Journal of the American Medical Association, 269,* 2749–2753.

Cook, T., Cooper, H., Cordray, D., Hartmann, H., Hedges, L., Light, R., Louis, T., & Mosteller, F. (Eds.). (1992). *Meta-analysis for explanation: A casebook.* New York: Russell Sage Foundation.

Cooper, H. (1987). Literature searching strategies of integrative research reviewers: A first survey. *Knowledge, 8,* 372–383.

Cooper, H. (1989). *Integrating research: A guide for literature reviews.* Beverly Hills: Sage.

Cooper, H., & Hedges, L. (1994) *The Handbook of Research Synthesis.* New York: Russell Sage Foundation.

Crane, J. (1969). Social structure in a group of scientists: A test of the "invisible college" hypothesis. *American Psychological Review, 34,* 335–352.

Fernandez, E., & Turk, D. (1989). The utility of cognitive coping strategies for altering pain perception: A meta-analysis of pain. *Pain, 38*(2), 123-135.

Fleury, J. (1996). Wellness motivation theory: An exploration of theoretical relevance. *Nursing Research, 45*(5), 277-284.

Ganong, L. (1987). Integrative reviews of nursing research. *Research in Nursing and Health, 10*, 111.

Glass, G.V. (1976). Primary, secondary, and meta-analysis of research. *The Educational Researcher, 5*, 1083-1088.

Hasselblad, V., Mosteller, F., Littenberg, B., Chalmers, T., Hunink, M., Turner, J., Morton, S., Diehr, P., Wong, J., & Powe, N. (1995). A survey of current problems in meta-analysis. Discussion for the Agency for Health Care Policy and Research inter-PORT Work Group on literature review/meta-analysis. *Medical Care, 33*(2), 202-220.

Hedges, L., & Olkin, I. (1985). *Statistical methods for meta-analysis*. Orlando: Academic Press.

Internet Health Care Network (1997). Newsletter. URL *http://members.aol.com/wperry/ihn.htm.*

Kerlinger, F. N. (1973). *Foundations of behavioral research* (2nd ed.). New York: Holt, Rinehart & Winston.

Kirkevold, M. (1997). Integrative nursing research—an important strategy to further development of nursing science and practice. *Journal of Advanced Nursing, 25*, 977-984.

Lynn, M. (1989). Meta-analysis: An appropriate tool for the integration of nursing research. *Nursing Research, 38*, 302-305.

Novallo, A., Alampi, M., & Nolan, K. (1997). *Gale directory of databases.* Detroit, MI: Gale Publishing.

Pealer, L., & Dorman, S. (1997). Evaluating health-related web sites. *Journal of School Health, 67*(6), 232-235.

Rosenfeld, R. (1996). How to systematically review the medical literature. *Otolaryngology—Head and Neck Surgery, 115*(1), 53-63.

Rosenthal, K. (1984). *Meta-analysis procedures for social science research.* Beverly Hills: Sage.

Sachs, H., Reitman, D., Pagano, D., & Kupelnick, B. (1996). Meta-analysis: An update. *The Mount Sinai Journal of Medicine, 63*(3-4), 216-224.

Sandelowski, M. (1997). To be of use: Enhancing the utility of qualitative research. *Nursing Outlook, 45*, 125-32.

Smith, M. C., & Stullenbarger, E. (1991). A prototype for integrative review and meta-analysis of nursing research. *Journal of Advanced Nursing, 16*, 1272-1283.

Smith, M. C., & Stullenbarger, E. (1995). An integrative review and meta-analysis of oncology nursing research: 1981-1990. *Cancer Nursing, 18*(3), 167-179.

Thomas, S., Liehr, P., DeKeyser, F., & Friedmann, E. (1993). Nursing blood pressure research 1980-1990: A bio-psycho-social perspective. *IMAGE: Journal of Nursing Scholarship, 25*(2), 157-164.

University of Wisconsin-Milwaukee. (1997) *Databases available for a fee at the Golda Meir Library.* Golda Meir Library-Reference Department. Milwaukee, WI: Author.

Weisberg, J., & Keefe, F., (1997). Personality disorders in the chronic pain populations: Basic concepts, empirical findings and clinical implications. *Pain Forum, 6*(1), 1-9.

Wolf, F. (1986). *Meta-analysis: Quantitative methods for research synthesis.* Beverly Hills: Sage.

14

A Multiphase Approach to Concept Analysis and Development

Judith J. Sadler

Concepts are said to be the "building blocks of theory." Relationships between and among them form the simplest to the most complex theories. Whether isolating factors, describing relationships, predicting relationships, or prescribing relationships in a theory, a clear understanding of what is meant when a concept is used is necessary. This has not been the case for the concept of caring; indeed the lack of clarity continues to plague scholars as they struggle to answer the questions and problems facing the discipline of nursing.

Crigger (1997) described the "Trouble with Caring," stating that "the current conceptualization of caring is too vague to support any substantial theory of nursing" (p. 217). She reiterated what Morse, Solberg, Neander, Bottorff, and Johnson (1990) stated seven years earlier as their conclusions to a concept analysis of caring using an integrative review method:

> . . . knowledge development related to caring in nursing is limited by the
> lack of refinement of caring theory, the lack of definitions of caring
> attributes, the neglect to examine caring from the dialectic perspective,
> and the focus of theorists and researchers on the nurse to the exclusion of
> the patient. (p. 1)

Morse, Bottorff, Neander, and Solberg (1991) further argued that not only was the concept of caring limited from a theoretical perspective, but also in terms of defining the use of caring in clinical practice. According to these authors, "presently the concept is poorly developed, and as a result it may not be comprehensive enough to encompass *all* the components of caring that are necessary to guide clinical practice" (p. 125).

Despite this lack of clarity there has been increased attention to the concept of caring in the discipline of nursing. Because of the increasing use of the concept throughout the professional nursing literature, analysis of the concept of caring demanded a broader approach, solidly founded upon a philosophical base that explored multiple perspectives to begin to answer a conceptual problem for the discipline of nursing: "What is *caring*?"

METHODOLOGICAL BASIS: PHILOSOPHY

Rodgers (1993b) described how concepts develop in an evolutionary fashion. As they are found to solve the problems of the discipline, they become significant to the discipline. As a concept is more widely used, new and different areas are found where the concept can be applied and the use of the concept expanded further. Thus the significance that a concept has, based on its ability to solve problems of the discipline, leads the concept to enjoy a wider use, with this expanded use leading to wider application of the concept in the discipline.

One measure of the significance of a concept to a discipline can be found in the published literature where, Rodgers (1993b) stated, concepts are institutionalized. It follows that a concept of little significance in a discipline would have little published about it and, conversely, a concept of growing or greater significance would have more written about it. Caring is a concept that powerfully supports this evolutionary cycle described by Rodgers (1993b). In the 1970s there were few articles written about caring in nursing. By the 1990s these few articles were joined by thousands of articles in print about caring. Thus one could argue that caring was of growing significance to nursing, yet the question remained, What is *caring*? What are the characteristics of the concept of caring? What significance does *caring* have for the discipline of nursing?

Rodgers' (1993a) contribution to the underpinnings of this study of caring was related to the view of a dynamic process of evolutionary development of a concept. This approach was applied through Schwartz-Barcott and Kim's (1993) "hybrid model" of concept analysis, in which analysis of a concept using data from published literature is combined with observation to support a more refined definition of a concept. To lend additional support to the convergence of findings, a third source of data was used. Nurses practicing on medical surgical units of general hospitals in the Midwest were interviewed. This analysis of the concept of caring in professional nursing was undertaken from an evolutionary philosophy, using multiple data sources to allow for a comprehensive investigation of a concept that was gaining in significance in the discipline of nursing, yet lacked clarity.

METHODOLOGICAL BASIS: PROCEDURE

A procedural map of the process followed to conduct this study is presented in Figure 14-1. The first phase of the study was to conduct an analysis of the concept of caring using the professional nursing literature. The professional nursing literature has been described by Rodgers (1993b) as a way of institutionalizing the use and definition of a concept. The second phase was to conduct an analysis using data generated from interviews with practicing nurses to gain a professional practice perspective. The results of these two phases were then critically compared and analyzed to discern similarities and differences and to develop a refined set of attributes, antecedents, consequences, and references of the concept. Definitions were developed for these refined attributes, antecedents, consequences, and references of the concept and used as a frame for the fourth phase. This phase of the study was conducted to confirm and refine the attributes, antecedents, consequences, and references of the concept through field observation of professional nursing practice. Upon completion of this phase, a final analysis was conducted based on Rodgers' (1993b) evolutionary view of concepts. During this phase the use, application, and significance of caring were identified. Each of these phases of analysis had portions of independence from the previous phase to maintain openness to the findings, yet were guided by and built upon findings from the previous phase. These phases can be viewed as overlapping circles of independent data in each phase, yet yielding areas of overlapping analysis that define and refine the understanding of the concept.

Phase One—Professional Nursing Literature

The first set of data was collected from the professional nursing literature using Rodgers' (1993b) guidelines for population and sample selection. There were 1,801 written works published between 1988 and 1992 selected by using the keyword "caring" in a search of the computerized data base of the Cumulative Index of Nursing and Allied Health Literature. A 20 percent random sample (Rodgers, 1993b) of the population was identified and retrieved.

This population of literature included both books and articles published in professional nursing journals. In an effort to assure that "essential works on [the] topic" (Rodgers, 1993b) were included in the sample, a careful review of the sample was conducted. Through the conduct of this review, it was determined that the random selection included an adequate representation of the books, and chapters within those books,

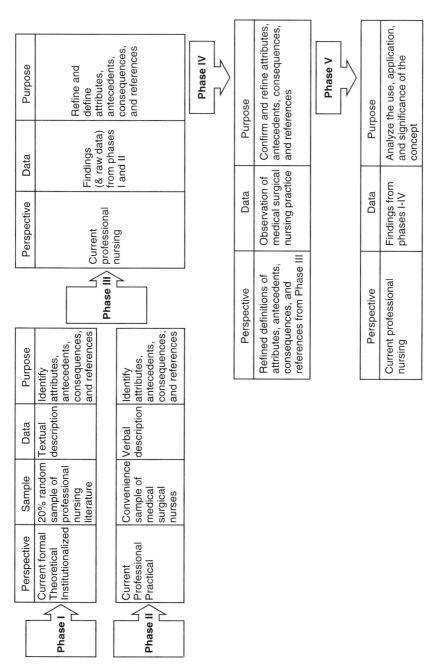

Phase I

Perspective	Sample	Data	Purpose
Current formal Theoretical Institutionalized	20% random sample of professional nursing literature	Textual description	Identify attributes, antecedents, consequences, and references

Phase II

Perspective	Sample	Data	Purpose
Current Professional Practical	Convenience sample of medical surgical nurses	Verbal description	Identify attributes, antecedents, consequences, and references

Phase III

Perspective	Data	Purpose
Current professional nursing	Findings (& raw data) from phases I and II	Refine and define attributes, antecedents, consequences, and references

Phase IV

Perspective	Data	Purpose
Refined definitions of attributes, antecedents, consequences, and references from Phase III	Observation of medical surgical nursing practice	Confirm and refine attributes, antecedents, consequences, and references

Phase V

Perspective	Data	Purpose
Current professional nursing	Findings from phases I-IV	Analyze the use, application, and significance of the concept

Figure 14–1 Procedural map of caring concept analysis.

Table 14–1 Description of the Sample Selected

Category of Selection	Frequency
Articles from professional nursing journals	200
Articles from *Caring* Magazine	91
Books	5
Chapters in books	23
Dissertations (complete)	16
Dissertations (abstract only)	3
Selections deleted	
Computer program	− 1
Australian nursing journal articles not retrievable	− 2
Allied health selections	− 15
Unidentifiable source	− 1
TOTAL SAMPLE	341

frequently referenced in the literature. A summary of the types of publications selected through random sampling and the resulting sample is presented in Table 14-1.

The primary reason for selection of a publication for inclusion in the sample was that the word "caring" appeared in the title (28%). The second highest selection (25% of the sample) was based upon "caring" appearing in the source (book or journal title). This was of concern inasmuch as the magazine titled *Caring* was the reason that many of these were selected, and in many cases, the author of the article did not use the word "caring" in the article. Rodgers' (1993b) position on the role of socialization in the development of concepts supports the use of these sources. She stated, "although concepts are individual in nature, the process of abstraction, clustering and association of the concept with a word (or other means of expression) is heavily influenced by socialization and public interaction" (p. 74). This supported the inclusion of these articles in the sample because the analysis of data from these sources represented a process of socialization and public interaction between the writer and the reader with regard to *caring*, and thereby development of the concept of caring in nursing.

Literature Data Analysis

Literature analysis followed Rodgers' (1993b) method. Each publication was read and reread to extract the attributes, antecedents, consequences, and references of caring, which then were entered into a computer data base. In consultation with researchers who were expert in the handling of qualitative data and in concept development, two additional categories for coding the data were added. These categories were, "Caring nurses do . . ." and "Caring nurses are . . ." This addition was made on the basis of the large number of instances in which "caring" behaviors or attributes of "caring" nurses or others were described. After coding of the sample was completed, all data in each of the categories were placed into a new data base document that allowed the investigator to work with the data, organizing the data into themes and descriptive categories. Once these groups of similar data were developed and structured into recurrent themes, a short label was created to describe the content of each particular group. This process continued until all relevant data were categorized. From this labeling, a definition of caring was developed along with a description of antecedents, references, and consequences. The final step was to review and critique the category of "related concepts" to determine if the data in this category really reflected concepts that were different from the concept of caring or were surrogate terms for caring.

Literature Analysis Findings

A preponderance of authors referred to the centrality of the concept of caring in nursing. Whether they noted it as the "essence of nursing" or a central component of nursing, the importance that these authors placed upon the concept in professional nursing was clear. Despite this consistency in emphasis, there were wide variations in the presentations of the concept of caring in the literature; it was possible to identify the predominant attributes of the concept. In several instances, data in antecedent categories were similar to data found as attributes, and in a few instances, consequences were described by similar data. These similar descriptive categories of data found in conditions that precede caring, describe the characteristics of caring, and are outcomes of caring could be presented as forming a spiral (rather than circular) and weblike nature to the concept. It is difficult to discuss and describe one aspect of the concept without crossing and becoming intertwined in another thread of the web. Brief descriptions of the findings from the first two phases are presented with a more detailed discussion presented for phase three. A detailed presentation of the development of the definition from the attributes, consequences, antecedents, and references found in the literature can be found in previous publications (Sadler, 1995, 1998).

Attributes. The attributes or characteristics of the concept "constitute a real definition, as opposed to a nominal or dictionary definition . . . and make it possible to identify situations that fall under the concept" (Rodgers, 1993b, p. 83). The attributes identified in the literature for *caring* were labeled: *process, presence, creative, contextual,* and *transformational relationship.* Authors consistently presented caring as a process. Caring was discussed as interactive in nature and developed with intentional action of the nurse. Caring was referred to as *work* in several instances, lending support to the attribute of process.

From the literature analyzed, caring as a process is developed through *presencing*. The nurse created a relationship with the patient through the use of self in a particular manner, described as *presence*. In the process of caring, the therapeutic use of self included the learned instrumental, physical interventions to meet patients' needs, as well as the more traditional psychosocial approaches the nurse used to create a therapeutic relationship. The *presence* label was descriptive of a category of data that included physical interventions, as these physical interventions were accomplished in a specific manner, with therapeutic intent, in a particular relationship.

Although the attribute labeled *creative* was underdeveloped in the data related to caring, it was present to a sufficient extent to consider it an attribute. An intuitive, intersubjective knowing of what to do and how to do it is reflected by this attribute. The relationship formed through caring itself can be viewed as an individualistic *creation*, something of unique beauty, much like a work of art. The attribute *creative* also describes what might be called the *expressive* form of nursing, sometimes noted by authors as going beyond the usual.

From a philosophical perspective that concepts are individual, private in nature, and developed with guidance from the social context in which the person interacts (Rodgers, 1993b), it was not surprising that the concept of caring was contextual in the literature analyzed. The expression of caring was described differently depending upon the context. The contextual nature of caring was noted in the different descriptions given by people in different roles and positions within an organization, between different populations and cultures, and in the various approaches used in different situations. Caring interactions vary with the time available to the nurse, the responsiveness of the patient (Samarel, 1991), and the need that the patient presents (Chase, 1990).

The attribute of *transformational relationship* is the core of the concept of caring. The key to caring is the process of forming this relationship. This type of relationship is unique in that it is formed with deliberation. There is a moral commitment for the nurse/teacher to achieve some end, such as the meeting of a patient's/learner's need. The relationship is holistic in that both participants are wholly present in the relationship, bringing with them their unique backgrounds, experiences, and being to the current relationship. The relationship also is transformational in that both participants in the caring occasion are changed. The condition or need calling forth the caring process is met and moral growth occurs for both. The attributes explicated in this analysis show that caring can be defined as a particular kind of process characterized by creativeness, context, presence, and the formation of a transformational relationship.

Antecedents. The antecedents of caring derived through the analysis of the literature included knowledge-based competence, resources, and intentional moral commitment. Caring as discussed by authors of the literature examined was founded upon a knowledge base that includes skills, cognition, attitude, and behavior. Examples such as technical knowledge, scientific knowledge, communication skills, professional values, and learned skills were found in the literature. In addition, there was an assumption in much of the literature that the nurse needed to possess a basic skill level to be caring. The context specificity of caring commands that the nurse possess a broad knowledge base that includes which intervention to use and competence in the practice of the specific skills to be applied. In particular, when authors wrote about the instrumental acts of caring, structured education for the nurse was described as preceding caring.

Consequences. Consequences, what happens after an instance of the concept of *caring* occurs, or what results from *caring*, included the promotion of health and healing, mutual moral growth, human survival, and burden. The theme *promotion of health and healing* was recognized easily in the literature. For example, *alleviation of suffering*, improved functioning, and relief of tension and pain were described as outcomes of caring. Whereas moral maturity was a precondition for caring, moral growth was discussed as an outcome. The moral aspect of caring was a particular aspect that described caring as a process with a spiraling effect. Although caring was preceded by a state of moral maturity and was characterized by a mature moral response, the process of caring was characterized as leading to moral growth. Moral growth was described as a developmental process noted similarly in the descriptions given by various authors. Authors wrote about this growth as knowledge of self, particularly as it related to knowing oneself as a caring being. Moral growth included mental and spiritual growth and knowledge of oneself, which in turn, led to a new higher level of caring potential.

References. References describe the contexts or situations in which an instance of the concept might occur (Rodgers, 1993b). In this study, they describe actual situations where one would expect to observe caring. From the literature, the data were coded into the following categories: multiple sociological contexts, multidimensional relationship, and person in need.

Surrogate Terms

Care was the only consistently used surrogate term for caring. This may be related to the grammatical form of the term *caring*, which may be used as a gerund for the concept of care. Care, as a noun, was defined for example, as "a variety of interventions designed to resolve a problem related to the health of the patient" (Norris, 1989, p. 546). However, the term did not relate the process, the interactive nature of caring, and tended to be used to describe only the physical acts, or nursing interventions. In this instance one can provide *care* or *nursing care* or *HS (hour of sleep) care*. The terms *care* and *caring* were used interchangeably by some authors, although other authors noted some distinction between these ideas. The interchangeability is best illustrated by a description of how one widely referenced author, Leininger, who has continued to write about care/caring over a prolonged period, has changed in how she used the two terms.

In one of her earliest writings Leininger (1977) stated, "For me *caring* [emphasis added] is the essence of nursing and is the most central and unifying focus for nursing decisions, practices, and goals" (p. 2). In this selection, Leininger distinguished between care and caring and often used both terms in the same sentence. "While I have found no universal definition of caring, nursing care, or care to date. . . . To date I have identified seventeen major constructs related to care, caring behaviors and caring processes" (p. 14). She used caring as an adjective to describe behaviors, processes, and rituals. However, in the second set of National Caring Conference papers, Leininger (1984/1988), with almost the same words that she had used earlier to define caring, defined *care* [emphasis added] as "the essence and the central, unifying, and dominant domain to characterize nursing . . . postulated to be an essential human need for the full development, health maintenance, and survival of human beings in all world cultures" (p. 3). Because many of the authors selected in the literature sample for this study quoted Leininger as the basis for their definition of caring, there were variations in definitions, descriptions, and use that depended upon which of Leininger's publications they referenced.

Related Concepts

Related concepts are those concepts that bear some relationship to caring, but do not share the same set of attributes. In this analysis the following were identified as related concepts and, because of their similarity, tended to fall into clusters: care, caretaking, and caregiving; work and help; virtue and ethics; stress and coping; presence, advocacy, and empathy. When *care* was used as a surrogate term, it was used most often (but not exclusively) in regard to physical acts performed by a person to meet another's need. When used to indicate a related concept, however, there was not a clear distinction between the terms *care* and *caring*. The term *caregiver* was used most often to describe a person giving physical care. Caregiving was used similarly to reflect acts and activities done by a caregiver, which, in the majority of this literature, referred to a person other than a professional nurse.

A cluster of related concepts were those described as *virtue* and *ethics*. Many authors frequently used the phrase "an ethic of care," with these concepts related to the idea that *caring* involved values associated with morality and ethics. This value guided the actions of the nurse and sometimes was described as an ideal to which the nurse aspired.

Various authors presented the concepts of stress and coping together. Codependency and burnout were concepts also included in this cluster. Coping was a positive concept related to the stresses of caring, whereas burnout and codependency were presented as negative concepts.

Presence, advocacy, and empathy were used by the authors to describe acts of the nurse in providing care or establishing the caring relationship. They were further described in some instances by other adjectives such as *existential advocacy* and *disciplined presence*. The related concepts described in some instances, for example *work*, tended to be used to describe actions that were like caring, whereas others related to acts and activities in forming caring such as advocacy and presence.

Caring People and What They Do

The data coded in the two categories of "caring people are . . ." and "caring people do . . ." were analyzed after preliminary analyses of the attributes, references, antecedents, consequences, surrogate terms, and related concepts were completed. These data involved the reporting of peoples', especially nurses', outward manifestations of the concept of caring. Data coded in the category "caring people do . . ." supported the labels assigned to the attributes and further clarified caring as a process.

The category of "caring people are . . ." described what caring people are like, or the outward manifestations of a "caring" person. Authors consistently described caring people as morally mature, honest, unselfish, acting as advocates, empathic, and sensitive in preserving the care recipient's dignity and integrity. The data coded in the categories of "caring people are/do . . ." supported the attributes by using many of the same terms to describe the outward manifestations of the concept in the way a caring person acted and responded to an "other."

From this analysis of the literature, a definition of caring was developed: Caring is a contextually defined, creative process whereby the nurse uses presence in a transformational relationship. Development of a definition based on analysis of the literature can be considered an end point in an investigation to clarify a concept (Rodgers, 1993b). Consistent with a goal of exploring other areas for development of the concept (Rodgers, 1993b), however, the findings from analysis of the literature served as a source for comparison and critique of the findings from analysis of interviews with nurses practicing on medical surgical units in acute care hospitals, which was the focus of the second phase of the study.

Phase Two—Caring as Reported by Practicing Nurses

Although Rodgers (1993b) primarily described use of the literature as the source of data for analysis of the concept of interest, she stated that the "ultimate goal is to generate a rigorous design consistent with the purpose of the study" (p. 79). Rodgers (1993b) also has advocated the use of other forms of data, such as from interviews, to expand efforts to develop concepts. Inasmuch as the purpose of the study was to analyze the concept of *caring* from a broad base, a second data set was formed from verbal descriptions of *caring* obtained through interviews with practicing medical-surgical nurses. Similar to the broad population selected for the analysis based on the literature, the area of medical surgical nursing was selected because this continues to be a predominant area of practice for nurses. Further, this area represents the generalized nature of nursing practice within hospital settings and involves a more diverse patient population than the specialized areas of practice. This supported the potential for more varied responses from the nurses interviewed, which in turn enhanced the richness of the data.

The 20 nurses who volunteered to be interviewed were currently practicing nursing on a medical surgical unit at one of three hospitals contacted by the researcher and worked at least 16 hours per week. Although other demographic data were collected from each interviewee (Table 14-2), they were not used as selection criteria. Following informed consent procedures, each nurse participated in a focused interview lasting 20 to 45 minutes. These interviews were structured ac-

Table 14-2 Frequency of Selected Demographic Characteristics of the Sample

Age		Gender		Highest Nursing Education		Years of Nursing Experience	
25–29	2	Male	4	Diploma	6	1 or less	1
30–34	4	Female	16	Associate Degree	1	2–3	2
35–39	3			BSN	7	4–5	1
40–44	6			MSN	2	6–10	4
45–49	3			MSN (student)	4	11–15	4
50–54	1					16–20	0
55–59	1					21 & over	8

cording to the characteristics of concept analysis described by Rodgers (1993b).

Interview Data Analysis

These interviews were then transcribed verbatim and accuracy was assured by carefully reading each transcript while listening to the corresponding tape. The text was imported into the Data Collector (Turner & Handler, 1992), a qualitative data management computer program.

Once the coding of the data from the interviews was completed, placing each unit of text into appropriate categories consistent with the analysis of a concept (attributes, antecedents, consequences, references), data represented by the code words were organized into categories and analyzed for similarities to discover recurrent themes. A short label was created to describe the particular attribute, antecedent, consequence, or reference. This process continued until all relevant data were categorized. From the identification of the attributes, a definition of caring was developed, comprised of a list of antecedents, references, and consequences. The final step was a review and critique of the category of related concepts to determine whether these ideas were really different concepts or were actually surrogate terms for *caring*.

Interview Findings

Of these 20 nurses, 11 worked at one hospital, four at one hospital, and five at a third hospital. All interviewees worked on units where patients with medical surgical conditions were placed for care. Patients on these units had been diagnosed with a wide array of medical or surgical conditions including cardiac, orthopedic, oncological, surgical, and neurological diagnoses. In general, the nurses interviewed found it difficult to offer a clear definition of caring. They offered varying descriptions and definitions of what caring was for them. However, despite the variations in the definitions, there were common themes and attributes that could be extracted. From the analysis of the data generated in these interviews, a definition of the concept of *caring* was formed. For these nurses, *caring* is individually and socially defined multidimensional work where a holistic connection is made with a person to meet a recognized need.

Attributes. Attributes identified from the interview data were *multidimensional work, holistic connection, individually and socially defined*, and *recognition of need*. Caring, for the nurses interviewed, was the multidimensional work of meeting patients' recognized needs. According to these nurses, caring was not universal, but depended upon the ability and competence of the nurse. Caring was further described by the attribute of holistic connection. This connection was characterized by a nonverbal psychic link with the patient and included giving and touching. Nurses also described this connection as including trust, feeling, and intimacy. Although there were descriptions of this attribute including individual aspects of the person such as physical, spiritual, psychological, and emotional, these were combined with the wholeness of the nurse and patient in making this connection. The nurses described holistic connection as a requirement for caring, a responsibility to recognize if this connection could not be made, and a responsibility to find another nurse who could make the connection with the patient.

Individually and socially defined was a label given to data that described caring as having a characteristic of being defined by the individuals in the situation as well as formed by social expectations. Nurses described how individual patients had different expectations of what they considered caring and the nurse had to explore the patient's definition to meet his or her expectations. Nurses also described how caring was socially defined and varied among hospital contexts and also changed over time.

Antecedents. The antecedents of caring identified from the interviews of medical surgical nurses were intentional moral commitment, time/ resources, and experiential learning. Several themes within the data were collapsed to form the antecedent of intentional moral commitment. These themes were labeled *intent, moral maturity, respect for person, choice,* and *commitment.* Interviewees described making a choice as preceding caring. The idea of choice included the choice of *caring* as life work or career and in the choice involved in each individual encounter. Nurses described weighing alternatives and options to reach a decision of whether to be caring or not. One stated, "There's going to be choices because, number one, you're only human and you react to people."

The category of data labeled *time/resources* was discussed by participants in regard to *staffing levels* and *time constraints* and what happened when these were limited rather than the nurse having enough time and resources. Time constraints were related to the nurses' need to prioritize and revealed *work* as a characteristic of caring. Because of time constraints, the interviewees noted the need to prioritize the needs of the patients that they were responsible for to be able to meet as many needs as possible within the time constraints of the day. Interviewees described staffing levels and patient census as affecting the time available for caring. Although time was noted to be necessary for caring to occur, a specific amount was not described other than a description of how more time would be helpful.

Consequences. Data from the interviews clustered into the consequences of met need, satisfaction, health/healing, and sustain/develop humanity. Generally, the nurses interviewed spoke of the consequence of caring in rather simplistic terms of meeting the identified need, whatever it happened to be. Some described it in regard to patient progress or the patient "getting better." Nurses used phrases that described a process of healing using descriptions such as *more relaxed, comfortable,* and *relief from pain*, with these phrases often related to a particular disease process.

References. Because the interviews were limited to nurses practicing on medical surgical units in acute care hospitals, there was little distinction made by the interviewees of particular contexts or patient types where caring occurred. Situations involving suffering and dying were discussed specifically by the interviewees. However, the primary context in which caring occurred for these nurses concerned any patient in need.

Surrogate Terms and Related Concepts. With the exception of the word "nurturing" used by one interviewee, these nurses did not describe any words that they would use interchangeably with caring. Some interviewees identified that *nursing, love, touching, helping,* and/ or *kindness* would be considered in some situations to be the same as caring. However, interviewees were clear that caring was the umbrella concept that encompassed the words that they offered as similar. None of these other terms were thought to capture adequately what the interviewees described as the concept of caring. The interviewees were explicit in stating that these words were not the same as *caring*, but rather were parts of *caring*.

The definition of caring developed from this phase of the analysis was "Caring is individually and socially defined multidimensional work where a holistic connection is made with a person to meet a recognized need." Caring was described as happening in a relationship with a patient in need. Interviewees reported that caring interactions with others promoted a process of development of the nurse as a person.

Upon completion of this phase, a comparison and analysis of the findings of the first two phases using the professional nursing literature and interviews with nurses practicing on medical surgical units in acute care hospitals was conducted. At this stage of the investigation, the two sources of data revealed similar, yet distinct, definitions of the concept of *caring*. Phase three was conducted to analyze further these differences and similarities and to develop a refined set of attributes, antecedents, references, and consequences.

Phase Three—Literature and Interview Analysis

A table was constructed listing the attributes, antecedents, consequences, and references identified in each of the first two phases to facilitate a side-by-side comparison. Beginning with the attributes, each of the categories of data was analyzed further to find the areas of agreement. Second, differences in the data obtained in each phase were identified and comparisons made across the data. There was a back-and-forth analysis of the data in each data set to answer questions concerning why there were differences. The first question asked was whether the data were similar, but merely labeled differently. This analysis at times included a review of the text of the interviews or rereading the source of the data from the literature to analyze the differences or similarities. If the investigator found that the data were similar, but labeled differently, further analysis was completed to determine a label that best described the data. At times, data that had been placed in a particular attribute from one or the other data set were more supportive of a differently labeled attribute in the other data set. The investigator found in several cases that a theme within a particular attribute was supportive of and clarified similar data in the other data set. This process of analysis helped to elucidate the particular attribute.

This procedure was followed for each attribute, antecedent, reference, and consequence. From this analysis, a current definition of the concept of caring as used in the professional nursing literature and in the practice of nursing was constructed, and areas of agreement and disagreement between the definitions derived from the literature and from practicing nurses were identified. The attributes, antecedents, consequences, and references of the concept from the first two phases and the resulting refined ones are presented in Table 14–3.

Attributes. The refined attributes were: individually and socially defined, holistic connection, recognition of need, and creative process of using presence (multidimensional work). Although there were many similarities in the attributes in the two data sets, there also were variations. The opportunity to ask questions to probe the responses of the nurses who were interviewed allowed for explication and refinement of the attributes. *Individually and socially defined* described data that were similar to data from the literature analysis that were labeled *contextual*. Both sets of data defined a characteristic of caring as varying in context, defined by the individuals in the situation and also defined by society. A careful review of both data sets supported the label *individually and socially defined* to capture the richness of both data sources.

The label *holistic connection,* identified through analysis of the interview data, was retained as the refined attribute. This attribute captured

Table 14–3 Development of the Refined Attributes, Antecedents, Consequences, and References

	Attributes	
Literature	*Interviews*	*Refined*
Contextual Transformational relationship	Individually and socially defined	Individually and socially defined
	Holistic connection Recognition of need	Holistic connection Recognition of need Creative process of using presence
Creative Process Presence	Multidimensional work	Multidimensional work

	Antecedents	
Literature	*Interviews*	*Refined*
Competence	Experiential learning	Experiential learning
Resources	Time/resources	Time/resources
Intentional moral commitment	Intentional moral commitment	Intentional moral commitment

Consequences

Literature	Interviews	Refined
Promotion of health/healing	Met need	Promotion of health/healing
	Health/healing	
	Satisfaction	Satisfaction
Human survival	Sustain/develop humanity	Sustain/develop humanity
Mutual moral growth		
Burden		

References

Literature	Interviews	Refined
Multiple sociological contexts	Relationship	Multiple sociological contexts
Multidimensional relationship	Person in need	Multidimensional relationship
Person in need		Person in need

the descriptions of caring as occurring in a person-to-person relationship where change resulted. The nurses interviewed consistently described a *connection* with a patient, rather than a relationship, when caring occurred. Further analysis confirmed that this was also characteristic of the *relationship* as it had been described in the literature. Further clarification of this connection was derived from the nurses' descriptions of the connection as occurring on various levels including physical, emotional, psychological, and, at times, spiritual. The term *holistic* was used to describe this characteristic of the relationship.

The term *transformational* was used as a descriptor of the attribute *relationship* found in analysis of the literature to capture the idea that the relationship was formed for some reason or to meet some identified need and that some change or transformation occurred. The interview data helped to clarify that the idea of purpose was an attribute by itself. Interviewees described a connection with the patient and a separate attribute of *recognition of need*. The interview data also provided clarification in describing that the transformation or change that occurred was an outcome or consequence of caring, rather than embedded in the attribute. The idea of both persons being changed through the caring relationship was not described by the nurses in the same depth as described by the authors of the literature. The nurses interviewed focused more on the changes and growth as an outcome, or consequence, of caring in terms of their own personal development.

Although similar questions could be asked of the data during analysis of each data set, the investigator was able to ask the nurses directly what were the characteristics of caring, and to ask for clarification, thus enabling a more exact distinction between the attributes, antecedents, consequences, and references. The distinction of *recognition of need* as separate, rather than combined with the purpose of the relationship, as it was in the data labeled *transformational relationship*, added descriptive power to the findings. Data in both the literature and the interviews described a characteristic of caring as an ability of the nurse to perceive, know, recognize, determine, or sense the need of the person. This characteristic was labeled *recognition of need*.

The last attribute identified from the analysis of the literature and interview findings was labeled in two variations to more accurately reflect the data in the two sources. The data extracted from the literature tended to support a more theoretical approach that separated out the nuances of caring into creativity (the artistic or expressive form of nursing) and the process of using presence. While authors of the literature reviewed more often described caring as a process, there were a few instances of caring being described as *work*. The nurses interviewed, however, were more explicit in describing this process as *work*. Where, in the literature, authors further described this process in terms of creativity, the interviewees tended to use more practical terms to describe this characteristic. These practical terms were captured more fully through the use of the label *multidimensional* to describe this aspect of the concept of caring. Interviewees used terms such as *meeting physical care needs or emotional needs* to describe this characteristic. The process described in the literature included some reference to competence and skills, but the interviewees were very clear that competence and skills were part of, rather than distinct from, the work of caring.

In the data from the literature, the attribute labeled *presence* included data that described that the nurse used *self* in a relationship with a patient in meeting some need. Again, this is a more theoretical description of what one interviewee stated as [the nurse in caring] "puts herself into her work, uses herself as an instrument, probably the main instrument."

Further analysis of both data sets revealed that, although there were different emphases in each source, the attributes really were parallel. The primary difference may be linguistic only, but there seemed to be a more theoretical approach to the attributes in the literature and a more pragmatic orientation in the nurses' descriptions of the *work* of caring. These labels were maintained to provide the theoretical and the pragmatic perspectives on the definition that was developed as a final step in this analysis. The attributes that describe caring from both data sources are *individually and socially defined, holistic connection, recognition of need,* and *multidimensional work* (or a creative process of using presence). These attributes were used to develop a refined definition of caring. The refined definition is: Caring is an individually and socially defined creative process of using presence, described by practicing nurses as multidimensional work, where a holistic connection is made with a person to meet a recognized need.

Antecedents. The refined antecedents were: *experiential learning, time/resources,* and *intentional moral commitment.* The refined antecedent *experiential learning* was formed from the data that were labeled *competence* from the literature analysis and *experiential learning* from the interview analysis. This antecedent described a level of skill and ability that precede caring in the literature, which was refined with the ideas of personal knowledge in terms of the nurse's *being,* his or her life experiences, as well as educational base from the interviews. The idea that caring developed through lifelong learning and experience was presented clearly by the nurses interviewed. Although competence was described in the literature as preceding caring, skills and knowledge were described by the nurses interviewed as being part of the multidimensional work of caring as an attribute. The idea of learning by building on both formal education and life experiences was described by the nurses interviewed rather than describing competence alone.

The antecedents of *time/resources* and *intentional moral commitment* were found and labeled with the same descriptors in both data sets. In the interview data, time was referred to more often than other resources. In the data from the literature, it was clear that certain structures and processes supported caring. Authors described that time, organizational structure, and supplies were necessary for caring to occur. However, the nurses interviewed described resources more as accounting for the differences in approaches when caring occurs. All three hospitals from which the interviewees were drawn were in some stage of "work redesign." Whereas some hospitals were using *patient focused care*, a trend found in the current literature in health care management as a framework for their redesign, others were in the process of a more generic redesign of the work in the hospital. However, in each case the redesign was in the planning stages or beginning implementation stages and the interviewees were uncertain as to the impact on caring. In both data sets, time was a consistent theme and based upon an analysis of both data sets, and the fact that the data did indicate other resources were important as well, it was determined that the best descriptor of this antecedent was *time/resources*.

Consequences. The consequences refined from the literature and interviews were: *promotion of health/healing, sustain/develop humanity,* and *satisfaction*. The *promotion of health/healing* explicated from the literature analysis was retained as the refined consequence. Interviewees once again were more pragmatic in their descriptions of what occurred following an instance of caring: They rather simplistically described that the identified need was met. In the literature, this idea of met need was embedded in the consequence of promotion of health and healing, although the nurses interviewed also described that health and healing followed caring. By retaining the consequence labeled *promotion of health/healing*, a clear distinction is warranted that this consequence also includes the practical aspect of *met need*, as well as health and healing.

The consequence referred to as *sustain/develop humanity* was retained from the interview data. Whereas in the literature there was a consequence of caring labeled *mutual moral growth*, the nurses interviewed focused on the personal impact and the development of self. There was a theme of moral growth for the nurse in the interview data, but these nurses did not describe moral growth as being mutual, affecting both the nurse and the patient. However, interviewees did describe the aspect of human survival noted in the literature. The label *sustain/develop humanity* captures the data labeled as two separate consequences in the literature: mutual moral growth and human survival. Sustain and develop humanity described the data from both sources that indicated that an outcome of caring is an individual personal change having potential societal or global significance.

The one consequence not found in the literature, but found in the interview data was labeled *satisfaction*. Interviewees were clear that they achieved satisfaction from the work of caring. This supported the idea that the interviewees in general liked what they did as life work and received rewards most often described as nonmonetary rewards and personal fulfillment.

The nurses interviewed did not describe the consequence of *burden* found in the literature. In the literature, this consequence described outcomes related to informal, family care-giving situations. The idea of the work of sustaining caring day after day, with the constraints in the hospital and the intensity of the illnesses of the patients, was embedded in the attribute of multidimensional work and the antecedent of intentional moral commitment. Although interviewees also described how hard it was to continue day after day, they described the rewards as well and no one used the term *burden* to describe a consequence of caring. Thus, burden was not supported either in the literature or by practicing professional nurses as a consequence of the concept of caring in professional nursing practice. The consequences of caring in professional nursing that remain after the analysis of both data sets are *promotion of health/healing, sustain/develop humanity,* and *nurse satisfaction*.

References. The references found in the literature and the interviews were parallel. Where the literature described caring as occurring in multiple sociological contexts, the limitation of the interviews to nurses practicing on medical surgical units of hospitals narrowed this distinction. There was an assumption that the context of caring in this situation was with the hospitalized ill person. Although the literature was also broader in describing caring as happening with a person in need, again the limitation of the interviews to medical surgical nurses narrowed the data in the interviews to primarily "patients in need," with a few references to other persons in need.

In the literature, one reference was labeled *multidimensional relationship* and in the interview data, it was labeled as *occurring in relationship*. The multidimensional nature of caring was embedded in the *holistic connection* and the *multidimensional work* attributes found in the interviews. However, upon a review and analysis of interview data regarding this reference, there were examples that supported the descriptor of *multidimensional* for this relationship. For example, one interviewee described the multidimensional nature in terms of how well one knows the other person, from strangers that one greets in passing to families of patients, and then a deeper level with patients that one works with more and gets to know better. Several interviewees described the multidimensional relationship similarly to the descriptions found in the literature in terms of levels of emotional, physical, and physiological aspects. One interviewee described how the relationship was limited in her previous experiences as an operating room nurse to the level of technological caring. Thus, a conclusion was reached that the relationship can be described as multidimensional in both data sources. Based on analysis of the combined data sets, the references of *caring*, or the situations in regard to which the concept of *caring* is used, are *multiple sociological contexts, multidimensional relationship,* and *person in need*.

Conclusion

The similarities in the findings from the two data sources are substantial. Several of the differences relate primarily to limiting the source of the interview data to practicing medical surgical nurses. Thus, a conclusion can be made that the literature offered a broad theoretical definition, whereas the practicing nurses offered a more practical definition specific to the nurses' experiences. The main difference was found in one attribute. This attribute was labeled *multidimensional work* in the data from the interviews. In the analysis of the professional nursing literature comparable attributes were labeled *process, creative,* and *presence*. The three attributes could be combined into the more descriptive phrase *a creative process of using presence*, which captures the theoretical, idealistic nature of the attribute. Although these two attributes could be combined into one, each of the perspectives would suffer. The idealistic, theoretically rich descriptors would be embedded into the "work world" definition of the practicing nurse, which has its own unique richness. Thus, the definition of caring formed from the analysis of the two data sources is: *Caring is an individually and socially defined creative process of using presence (described by practicing nurses as multidimensional work), where a holistic connection is made with a person to meet a recognized need.*

The analysis combining the findings from the literature and interviews served to provide a deeper understanding of caring in professional nursing. Either source alone would have limited the understanding to one perspective—what the researcher has termed *theoretical* contrasted to the *practical*. Although the findings from either of the first two phases can be considered "final products," there are obvious limitations that become evident when the two sources are analyzed concurrently. The refined findings provide depth and breadth of understanding and served as a base for the researcher to conduct phase four—a field observation of nursing practice on medical surgical units in acute care hospitals.

Phase Four—Field Observation

While Schwartz-Barcott and Kim (1993) described this phase as "aimed at refining a concept by extending and integrating the analysis begun in phase one with ongoing empirical observations" (p. 113), the aim of the field observation phase of this study was to observe for the occurrence of caring in practice as defined from the literature and interviews of practicing nurses in the first two data sets. Rodgers' (1993b) framework was used to guide the observation.

Rodgers (1993b) described the identification of attributes as the primary accomplishment of the concept analysis. These "attributes . . . constitute a *real* definition . . . [and] . . . make it possible to identify situations that can be characterized appropriately using the concept of interest" (Rodgers, 1993b, p. 83). With this framework as a guide, the investigator sought to identify the characteristics of caring that were observable in the setting of medical surgical nursing practice.

The researcher chose medical surgical units in an acute care hospital as the site for the observation to continue building on the understanding of the concept of caring gained from the first analyses. This setting represented the generalized nature of nursing practice in the hospital, a relatively large, diverse, patient population, and a high number of nurses working at any one time, which increased the potential for observing occurrences of caring. Further, the investigator's familiarity with nursing practice in these areas helped to create and sustain observation in the setting. A participation level for the investigator was chosen where the participants were aware of the role of the investigator as interested in the situation and able to ask questions for clarification. This allowed the observer to be " 'kind of' a member of the group allowing them to quickly minimize, even temporarily forget [the researcher's] presence, and thus return the situation to nearly 'normal' " (Schatzman & Stauss, 1973, p. 60).

Once the hospital had given permission for the conduct of the observation, mapping of the chosen unit was completed over a period of seven hours over five different observational times. An intensive interview was conducted with the Assistant Nurse Manager of the unit to obtain background data and a detailed description of the unit. The researcher attended a staff meeting where introductions were made by the Nurse Manager prior to beginning observation to facilitate entry and gain the trust of the nursing staff.

Observation started after that meeting and was facilitated when the investigator began at the time that the particular shift started. Once the assignments were made for the shift, the investigator selected a geographic area to begin observation and requested permission from the nurse to observe her practice. The investigator reminded the nurse that the purpose of the observation was neither for evaluation nor judgment of nursing practice. Only one nurse declined to be observed. All the nurses in this setting were female with the exception of the Assistant Nurse Manager. Therefore, the feminine pronoun is used in references to the nurse.

Periods of time beginning with two hours and building to complete eight-hour shifts were used for observation during daytime and evening shifts. The researcher observed during 12 different time periods over a span of two months. Seven nurses were observed by following them during part or their entire shift for a total observation time of 60 hours. Schatzman and Strauss's (1973) notation format was used including observational notes, theoretical notes, and methodological notes.

Observation Analysis

Data analysis was concurrent with data collection. Theoretical notes served as preliminary analysis for the investigator, helping to chronicle thoughts, and to check and test ideas (Schatzman & Strauss, 1973). Preliminary analysis began with the writing of the field notes after each observational period. The field notes were exported into the Data Collector (Turner & Handler, 1992) qualitative data management computer program. At the suggestion of a consultant who is an experienced field researcher, short working definitions were developed for each of the attributes, antecedents, consequences, and references that were found in the literature and the interviews as an aid to the investigator in the analysis. These definitions assisted the investigator to analyze the data and determine appropriate placement of the field data into predefined categories. The computer program was used to collect the coded data into one document for each attribute, antecedent, reference, and consequence for further analysis. This provided for a back-and-forth analysis process that was similar to the procedures followed in the analyses of the literature and interview data.

Fieldwork data were compared and contrasted with the definition developed from the first phases to find areas of similarities and areas of dissimilarities. Definitions and themes that described the antecedents, consequences, references, and related concepts from each phase were analyzed. Analysis included whether there were incidents in the fieldwork that were similar to findings from the analysis of the theoretical and empirical interface phase. Characteristics of caring that were observable in nursing practice and characteristics that differentiate caring from other similar concepts were identified.

Observation Analysis Results

Based on 60 hours of observation of nursing practice on a 50-bed medical surgical unit in a religiously affiliated community hospital, the investigator came to agree with previously published authors. The ideas that caring is invisible work (Baines et al., 1991; Roberts, 1990; Watson, 1990) and is frequently conspicuous in its absence (Rieman, 1986) were supported. Although certain characteristics of caring were observed, frequently when the investigator would have expected to observe caring, characteristics of the concept were notably absent.

An overarching attribute, that of *individually and socially defined*, was evident in the overall milieu of the unit and the manner in which nursing care was organized and delivered. Organization of the tasks of nursing were supported by structures for reporting patient information that included written summaries by the nurse from the preceding shift, supplies and medications located in each patient room, and clear assignment of responsibility. Nurses would offer assistance to other nurses who had demonstrated caring behaviors when those nurses appeared to be falling behind in meeting their schedule. This overall sense of the organization of work supported the definition of caring for the nurses.

The characteristic of caring as multidimensional work was evident during much of the observation time and in many ways was embedded in the ordinariness of the workday. The theoretical characteristic found in the literature labeled *creative process of using presence*, which parallels the attribute of *multidimensional work* described by practicing nurses through interviews, was observed in a few, arresting, extraordinary occasions. Although *recognition of need* and *holistic connection* were observed, these two attributes were noticeable particularly when they were absent.

The antecedents of *experiential learning, time/resources,* and *intentional moral commitment* were observed in variations in levels of caring. The investigator attempted to ascertain, when possible, which of the antecedents were missing when one would expect to see caring and did not. There were a few occasions observed that could be considered "negative" intent. These included an instance where a nurse loudly announced that just because she admitted the patient did not mean that she was the primary nurse. While one nurse observed had time available to respond to a patient, she was observed to tell the Diabetic Educator that she did not know why the patient was not responding, and stated, "Why don't you just come back tomorrow?"

Demonstrating the antecedent of experiential learning, nurses routinely used resources on the unit and each other to find the answers to questions and review procedures before attempting them. This quest for learning did not stop for nurses with more years of experience. One of the nurses with the longest employment history on the unit was observed frequently seeking out additional information. This nurse also repeatedly asked the investigator how she could improve her nursing practice.

Consequences were difficult to observe as they often are defined from the perspective of the one who receives *caring*, and patients were not interviewed in this study. What could be considered to be consequences tended to be observed in the themes that were identified in the first two data sets such as *relaxation* and *relief of pain*. Thus, the investigator could observe that needs were met or relaxation occurred, while the consequence of *promotion of health/healing* could not be determined to occur as consequences of occasions of caring. Similarly, *satisfaction* was difficult to observe. Satisfaction tends to be conveyed to another by verbal comments or written communication. The consequence of satisfaction was not observed in this setting because the investigator neither saw written communication reporting satisfaction nor heard verbal comments reporting satisfaction. However, a few instances could be construed to indicate satisfaction from caring occasions. Patients were observed to be resting comfortably after occasions of caring were observed. A patient who had demonstrated nervous shaking of her legs and yelling at the nurse was observed to be resting quietly in bed and would smile upon the nurse's return to the bedside.

Although the aim of this observation was to find what characteristics of caring were observable in nursing practice, the investigator found that the field notes developed during observations tended to chronicle what the nurse did and her behaviors in her interactions with patients over the time observed. This supported the characteristics of caring as a part of the nurses' *being* and the use of self as the instrument of caring. This was also found in the literature in the data that the investigator had labeled *caring people do* and *caring people are*.

In observations, the *caring* nurse was seen to be accessible to her assigned patients. She responded to the patient when she was paged and often met needs of the patient so that she had few, if any, calls for assistance from her assigned patients. While the nurse who demonstrated caring put the patient first, she also was skillful in organizing her work so that she had time for breaks and meals.

The findings in this phase confirmed what was described by authors of the literature and by practicing nurses and formed the attributes, antecedents, consequences, and references of caring. This phase was particularly helpful in determining the use, application, and significance of the concept of caring in nursing, the focus of phase five, the final analysis.

Phase Five—Final Analysis

The final analysis was completed using Rodgers' (1993b) evolutionary philosophy of concepts. The significance, use, and application of the concept were analyzed from the data gathered and analyzed for this study.

Significance

A preponderance of authors referred to the centrality of the concept of caring in nursing. Whether they noted it as the "essence of nursing" or a central component of nursing, the importance that these authors placed upon the concept in professional nursing was clear. From the aspect of defining attributes or characteristics of a concept, one cannot defend with certainty that caring is the central focus of nursing, or the essence of nursing. One could argue that embracing *caring* is the latest in the search for legitimacy and a scientific knowledge base to define the practice realm of nursing. Leininger (1981/1988) reported in the foreword to the proceedings of the first three national caring conferences that:

> Prior to the mid-1970s, there had been virtually no specific focus on caring phenomena and its [sic] relationship to nursing care. Instead, topics at most national meetings were about nurse shortages, unions, economic welfare, legislation, and entry into professional practice and related concerns. There was nothing about the sources of caring knowledge and how caring might distinguish nursing from other disciplines. (Foreword)

In the literature published between 1988 and 1992 and selected for this analysis, the concept of caring received substantial support as a deeply held value and a developing focus for the study of nursing. This finding demonstrates the growing significance and, thus, the increasing use of the concept during the last decade.

The significance of the concept of caring was evidenced by the volume of professional nursing literature published and indexed in one nursing literature index over the selected five-year period. This population of literature was evidence of an emphasis on studying and writing about the concept and included selections about how to teach caring in nursing. Significance was likewise supported by the interviewees who volunteered their time to contribute to an explication of a definition of caring. Although observation of the practice of nursing did not uncover pervasive use of the concept of caring, there were occasions observed of the significance of caring in the setting of medical surgical nursing.

The concept of caring is relatively new in terms of significance in nursing. Earlier in the development of the discipline of nursing, attention was focused upon building a "scientific" basis for nursing practice; concepts of significance to resolve the problems of the discipline were concepts that could be studied "scientifically." Thus, emphasis was placed upon concepts that were measurable, observable, and "concrete." Concepts such as caring may have been believed to be too "soft" to warrant attention because they did not possess "significance" for nursing as defined by Rodgers (1993b).

In the literature there was a predominance of references that cited the early pioneers in the study of caring, particularly Leininger, who began to publish articles about caring in 1976. Of particular importance is that Leininger (1981/1988) described that in 1976 she and Dr. Jody Glittenberg presented a program on the general subject of caring as the "essence of nursing" during the 1976 American Nurses Convention. This event was followed by the National and now International Caring Conferences beginning in 1978 (Leininger, 1981/1988, 1984/1988, 1988; Gaut, 1992, 1993; Gaut & Leininger, 1991; Leininger & Watson, 1990). Leininger was visionary in her identification of the potential of the concept of caring to address "a critical need to establish caring as our *central and unique focus of the discipline* . . . [which] could greatly advance the profession and help the public more fully understand nurses' contribution to society" (Foreword). From a historical perspective, these events could be considered the initial identification of the potential for the significance of caring in nursing.

This position of significance is further supported by recent publications. Jacques (1993) described the project of theorizing caring work as "important, not just to the future of nursing, but to our fundamental understanding of work, organizing, and social experience of our time" (p. 10). Similarly, Sullivan and Deane (1994) called for nursing's reinvestigation of caring—"the moral value which their predecessors cherished, protected, and passed on" (p. 9). Chinn (1994) described the significance of caring in terms of balancing "technocratic materialism" in society in the foreword to *Being Called to Care* (Lashley et al., 1994). Chinn (1994) stated, "Caring, a notion that is sometimes trivialized as merely something everyone can do, requiring little or no educational prowess, cannot be easily dismissed in a world that has been rendered spiritually bankrupt by a century of run-away technocratic materialism" (Foreword). These publications are additional evidence of the continued significance of the concept of caring to nursing and are quite clear in stating that caring currently holds a central role in nursing.

Use of the Concept of Caring in Nursing

In 1981, Gaut defined the concept of caring in terms of action. Benner and Wrubel in 1989 claimed that caring is primary in the "relationships between caring, stress and coping, and health" (p. xi). Benner and Wrubel further described caring as setting up "the condition that something or someone outside the person matters and creates personal concern" (p. 1) and that caring is "the enabling condition of nursing practice (indeed, of any practice)" (p. 7). Ten years after Gaut's analysis of caring, and in contrast to Benner and Wrubel's position, Bishop and Scudder (1991) and Bottorff (1991) argued that nursing is the practice of caring, combining practice and feeling, caring and concern. Swanson (1993) has refined that argument to propose that "nursing is the informed caring for the well-being of others" (p. 352). Although Bishop and Scudder did not use the term *informed* in their definition of the practice of caring, they clearly described that caring has an aspect of competence that is integral to the practice. In this study, the attribute of *multidimensional work*, which had a clear component of knowledge-based competence, was similar to these authors' positions of a knowledge base for caring in nursing. Using Rodgers' (1993b) definition of *use* as "the common manner of employing the concept and the situations appropriate for its use" (p. 76), a conclusion could be reached that several authors (Bishop & Scudder, 1991; Bottorff, 1991; Swanson, 1993) present nursing as the *use* of caring. However, from the analyses in this study, there was only some beginning support for caring holding that position (nursing is the practice of caring) within the discipline of nursing.

Based on the vast support for the significance of caring in nursing from the literature and the widespread description of the use of caring in nursing by authors and interviewees, it was surprising to find that the use of caring in the setting of medical surgical nursing practice was limited. Although the use of caring was observed, it was not observed to be pervasive in the practice of nursing in this setting.

The finding from the interviews was similar to the finding in the literature of descriptions of *caring* nurses and what *caring* nurses do. The descriptions of what behaviors and demeanor nurses use when they use caring were similar in the literature, the interviews, and the observations. This leads to the conclusion that caring has certain defined characteristics that are evident when one uses it. This finding of descriptive characteristics of the person using caring promotes further development of the concept of caring.

Application of the Concept of Caring in Nursing

In the literature, there were descriptions of the application of caring that ranged from use in the teacher-student situations to use with particular patient populations. Beginning with Bevis and Watson's (1989) publication, *Toward a Caring Curriculum: A New Pedagogy for Nursing*, primarily a theoretical presentation to "create a new curriculum-development paradigm for nursing education" (p. 1), there was a beginning description in the literature of the application of caring in the nursing educational setting. Descriptions of the use of the concept of caring in those situations tended to reflect a description of situations, classes, courses, and techniques where teachers had been successful in using and teaching caring.

There also was a beginning application of caring as a moral base for the practice of nursing in the literature examined. Although some authors proposed that caring could be a balance for the technology in health care (caring as "high touch" to balance "high tech"), other authors were more specific in describing caring as providing a moral base for decisions and actions. However, since the completion of this analysis, there have been challenges to this perspective (Crigger, 1997).

Although the nurses who were interviewed worked at three different hospitals on 12 different units, all units where the nurses worked were some variation of areas where patients with medical and surgical conditions were placed for care. The investigator did not ask, but several nurses volunteered that they had worked in other areas of nursing including the operating room, intravenous therapy, intensive care, and obstetrics. In each case, they gave reasons that they had moved to a different area of nursing. In some cases these related to the areas identified in the literature where caring was inhibited. For example, one nurse described what would be considered "existential anxiety" (Holden, 1991). She described how after she had her children she could not work in obstetrics any more. She said:

> I started out in OB and I could eat and sleep and breathe it. And then after I had kids I couldn't stand it. I was just so turned off by the whole thing because my biggest thing was I couldn't imagine being pregnant for nine months and being responsible for something if it went wrong. It was just too nerve wracking for me. I just couldn't do it. So that was it. I couldn't be responsible—that part of it. I couldn't watch that person carry that baby for nine months and have a stillborn or something that if, or feeling like I could have caused it. I never had any kind of situation like that. I just kind of freaked and that was it for OB.

A conclusion can be drawn that there are areas where the use and application of caring are limited in the hospital setting. The nurses interviewed, however, did describe using caring in their everyday practice. They described specific patient conditions such as suffering or dying where caring was particularly applicable. Nurses also described the application of caring to situations with peers and coworkers in their work setting, as well as in their personal lives.

The findings from observation of nursing practice support a conclusion that the individual nurse, through using caring, learns when and where caring is successful and then can apply it in new situations. However, the nurse must have intent to use caring in the situation for him or her to be able to develop knowledge of where and when it works and then to expand the use and application to new situations.

CONCLUSION

The philosophical position that formed the foundation of this study allowed the researcher to choose written works published in a recent time period to analyze the development of a concept of great interest in professional nursing. The development of the methods for this study that built upon Rodgers' (1993a) evolutionary philosophy of concept development and analyzed the concept of caring from the written works, the spoken words of practicing nurses, and observation of nursing practice provided a clear current conceptualization of caring. These multiple perspectives each had a valuable contribution to make in understanding the development of the concept of caring. Together, they promoted findings that were deep and credible descriptors of the current development of the concept.

The findings also form a sound basis for future research. With the knowledge of the context specificity of caring, an analysis of the concept of caring should be extended into other settings and with nurses practicing with different populations. The knowledge that caring involves a relationship provides a basis from which to explore understanding from the patient's perspective. An exploration of the outcomes of caring is needed to determine the efficacy of continued emphasis on this concept in nursing. Through the use of multiple data sources, based on evolutionary concept development philosophy (Rodgers, 1993a) melded with the ideas of hybrid concept analysis (Schwartz-Barcott & Kim, 1993), this study has made significant contributions to the understanding of caring in nursing. A current consensus was identified and the "state of the art" of caring in nursing was described, which provides a firm foundation for further study of caring in professional nursing.

REFERENCES

Baines, C., Evans, P., & Neysmith, S. (Eds.). (1991). *Women's caring: Feminist perspectives on social welfare*. Toronto: McClelland & Stewart.

Benner, P., & Wrubel, J. (1989). *The primacy of caring: Stress and coping in health and illness*. Menlo Park, CA: Addison-Wesley.

Bevis, E., & Watson, J. (1989). *Toward a caring curriculum: A new pedagogy for nursing*. New York: National League for Nursing.

Bishop, A., & Scudder, J. (1991). *Nursing: The practice of caring*. New York: National League for Nursing.

Bottorff, J. L. (1991). Nursing: A practical science of caring. *Advances in Nursing Science, 14*(1), 26–39.

Chase, S. K. (1990). Clinical judgment by critical care nurses: An ethnographic study. (Doctoral dissertation, Harvard, 1990). *Dissertation Abstracts International, 51,* 3170B.

Chinn, P. (1994). Foreword. In M. Lashley, M. Neal, E. Slunt, L. Berman, & F. Hultgren (Eds.), *Being called to care* (pp. vii-viii). Albany: State University of New York Press.

Crigger, N. (1997). The trouble with caring: A review of eight arguments against an ethic of care. *Journal of Professional Nursing, 13,* 217-221.

Gaut, D. (1981). Conceptual analysis of caring: Research method. In M. Leininger (Ed.), *Caring: An essential human need* (pp. 17-24). Thorofare, NJ: Charles B. Slack.

Gaut, D. (Ed.). (1992). *The presence of caring in nursing.* New York: National League for Nursing.

Gaut, D. (Ed.). (1993). *A global agenda for caring.* New York: National League for Nursing.

Gaut, D., & Leininger, M. (Eds.). (1991). *Caring: The compassionate healer.* New York: National League for Nursing.

Holden, R. J. (1991). An analysis of caring: Attributions, contributions, and resolutions. *Journal of Advanced Nursing, 16,* 893-8.

Jacques, R. (1993). Untheorized dimensions of caring work: Caring as a structural practice and caring as a way of seeing. *Nursing Administration Quarterly, 17*(2), 1-10.

Lashley, M., Neal, M., Slunt, E., Berman, L., & Hultgren, F. (1994). *Being called to care.* Albany: State University of New York Press.

Leininger, M. (1977). Caring: The essence and central focus of nursing. Nurses Foundation (Nursing Research Report), pp. 2, 14.

Leininger, M. (Ed.). (1981/1988). *Caring: An essential human need.* Thorofare, NJ: Charles B. Slack.

Leininger, M. (Ed.). (1984/1988). *Care: The essence of nursing and health.* Detroit: Wayne State University Press.

Leininger, M. (Ed.). (1988). *Care: Discovery and uses in clinical and community nursing.* Detroit: Wayne State University Press.

Leininger, M., & Watson, J. (Eds.) (1990). *The caring imperative in education.* New York: National League for Nursing.

Morse, J., Bottorff, J., Neander, W., & Solberg, S. (1991). Comparative analysis of conceptualizations and theories of caring. *Image: Journal of Nursing Scholarship, 23,* 119-126.

Morse, J., Solberg, S., Neander, W., Bottorff, J., & Johnson, J. L. (1990). Concepts of caring and caring as a concept. *Advances in Nursing Science, 13,* 1-14.

Norris, C. M. (1989). To care or not care—questions! Questions! *Nursing and Health Care, 10,* 544-550.

Rieman, D. J. (1986). Noncaring and caring in the clinical setting: Patients' descriptions. *Topics in Clinical Nursing, 8*(2), 30-36.

Roberts, J. E. (1990). Uncovering hidden caring. *Nursing Outlook, 38*(2), 67-69.

Rodgers, B. L. (1993a). Philosophical foundations of concept development. In B. L. Rodgers & K. A. Knafl (Eds.), *Concept development in nursing: Foundations, techniques, and applications* (pp. 7-33). Philadelphia: W. B. Saunders.

Rodgers, B. L. (1993b). Concept analysis: An evolutionary view. In B. L. Rodgers & K. A. Knafl (Eds.), *Concept development in nursing: Foundations, techniques, and applications* (pp. 73-92). Philadelphia: W. B. Saunders.

Sadler, J. (1995). Analysis and observation of the concept of caring in nursing. (Doctoral dissertation, University of Wisconsin Milwaukee, 1995). *Dissertation Abstracts International, 56,* 05B, p. 2564.

Sadler, J. (1998). Defining professional nurse caring: A triangulated study. *International Journal for Human Caring, 1*(3), 12-21.

Samarel, N. (1991). *Caring for life and death.* New York: Hemisphere Publications.

Schatzman, L., & Strauss, A. L. (1973). *Field research: Strategies for a natural science.* Englewood Cliffs, NJ: Prentice-Hall.

Schwartz-Barcott, D., & Kim, H.S. (1993). An expansion and elaboration of the hybrid model of concept development. In B. L. Rodgers & K. A. Knafl (Eds.), *Concept development in nursing: Foundations, techniques, and applications* (pp. 107–133). Philadelphia: W. B. Saunders.

Sullivan, J., & Deane, D. (1994). Caring: Reappropriating our tradition. *Nursing Forum, 29*(2), 5–9.

Swanson, K. (1993). Nursing as informed caring for the well-being of others. *Image: Journal of Nursing Scholarship, 25,* 352–357.

Turner, S., & Handler, M. (1992). *Data Collector* (Version 2.0) [Computer Software]. Santa Barbara, CA: Intellimation.

Watson, J. (1990). The moral failure of the patriarchy. *Nursing Outlook, 38*(2), 62–66.

CHAPTER
15

Methods and Application of Dimensional Analysis: A Contribution to Concept and Knowledge Development in Nursing

Chantal D. Caron and Barbara J. Bowers

The overall purpose of this chapter is to demonstrate how dimensional analysis (Schatzman, 1991) could be used as one alternative for conducting a concept analysis. Concept analysis has been proposed as a way to clarify meanings and uses of concepts in the nursing discipline, and ultimately, to enhance the theoretical soundness of nursing knowledge (Rodgers, 1993; see also Chapter 2). Various approaches to concept analysis have been suggested by nurse researchers; we hope this approach will offer one new avenue to researchers interested in clarifying and developing concepts important to nursing scholarship. Dimensional analysis is particularly relevant to nurse researchers who wish to understand how concepts of interest to nursing are socially constructed, and how they vary across perspectives and contexts. In other words, dimensional analysis offers new understandings about concepts by examining the processes by which they are constructed rather than by looking for essential, universal, or common criteria.

Our intentions with this chapter include: (1) to present a brief introduction to dimensional analysis, including a selective discussion of pragmatism and symbolic interactionism as the philosophical underpinnings of dimensional analysis; (2) to identify the procedures involved in conducting a concept analysis using dimensional analysis; (3) to illustrate, with a specific example, e.g., nurse/client relationships, how to use dimensional analysis in conducting a concept analysis; and (4) to discuss how dimensional analysis can contribute to the development of nursing theories and knowledge. In selecting and using dimensional analysis as a way to explore, and to better understand concepts in nursing, researchers commit themselves to some fundamental premises about the nature of social reality and the purpose of their analysis. The following sections are intended to explicate those premises.

The intellectual roots of dimensional analysis can be found in pragmatism (Dewey, 1938; Schatzman, 1991; Shalin, 1986) and symbolic interactionism (Blumer, 1969; Shalin, 1986). Therefore, an understanding of the philosophy, operations, and implications of dimensional analysis will be enhanced by situating it within this larger intellectual context. The following section provides a brief summary of symbolic interactionism and pragmatist philosophy as they relate to the current discussion only. (The limitation of space and the focus of the current discussion necessitate a very brief and selective presentation of both intellectual traditions and their relationship to dimensional analysis.)

THE INTELLECTUAL ROOTS OF DIMENSIONAL ANALYSIS

Pragmatism

There is general agreement that pragmatism was a major influence on the development of symbolic interactionism. The nature of the impact, however, continues to be the subject of debate (Lindesmith et al., 1975; Shalin, 1986; Stryker, 1980). Specifically, the areas of pragmatism with the most profound influence on symbolic interaction (and therefore on dimensional analysis) include:

1. The pragmatist commitment to reality as always in a state of flux, as created through the human action of selectively attending and carving out reality ("Knowing as carving," Shalin, 1986, p. 10);
2. The pragmatist understanding of social structure as emergent process;
3. The pragmatist view of reality, definitions, and social "objects" as created through and discovered in action;
4. The pragmatist understanding of the person and the environment as mutually constitutive.

Pragmatism is an expansive and complex intellectual tradition having influences on symbolic interactionism, generally well beyond these simple selected areas. The influences on pragmatism indicated here have, however, been identified as those most significant to the development of symbolic interactionism. The nature of these influences can be quickly discerned in symbolic interactionism.

Symbolic Interactionism

Symbolic interactionism, or Chicago School Sociology, is a social psychological theory of human action that is generally associated with the work of Herbert Blumer (Blumer, 1969; Charon, 1997; Lindesmith et al., 1975; Shalin, 1986; Strauss, 1987; Stryker, 1980). Although there are other forms of symbolic interactionism, both currently and historically, the discussion in this chapter assumes symbolic interactionism as articulated by Blumer and the Chicago School Sociologists. The central tenets of symbolic interactionism include:

1. *Reality is socially constructed.* There are no social realities apart from our constructions of them. Interactionists define social objects as anything that humans can think about, the object of thinking. This must be distinguished from the more usual meaning of an object or as anything objective.
2. *Humans act based on constructed meanings, e.g., their definition of the situation or their understanding of the social object.* It is in action, or how individuals and groups act toward something, that the meaning or definition of the situation can be discerned.
3. *Realities, meanings (including social structures) are emergent.* They are constructed, maintained, and changed through human interaction. Human group behavior, including interaction, proceeds by "constant interpretation of each other's ongoing lines of actions" (Blumer, 1969, p. 66). We interact by "taking the role of the other", and seeing the situation and ourselves from the perspective of the other. Social action and interaction is based on the ability to take the role of the other, both generalized and particular other. This is a process defined by Blumer and elaborated by many later interactionists. Taking the role of the other allows us to see ourselves from the perspective of the other (as we have constructed that perspective), to "see" what the other understands, to interpret the meaning of the other's actions, and to anticipate how the other is likely to proceed.
4. *Interaction, as well as social action, all presumes the ability to create and use symbols.* Humans use symbols, primarily language, to communicate. Shared symbols (primarily but not exclusively language) are the basis upon which action and interaction proceed and are understood. Given this, human action can only be understood through an understanding of how the situation is defined by the actors in question, the meanings they attribute to the situation, and the interacting process.

5. *Context is inherent in meanings and realities, not separate from surrounding or containing realities.* Therefore, definitions/realities/meanings cannot be understood apart from context. Context is not simply what can be identified by the actor, or even the researcher, in "the situation." It is, rather, what Mills (1967) identified as "the intersection of history and biography." Context is a complex notion comprised of influences brought by the personal biography of the individual, more immediate influences found in the environment, and more distant and less obvious social, cultural, historical forces. Thus, the construction of reality is never an isolated or individual endeavor. All action and meanings are inherently contextual and therefore social.

Hence, for an interactionist, context includes both immediate and larger social context. This includes history, culture, and other circumstances that systematically contribute to widely shared symbols and perspectives. Most interactionist work has focused on the micro level or context that is close to the actors. There is, however, an opportunity within the interactionist framework to move beyond immediate context and examine the relationship between macro context (including class, race, gender, and other social and historical constructions) and the generation of symbols (Shalin, 1986; Strauss, 1978).

Dimensional Analysis

Dimensional analysis was initially developed by Schatzman (1991) as "a methodological approach to the grounding of theory in qualitative research" (p. 303) and has since been extended to a more general theory of analysis. Dimensional analysis, as a method or set of procedures, is built on and consistent with both pragmatist philosophy and symbolic interactionist theory and "is generally informed by the core ideas and practices in grounded theory." (Schatzman, 1991, p. 303). As such, dimensional analysis incorporates the following assumptions. Reality is (1) socially constructed; (2) always defined from a particular perspective; and (3) contextually situated. Perhaps one of the most important contributions of dimensional analysis is an articulation of the social construction of reality or "defining the situation." Dimensional analysis offers an elaboration of how situations are defined and demonstrates the process by which perspective and context are integrated into the definition of the situation.

The theory suggests that human understanding, the constructing of meaning, or defining the situation proceeds by a process of dimensionalizing, a basic characteristic of human thinking. Dimensionalizing, or defining the situation, involves a process of selecting (implicitly or explicitly) the dimensions that are relevant to the concept (i.e., the social object in symbolic interactionist language). Dimensional analysis explicates the process of selecting and organizing dimensions that are used to define the situation or construct meaning. As part of the selecting and organizing of dimensions, attributions of irrelevance, relevance, and salience are made. These attributions are central to the meanings or definitions that result. In other words, some characteristics, attributes (dimensions), are seen as central to the meaning while others are of less significance or insignificant. The selection of dimensions and their organization is directed by both (1) the perspective of the actor and (2) the context. In this way, both context and perspective are integrated into defining the situation and become part of the situation. Changing the context therefore alters the definition or meaning of the social object. A new perspective can do the same. Hence, both context and perspective influence which dimensions are most significant. This resulting shift alters the organization of dimensions (dimensional reconfiguration).

Dimensionalizing as a way of constructing meaning refers to the process of selecting dimensions, characteristics, or qualities of situations and organizing the relationships among these dimensions. The result of this process is a particular understanding or definition. A more elaborate description of dimensional analysis in Schatzman's (1991) theory of analysis can be consulted for more detail.

In dimensional analysis, natural and scientific approaches do not reflect different forms of thinking, but instead share basic characteristics and procedures. What distinguishes these types of thinking from one another is purpose and audience rather than the basic structure or process of analysis. Therefore, the same analytic procedures can be applied to an explication of human thinking across domains. Further, human analysis can be characterized as either (1) recognition-recall (quick recognition of something familiar) or (2) scientific.

Dimensionalizing as a way of constructing meanings is most visible in an explicit formal problem solving mode. At such a time dimensions are likely to be explicitly identified and considered. For example, when habitual action suddenly does not lead to the usual outcomes, the actor is likely to become more aware of the dimensions of the situation and considers their relationships to each other in order to solve the problem. This occurs "when recognition-recall does not provide a situationally sufficient understanding" (Schatzman, 1991, p. 309). On the other hand, action that is habitual, and not experienced as problematic, proceeds at a lower level of awareness. Therefore, a less active considering of dimensions and their interrelationships is called for. Thus, in these instances, thinking can remain relatively unexamined. It is generally believed that formal problem solving, and more explicit thinking, is characteristic of formal scientific analysis, whereas superficial and less critically examined thinking is related to more mundane activities. Schatzman suggests that both types of thinking are characteristic of mundane as well as scientific explanation and understanding. The construction of meanings as situationally sufficient requires an awareness of what the audience assumes and expects, and what the purpose demands. Thus, the distinction between natural and scientific or "formal" analysis lies in the audience and purpose of the analysis rather than in the structure, process, or complexity of analysis.

Recognition-recall refers to understanding and consequent action that arises from defining a situation as familiar, predictable, unproblematic, and requiring little analysis for action to proceed. Although the ability to recognize a situation as familiar requires some analysis, this type of analysis is often brief and unproblematic enough to be barely perceptible to the actor himself or herself. This situation occurs "when recognition-recall is sufficient to his or her situated requirements" (Schatzman, 1991, p. 309). Much of our actions proceed in this manner and therefore do not lead to explicit and systematic analysis about the definition of the situation or the identification of actions that might be used to proceed. Recognition-recall is characteristic of some natural analysis, as part of daily routines and actions at a mundane level. However, recognition-recall is also characteristic of scientific work in which analysis proceeds by simply applying familiar concepts to academic situations or data (Schatzman & Bowers, unpublished manuscript).

The consequences of using recognition-recall in academic work is that assumptions about the presence, relevance, and salience of dimensions defining the situation are often integrated into the researcher's understandings unproblematically. Each discipline uses its own categories to construct an understanding of situations that are the object of study. The understanding of a situation, as well as what the data reflect, depends on the discipline of the researcher(s). Recognition-recall is likely to be interrupted if the understanding and/or resulting action become problematic. Otherwise, action generally proceeds unproblematically, not inviting any interrogation of the accuracy or usefulness of the understanding.

If the situation is determined to be problematic, unfamiliar, or for any reason requiring further analysis, a more elaborate and deliberate analytic process is often initiated. This is true of both natural analysis (involving the mundane or personal) and "formal" analysis of scientific or scholarly activities. Both natural and scientific analysis rely on dimensionalizing. An example described by Schatzman (1991) is the analysis of nurse graduates assessing job opportunities. A "good job" can only be understood by knowing the dimensions incorporated into the definition and how they relate to each other, the context, and the perspective taken. A good job may include a dimension related to compensation.

Compensation can be further dimensionalized (sub-dimensionalized) into philosophy of the organization, product or service produced, monetary dimensions, benefit packages, status, security, etc. Which of these dimensions is most salient depends on the context of job seeking, including, for example, whether there is a shortage or an oversupply of similar applicants, the availability of benefits from other sources, the size of one's savings account, and other sources of income or support to cover until the right job is found.

Perspective is also incorporated into the logic of seeking and assessing (determining relevance and salience of) the jobs available. Being a new graduate, highly ideological or having very little information about the economy, job opportunities or career possibilities would alter the attributed significance of the above considerations. Which is really the best job can be understood only through the integration of context and perspective, including how they influence the selection and organization of dimensions related to the jobs under consideration. The definition of a "good job" cannot be constructed apart from the context and perspective. In summary, dimensional analysis requires the researcher to explore (1) the dimensions conjured (both explicitly and implicitly); (2) the attributions of salience and relevance assumed (and designated); and (3) the influence of perspective and context on understanding (Schatzman, 1991).

CONCEPT AND KNOWLEDGE DEVELOPMENT IN NURSING AND DIMENSIONAL ANALYSIS

Consistent with pragmatist and interactionist thought, concepts (as social objects) are not seen as static or essential entities to be discovered, either as empirical reality or mental category (Rodgers, 1993). As Schatzman (1980) said in his discussion of dimensional analysis:

> . . . there is no single meaning to any concept or situation. The dimensional permutation of concepts through a variety of perspectives or contexts provides variety in interpretation, even within stated situations. Thus, reference to '*the* meaning' of things appears simplistic . . ." (p. 40),

and we would add, incomplete and misleading. Consequently, when using a dimensional analysis approach, concepts are assumed to be (1) socially constructed; (2) defined primarily by how researchers and scholars "act toward them" or how they are used; (3) contextually situated; and (4) defined from a perspective that is often implicit. These premises have clear implications for how a concept analysis, using dimensional analysis, should be carried out. Dimensional analysis can be used to understand the conceptual nature and evolution of concepts, and the fluidity of concepts across perspectives and contexts. The variations in meanings and uses of concepts are explored in order to gain insight into the relationships among the concept (as object or social definition) and the social, historical, cultural influences resulting in predictable and patterned variations. The variations and consistencies in concepts reflect socially situated understandings of what a given concept represents.

Assuming the interactionist view that concepts are defined by their use suggests that an understanding of any concept can only be gained by examining the many ways in which that concept is used. While explicit definitions are important, it is also crucial to examine the uses of the concept apart from their explicit definitions. Therefore, a dimensional analysis would include examining definitions implicit in the way the concept is used. This, specifically, assists the researcher to identify differences in explicit definitions as well as those left implicit but still integrated into theory, research, and/or practice.

If meanings are assumed to vary by context, then understanding the meanings of a concept requires an understanding of (1) the contexts in which it occurs; (2) any shift in meaning across contexts; and (3) the relationship between context and meaning. Consequently, searching primarily or exclusively for essence (universality or consistency) in meanings, as reflecting a concept's "real" substance or true definition, will necessarily result in the exclusion of any definitions or uses that are not universally shared. If meanings vary by context and perspective, then only attending to essences or consistencies will preclude the ability to understand the significance or nature of variations that are related to context and perspective. Attention to perspective and context directs the researcher to ask:

- Whose perspective is reflected in research and theory (and other scholarship) that forms the basis of nursing knowledge?
- What is the relationship between the definition of the concept, how it is used, and the perspective from which it is presented?
- If there are multiple perspectives out there, whose perspective has greater authority, and is consequently integrated into our knowledge base?
- Does our empirical work support our theorizing? For example, when we present "the clients" understanding, is that understanding based on the clients' perspectives, or are those perspectives attributed to clients by others?
- How do perspectives, other than our own, inform our use of concepts? For instance, when clients and nurses interact with each other, how are their respective definitions of the situation similar and different? What dimensions do they share and not share?

Understanding both nurse and client perspectives is crucial for nursing research and practice. Assuming and attributing a perspective (and therefore meaning) precludes the ability to understand the "other" perspective or experience. Without acknowledging and understanding these multiple perspectives, and the meaning related to them, it is impossible to develop meaningful knowledge that can contribute to the development and well-informed use of nursing theories. Consequently, important and relevant questions for a concept analysis informed by dimensional analysis relate to: (1) awareness of how concepts are used; (2) identification of whose perspectives are represented and whose are not; (3) understanding the relationship between the context described or assumed; and (4) how the concept is presented.

Dimensional analysis also differs from other forms of concept analysis in its focus on identifying implicit as well as explicit assumptions. Authors (researchers) frequently incorporate assumptions concerning the definition of a specific concept, its relationship to the dimensions of which it is comprised, and its consistency across contexts and perspectives. (The latter is often demonstrated by the absence of recognition of variation.) A dimensional analysis is based on the assumption that a concept is always defined within a perspective—and may have different meanings depending on whose perspective is reflected and in what context the concept is defined or used. As an example, in both empirical and theoretical accounts of nurse/client relationships, there is an assumption about the importance of *trust*, proficient care, and good outcomes (Pask, 1994; Repper et al., 1994; Thorne & Robinson, 1988a, 1988b; Washington, 1990; Wendt, 1996). A closer look at this literature reveals many inconsistencies and contradictions in regard to the meaning of *trust*, and the relationship of *trust* to quality of care. Although the significance, even centrality, of *trust* in nurse/client relationships is assumed, the relationship remains largely unexplored, both empirically and theoretically. The unexplored and unchallenged assumption about the significance of *trust* is reflected in the general absence in the nursing literature of explications about (1) the meaning of *trust* and (2) the nature of its relationship to both quality and outcomes of care, as well as the variations that might occur across contexts and perspectives.

Indeed, when a phenomenon such as "trusting nurse/client relationships" is taken for granted and consequently unexplored, many of the dimensions of this phenomenon, the relationships among these dimensions, and the context in which the concept is used remain obscure. Therefore, confusion in conceptualization and understanding of the phenomenon under study results. Paradoxically, the obvious centrality of *trust* in relationships—that *trust* is essential to effective nurse/client relationships, and hence to high quality care (Repper et al., 1994; Trojan & Yonge, 1993)—renders trusting relationships more challenging to study. This is so because it is difficult to identify, describe, and analyze what we take for granted in our day-to-day life; the things that are not problematic and not made visible to us on an ongoing basis (recognition-recall). This example will be presented in the last section of this chapter in detail.

METHODS OF DIMENSIONAL ANALYSIS

Dimensional analysis is not a linear process. Rather, the procedures we suggest in this chapter occur simultaneously and are adapted based on the texts under study. In accordance with Schatzman's work, the following four processes are essential to conduct a dimensional analysis: (1) describing the social construction of the concept; (2) describing the logic of a concept from multiple perspectives and as part of multiple contexts; (3) differentiating the relationship between perspectives; and (4) identifying and examining assumptions.

Describing the Social Construction of the Concept. This process requires the researcher to identify the dimensions used in constructing the concept and to describe the relationships among those dimensions. In addition, if appropriate, the researcher highlights conceptual inconsistencies. Describing the logic of a concept will clarify the different uses of the concept under study by uncovering what are the factors (perspectives, assumptions, and context) that relate to the different uses. In addition, examining how the author presents the logic of the conceptualization makes explicit the relationships among different dimensions of a concept. Accordingly, a dimensional analysis is more inclusive than other types of concept analysis because it asks the researcher to explore all the ways that the concept is used—where, when, how, by whom a concept is used, and what the consequences of its uses are. It is important to understand that the social construction of the concept can be ascertained by examining both the explicit definitions/descriptions of the concept as well as how the concept is used. Consistent with an interactionist perspective, the concept is best understood by how it is used. Therefore, including sources that explicitly define the concept, in addition to those that describe or refer to how it is used, allows the researcher to gain a more comprehensive understanding of the concept. Including and comparing both sources facilitates the identification of inconsistencies in uses of the concept.

Describing the Logic of a Concept from Multiple Perspectives and As Part of Multiple Contexts. Contexts and perspectives are neither eliminated, controlled for, nor simplified in the analysis. Rather, context and perspective are used to explain, with more precision, how a concept is constructed and under what conditions a concept varies in meanings. In doing so, the researcher presents a more inclusive and detailed schema of a concept including possible variations observed across contexts and perspectives. The purpose is to uncover the fluid and situational nature of concepts. To accomplish this, the researcher examines whether the assumptions are (1) explicit or implicit; (2) integrated into the author's conceptualization; (3) consistent and coherent throughout the text; and (4) taken for granted and unquestioned. One strategy to accomplish this is to examine the use of quotes, specifically, examining whether quotations are representative of the particular perspective they claim to represent.

Differentiating the Relationship Between Perspectives (e.g., Nurse vs. Client) and Use or Definition of the Concept. An important aspect of dimensional analysis is the careful examination of multiple perspectives—how perspectives are integrated into conceptualization. Identification of perspective will uncover various definitions of the concept under study. Variation in definitions can have important consequences. For example, nurse/client relationships may have different purposes for nurses than for clients. If nurses define their relationships with clients as a means to a specific end (e.g., patient independence, implementing a care plan, gaining compliance, etc.), then nurses' interactions with clients and their use of the relationship will reflect this particular purpose. On the other hand, if clients see the same relationship as having a different purpose (e.g., getting to know the nurse, obtaining a service, etc.), their view of nurse/client relationships will reflect this difference in purpose. When the purpose of the relationship, e.g., what it is used to accomplish and the strategies to be engaged in, differs for nurses and clients, there may be significant consequences for each. For instance, this could lead to confusion during nurse/client interactions, frustration, and/or difficulty achieving desired outcomes. Thus, giving particular attention into the analysis of "who" defines "what," and "how" it has been defined, gives the researcher better insights into "how" concepts get defined and how people use them according to the definitions they give to them. It does not make sense, in using dimensional analysis, to look for the essence of a concept since dimensional analysis defines concepts as being contextually embedded; understandings of multiple perspectives permit understandings of the shifts in definitions and uses of a given concept.

Identifying and Examining Assumptions. The researcher pays attention to which perspective is likely to be associated with which assumption. This will help in clarifying different uses of the concept and in explaining how the concept is socially constructed. In other words, the researcher identifies what are the assumptions underlying the various definitions given from various perspectives. For example, if nurses define trust in their relationships with clients as a means (instrumental) to help clients comply with their care, this definition may (or may not) carry the following assumptions: (1) clients must comply with their treatment; (2) clients who do not comply do not trust their nurse; (3) trust in nurse/client relationships facilitates compliance; and (4) without trust, reaching compliance is difficult (if not impossible). This example is rather simplistic, but does illustrate how poorly defined concepts can carry many assumptions that may or may not be conscious to the individual using the concept (in this example, trust).

Dimensional analysis calls for a questioning strategy that differs from other concept analysis methods. Most of the time, questions will help to define, in greater detail, the complexities of various contexts in which a concept is used, to uncover explicit/implicit assumptions that contribute to conceptualizations, and to describe the logic of the authors/researchers' conceptualization. Consistent with dimensional analysis, the generic questions (and sub-questions) displayed in Table 15-1 are proposed to serve as a guide when analyzing all sources of information that relate to the concept under study, such as literature (articles, books, popular literature, etc.) and interview transcripts obtained from participants sharing their understandings of that concept. An illustration of how these questions are applied when using a dimensional analysis to conduct a concept analysis will be presented later in this chapter.

Dimensional analysis involves two distinct analytic processes (Schatzman, 1991). The analysis is concerned with "identification and logistics" of what is important and meaningful about the concept, "what 'all' is involved here?" (Schatzman, 1991, p. 310). In other words, in the "identification" phase the researcher identifies as many as possible dimensions involved in the conceptualization without trying to interpret what meaning is attributed to these dimensions. Second, in the "logistic" phase, the researcher integrates the dimensions into a more sophisticated analysis. This second phase refers to the relationships among the dimensions found in the analysis, how these relationships vary across perspectives and contexts, and what are the consequences of using the concept. Most of the time, it is the second phase that is presented in writing. The first phase is more an inclusive process and is, in fact, an extensive listing of dimensions that relate to the phenomenon under study without careful attention to how they relate to each other.

To summarize, dimensional analysis of concepts seeks to make explicit the multiple ways in which the concept is constructed and used (i.e., the multiple meanings of the concept). Dimensional analysis can be used to (1) attend to the specific selection and organization of dimensions and (2) define the shifts in meanings across context and

Table 15–1   Questions to Ask When Applying Dimensional Analysis

I. **What are the dimensions of the concept and how are these properties related to each other?**
- What are the properties used to define a concept? What are the attributes used in articles and other texts to describe the concept? (e.g., level of intimacy, trust, and purposes can represent some of the attributes used to qualify the concept of relationships).
- How do these attributes relate to each other? (e.g., does the level of intimacy influence how one values a relationship? Does purpose of relationship influence how the relationship develops?)

II. **What is the perspective reflected in the text?**
- Whose perspective(s) is represented?
- Whose perspective is not included?
- How is the perspective presented?
- Are the quotes consistent with the author's interpretation and analysis?
- Are perspectives represented supported by quotes or other empirical data or are they attributed? If perspectives are not supported by empirical data, how are they attributed?

III. **What are the contextual elements that contribute to definition and use of the concept?**
- What are the contexts or conditions found or assumed to be related to variations in the logic or use of the concept? For example, does a relationship take on a different meaning if it develops within a long-term context, rather than a short-term context?
- Is trust as important in a brief encounter as it is in a long-term relationship?
- In what way is context relevant to the analysis?

IV. **What are the assumptions the author(s) integrate into the text? (Recognition-recall)**
- Are these assumptions consistent throughout the conceptualization?
- Are there relationships among the dimensions that are assumed?
- Are these assumptions implicit or explicit?
- Are these assumptions consistent with the overall logic of the discussion (study design) presented by the author? Do assumptions contradict each other, or the author's overall conceptualization?
- What questions do these assumptions raise regarding the development of the concept under study?
- What are the implications of leaving these as assumptions rather than as theoretical or empirical questions?

V. **What are the implications of how the concept is constructed and used?**
- Why is the concept important to nursing theory research or practice?
- Why is it important to study the concept?

perspective (including culturally and historically) and the relationship among dimensions (derived theoretically and empirically), as well as those derived through recognition-recall. It is an inclusive analysis, deliberately exploring and comparing a multiplicity of uses and meaning of a concept. The outcome of dimensional analysis is intended to provide a better understanding of systematically generated differences in meanings and uses of the concept.

Defining a Concept. Researchers generally study (nursing) phenomena that are of interest to them. Similarly, researchers are familiar with the concept they are examining and usually are or become immersed in the literature pertaining to the concept. Through research, practice, and other scholarly work, researchers have generally studied and have read widely about the topic. Their familiarity with the concept increases the likelihood that recognition-recall will be used by researchers to "analyze" the data or to define the concept. Consequently, it is almost impossible for researchers to identify many of the assumptions they bring to their discussion (or analysis of a concept). For this reason, it is important for the researcher to begin a dimensional analysis with a deliberate explication and review of what the researcher "knows" already. This includes the meaning and significance of the concept, its relationship to practice, and the inconsistencies between the theoretical and the empirical basis of their assumptions.

Questions pertaining to assumptions, dimensions, perspectives, and context should be applied initially to the researcher's knowledge about the concept. At this point, questions include: Why is it important to study this phenomenon/concept? How will the results of the dimensional analysis contribute to knowledge development in nursing? What do I know about this concept? Do I have a precise idea of what a concept should or should not be? And how does that idea influence my understanding of the phenomenon? Most importantly, one has to keep in mind that all knowledge is from a perspective, and as researchers, we hold a particular perspective on the phenomenon under study. It is always important, conceptually and practically, to examine the operation of perspective in the researcher's understanding of the concept. Such an exercise helps to demonstrate and make use (theoretically) of the researcher's implicit integration of assumptions and received categories (recognition-recall) into the analysis. For example, if a researcher strongly believes that *trust* is a central concept for nurse/client relationships, this researcher might unwittingly integrate that assumption into a concept analysis without raising questions about (1) its theoretical and empirical basis; (2) the nature of its relationship to other dimensions or contexts; and (3) its possible variation in presence, form, or significance across perspectives.

It is important to understand that perspective cannot be eliminated or minimized because it is integral to any definition of the situation. However, perspective can be made explicit and used to compare the shift in definitions across perspectives. It is theoretically useful to bring this perspective to a conscious level before starting any dimensional analysis. Doing so does not minimize the researcher's perspective; to the contrary, researchers might use their perspective to guide the analysis, increasing opportunities for comparison across perspectives (using their own perspective as one possible perspective). Such an exercise prevents the researcher from imposing or bringing assumptions into the analysis unreflectively.

Most of the time, integrating one's assumptions into an analysis is done without being aware of it. This process is a form of recognition-recall described by Schatzman, which has the effect of precluding or truncating the problem solving, explicit analysis mode. For example, as familiarity with a concept increases, our understanding of it seems less problematic and does not tend to initiate an explicit problem solving mode. One helpful strategy for making assumptions more visible is to work with a deliberately diverse research team, thus minimizing the use of recognition-recall to analyze data. Ideally, this group should include people who do not share the researcher's experience, hence perspective/assumptions about the concept in question. This research team can assist the researcher to identify assumptions and make the integration of these assumptions more conscious to the researcher. In bringing in new perspectives, the group can help highlight dimensions in the analysis that the researcher would have otherwise missed. If the group members are all in the nursing discipline, having on the team people involved in different clinical areas can have the same effect.

Selecting Sources of Information. It was previously stated that using dimensional analysis as a method to analyze concepts is not designed to discover the essence of a concept, or to identify the most "accurate" or best understanding of a concept. Rather, it is designed to inform the researcher about the complexity and contextuality of the concept as it is used. The analysis can also be used to compare multiple perspectives and to understand the consequences of holding those perspectives. Consequently, a comparison across multiple perspectives will require collecting data from multiple sources, such as articles, interviews with diverse groups, policy documents, popular literature, marketing material, text books, media, etc. An understanding of the public's perception of a concept, for example, will not be achieved by consulting professional or technical sources.

In addition, the selection of texts is guided by the ongoing dimensional analysis. For instance, if some texts under study reveal that "time" is a central dimension for understanding how relationships between nurses and clients develop, the researcher purposely seeks texts that highlight this dimension. This would mean thus selecting texts that discuss long-term (chronic illnesses, home care, etc.) versus short-term (emergency room, intensive care unit, etc.) encounters between nurses and clients/families. Thus, the researcher begins the analysis with a small number of texts. Continued selection and integration of texts is guided by the ongoing dimensional analysis. During this ongoing analysis, the researcher will make theoretical choices and will pursue specific directions relevant to the purpose of the analysis. For the above reasons, it is impossible to choose in advance, with exactitude, what texts should be the object of the analysis. Texts are, therefore, selected on a theoretical basis to enhance an inclusive understanding, maximizing the opportunity to explore the significance of contexts and perspectives.

A crucial consideration in selecting sources of text is that the selection should not be determined by the researcher's assumptions. We have already mentioned the importance for researchers to be aware of their own assumptions regarding the concept under study. It is very easy and common to look for texts that reinforce one's own conceptualization, and to disregard those texts that challenge our understanding. One makes a conscious effort to include in the analysis all possible ways of conceptualization, presented from diverse perspectives, and in various contexts. Indeed, presenting a more complete picture will make the analysis only more credible, meaningful, and significant to the reader.

In sum, after identifying a concept and exploring meticulously the researcher's assumptions regarding the concept under study, three elements are suggested to guide the selection of the appropriate sources of information to include in the analysis: (1) the purpose of the analysis; (2) the ongoing analysis; and (3) theoretical choices. The following section presents an application of dimensional analysis as an analytic method for concept analysis.

AN APPLICATION: DIMENSIONAL ANALYSIS OF NURSE/CLIENT RELATIONSHIPS

The concept to be examined is nurse/client relationships, although limited space precludes a comprehensive dimensional analysis of the concept. Using dimensional analysis to examine nurse/client relationships would lead the researcher to begin by addressing the following general questions.

- What is the nature (dimensions and sub-dimensions) of nurse/client relationships?
- Does the nurse/client relationship shift across contexts? If so, how?
- Does perspective alter the selection or the organization of dimensions? (nature of the relationships)

Analysis based on the above questions would likely reveal that "trust" is a central dimension in the literature about nurse/client relationships. "Trust" would therefore become one focus of analysis (e.g., the nature of trust, its links to and consequences for nurse/client relationships). In fact, a wider review of literature on nurse/client relationships reveals that "trust" is consistently specified (implicitly or explicitly) as a central dimension of the nurse/client relationship. Therefore, the nature of nurse/client relationship, specifically the dimension of "trust," will be used to illustrate how dimensional analysis can be used to conduct a concept analysis. For the present discussion, the reader is asked to accept the authors' conclusions that trust was found to be a central dimension in most nursing literature on nurse/client relationships. The actual analysis leading to that conclusion is not included here. Given that conclusion, however, the researcher would pursue an analysis of trust as a salient dimension of nurse/client relationships. Questions* relevant to this pursuit include:

- What are the dimensions (and sub-dimensions) of trust in nurse/ client relationships?
- What are the relationships among these dimensions?
- What is the evidence used for the presence and/or significance of trust?
- Are there different types (dimensional organization) of trust?
- Are some types more important or central than others? When?
- Are meanings/types of trust related to perspective or context?
- When is trust (from whose perspective, in what context, under what conditions) central or relevant to the development of nurse/ client relationships?
- When perspectives differ, whose has greater authority (in the literature) for defining the meaning of trust?
- How does the presence or absence of trust influence or change the nurse/client relationship?
- What is the empirical basis for answering any of these questions?

The centrality and consistency of trust found in the literature renders trusting nurse/client relationships and nurse/client relationships as equivalents. In a dimensional analysis, it would be important for a researcher to examine literature on nurse/client relationships that did not assume the centrality of trust and to compare them with those that do. This would assist the researcher in identifying how and under what conditions trust is assumed to be central. Another option for dimension analysis would be to explore nurse/client relationships that assume trust as a central dimension. The purpose of this would be to develop an understanding of how trust operates in nurse/client relationships, as

---

*We have suggested a list of generic questions in Table 15-1. These questions are translated, in this last section of the chapter, from generic to specific in order to give the reader a concrete example of how these generic questions can look when exploring/analyzing a given concept (in this case, trust in nurse/client relationships), using the dimensional analysis method.

presented in the literature. The following discussion will focus on the second of these options.

Several studies reviewed assumed the significance of trust in nurse/client relationships. Three have been selected to demonstrate some aspects of a dimensional analysis of *trust* in nurse/client relationships. Three articles may appear to the reader as a rather limited number of texts. However, it must be kept in mind that the example we present in this chapter represents an illustration of how dimensional analysis is conducted, and is not a complete dimensional analysis of nurse/client relationships. Our intentions here are to guide the reader through just a small part of the process of conducting a dimensional analysis. Including additional dimensions of nurse/client relationships would add levels of complexity to the analysis that space does not allow. The reader is reminded that the process demonstrated here would be used much more expansively to conduct a comprehensive concept analysis using dimensional analysis. A more adequate dimensional analysis of nurse/client relationships would require integration of each article more completely and selection of a much wider range of articles. In this illustration only a portion of the three articles are used for analysis. Although many questions relevant to dimensional analysis will be identified, only a few can be pursued. These questions could be used as guides in a continuing analysis of the literature. When reviewing the literature on nurse/client relationships, one could use the following questions to begin the analysis:

- What are the dimensions used to define (explicitly and implicitly) a nurse/client relationship? (How is the concept constructed?)
- How central is trust from the nurse *and* the client perspectives? (Relationship among dimensions and sub-dimensions as they vary by perspective.)
- How do nurses define trusting relationships—What are the dimensions nurses and clients use to identify trust in nurse/client relationships? (Perspective.)
- What is the purpose (and consequences) of having/not having trust in nurse/client relationships?
- What are the contextual factors that contribute to and/or impair the development of trust in clients/nurses relationships?
- How do nurses use trust in the context of their relationships with clients? (Consequences.)
- What are the implicit and/or explicit assumptions about trust? (Construction of the concept.)
- What is construed as evidence for presence or absence of trust, or various types of trust?
- What are the consequences of assuming a trusting relationship for the client, the nurse, their relationship, and the care?

- Is it assumed that both clients and nurses define and use trust in the same ways? How does trust influence nurse/client relationships, and how is it assessed? (Perspective.)
- Is there an empirical basis in research for the answers to the above questions or are they assumed?

This latter question, in particular, has important implications for research. The reader will note that these questions, which would be addressed in a review of literature on nurse/client relationships, are quite balanced in perspective. For each issue the perspective of the client, as well as that of the nurse, is sought. This illustrates the centrality of perspective and the relationship between perspective and meaning when conducting a dimensional analysis of a concept.

Hence, continuous searching for a comparison between the perspectives of the nurse and those of the client may reveal perspective-related differences in the construction and use of the concept. Despite the importance of perspective, the analysis presented here will focus primarily on the perspective of the nurse. This is so for two reasons. First, space does not permit an analysis of both perspectives and a comparison between them and the dimensions of each. Second, and theoretically more significant, there is very little research and theory development that has been done on nurse/client relationships from the client perspective. Therefore, the client perspective will be included in selected places but cannot be considered a comprehensive analysis of client perspective or how client perspective differs from the perspective of the nurse. The illustration will provide a starting point only.

An analysis of how trusting relationships are constructed in the nursing literature could inform the researcher about (1) what is known about trusting relationships between clients and nurses; (2) what is assumed but unexamined and consequently, inherently problematic to conceptualizations of trust in nurse/client relationships; (3) what needs to be explored for further explication of the concept; and (4) the influence of the context on the uses and definitions of trust in nurse/client relationships. Sections of the three articles included for review in this chapter articles (Pask, 1994; Repper et al., 1994; Trojan & Yonge, 1993) comprise the basis of this dimensional analysis. This review should not be considered a critique of these because much of the authors' discussion, as well as relevant data, is not included in our discussion. Selected sections from each of these articles, are used heuristically to demonstrate an analytic process. Therefore, our analysis of these sections is not an analysis or critique of the articles themselves, as such an analysis would be incomplete and much too selective.

Identifying Dimensions. Time (and its sub-dimensions) is frequently identified as a central condition for "developing a nurse/client relationship." In the Repper, Ford, and Cooke (1994) article, time is sub-dimensionalized (conceptualized) by duration (e.g., "having a long-term perspective"). As Repper, Ford, and Cooke state, a long-term nurse/client relationship promotes trust in the relationship. Thus, "long-term," as a sub-dimension of time, is identified as a facilitating condition for a trusting nurse/client relationship. This is illustrated by the following quote in which a nurse case-manager talks about one of her clients: "[She] didn't trust me in the beginning . . . it was months before she was really doing things or saying much" (p. 1101).

The quote suggests that the long-term nature of the relationship (duration) is directly related to trust. Whether "long-term" is sufficiently specific in itself, and the nature of the interaction between trust and duration of time, remains unspecified. A dimensional analysis would involve a search of additional literature to learn how time, specifically duration, is conceptualized as a condition for the development of a trusting nurse/client relationship.

In much of the literature reviewed, the existence and significance of a time/trust link is assumed. However, even when time is explicitly identified as a condition, the nature of the interaction between time and trust remains generally undefined. A dimensional analysis would direct the researcher to ask the following questions about this link.

- Is duration always a condition for the development of trust?
- How does this condition relate to the development of trust?
- What other conditions facilitate the development of trust?
- (How) does time influence trusting from the client's perspective?
- Is trust possible without duration of time?
- Are there other conditions that substitute for duration of time?

These questions would lead the researcher to search for evidence (in both theoretical and empirical work) of how trust develops over time. It would also be important to ask whether any shift over time in the client's perspective on trust is based on evidence (empirical work) or is assumed? If based on empirical evidence, what sort of evidence? If this shift is described in empirical work, is it demonstrated by including the client's perspective (quotes from clients) or is it attributed by the nurse or the author?

The questions raised above are primarily focused on the social construction of the nurse/client relationship, the relevance or salience of trust as a dimension of the relationship, and the links among context, perspective and the construction of the nurse/client relationship. A researcher conducting a dimensional analysis would pursue (selecting additional sources of text) an examination of *how* time (specifically duration, but also other sub-dimensions of time) relates to trust, in what context trust is (and is not) important, and from whose perspective.

The authors' (Repper et al., 1994) statements that time allows the nurse and the client to "take things slowly," to "be consistent," to "be persistent," to "be supportive," or to "go at the client's pace" are all relevant to this analysis.

Persistence, consistency, and pacing are uses of time that are possible under the condition of having a long-term relationship. A comprehensive dimensional analysis would further inquire into how these uses of time (as a sub-dimension of time) are themselves related to developing trust, when they are and are not involved in the development of trust, whose perspective of trust they represent, how they are demonstrated, and what are the sub-dimensions of each, e.g., what does it mean to be consistent, persistent, and appropriately paced? Also, empirical questions are raised, such as how does one discern "the client's pace" and alter intervention accordingly? What are examples of how to consider and respond to a client's pace?

Analysis of this literature also suggests that there are different purposes (e.g., providing services, demonstrating persistence and consistency, and being supportive) for client visits. One would then ask (searching the literature) if these various purposes require different types of intervention, or require additional conditions to be achieved. The quote above suggests that time might be used differently depending on the purpose. In the following example from a nurse manager, being consistent means visiting on a regular basis, even when the client does not need the service. The purpose of the visit for the nurse is something other than providing a service.

> I will see her twice a week no matter what her mental state or whatever her life is like. She actually finds that difficult at times because her experience in the past has been very different, so when she has been well no one has visited, when she's been ill she's had a lot of people, but now she has consistency. (Repper et al., 1994, p. 1100)

A dimensional analysis would explore how (whether) different types and purposes of "visiting" (also dimensions of the nurse/client relationship) relate to trust. The authors' statement that "being consistent" enables case managers "to remain positive in the face of rejection and when there was little evidence of achievement" (p. 1100) suggests an important use of consistency in facilitating the development of the relationship. Thus, being consistent becomes a strategy for enhancing trusting relationships, by allowing nurses to frame apparent rejection in a way that reduces the threat to trust. This also has implications for how visits should be understood and evaluated.

In addition, Repper, Ford, and Cooke (1994) report that from the client interviews conducted in their study the "clients valued the long-term nature of the relationship and were consequently able to trust their case manager, so it would appear that this persistence paid off"

(p. 1100). This quote ties persistence, made possible by a long-term relationship, to the development of trust. In a dimensional analysis the researcher would then ask how (whether) the client's perspective is integrated into how the meaning of persistence is constructed. The researcher would explore whether this construction is based on the client's view or on the nurse's view. In the above example, a dimensional analysis would seek clients' perspectives about: What persistence accomplishes, from the client's perspective? What it looks like? Under what conditions it is appropriate to be "consistent" or persistent, and when it is not appropriate? What is consistency or persistence used for? Does the client share the same assumption concerning how "being consistent" is perceived and contributes (or does not) to developing a trusting relationship? The following quote from the Repper, Ford, and Cooke (1994) article presents a client's view on this issue:

> I haven't seen so much of her [case manager], but I don't really want to see so much of her. I don't want to spend the time having appointments when I don't really need them . . . It's a lot of hassle to keep in touch for the sake of it. (p. 1100)

In dimensional analysis, the researcher would compare the nurses' and clients' perspectives on the meaning of consistency as separate from the provision of services. This quote raises questions about whether from the clients' view, consistency is useful in itself and, therefore, whether the clients' construction of consistency corresponds to that of the nurse. Questions about the consequences of specific conditions, and for whom the consequences are relevant, are thus addressed. There are consequences for both nurse and client. Returning to the nurses' perspectives, a dimensional analysis would lead the researcher to the following questions: Is consistency, as a use of time (sub-dimension), generally assumed to produce trust? Are "continuous time" and "repeated contacts" equivalent? Are both necessary for developing trusting nurse/client relationships? Under what conditions is this (is this not) the case? Can trust be the consequence of other dimensions?

These questions could be used to examine additional articles on trusting relationships. For instance, Pask (1994) also refers to time as potentially influencing trust. She states: "The longer that we trust, the stronger may be our sense of trust. Some relationships may take time to establish" (p. 191). In Pask's article, time is not the only condition for developing trust in nurse/client relationships. Pask (1994) also introduces an additional condition (past experience):

> . . . patients who in the past have had reasons to doubt the competence of health care professionals, or who fear that they will be hurt, may find it particularly difficult to trust when they are again in need of help. When

such fears exist, trust may only be achieved if regular indication is given of competence, sensitivity and care. (p. 191)

Past experience, therefore, becomes another condition for developing trust and, as a consequence, has implications for the significance and uses of time.

Trojan and Yonge (1993) highlight the importance of "getting to know the other" in developing trusting nurse/client relationships and state that "[o]ver a period of time, the relationship gets friendlier" (p. 1906). This suggests that "friendlier" relationships might be the same as "more trusting" relationships. A researcher at this point would examine whether "friendlier" is the equivalent of trusting and if not, how they are different. For example, it is not clear whether a "friendlier" relationship is a dimension of a trusting relationship, whether it is evidence for a trusting relationship, a condition for, or a consequence of a trusting relationship. In this example (p. 1906), time is conceptualized as a condition that allows clients and nurses to come to know each other, to "become friendlier," thus as being an important condition to developing trusting (through friendlier) relationships. Note: the majority of the discussion relates to conditions for developing trust rather than an explication (dimensional designation) of its meaning or substance, and its consequences for the care, the nurse/client relationship, and both the nurse and the client experiences. This has implications for research in the area as well as for theory development.

Time has been discovered to be an important condition for developing trusting nurse/client relationships in the literature reviewed. A dimensional analysis would lead the researcher to search the literature, and other sources, for all the ways that time, as a condition for the development of a trusting relationship, is conceptualized. Relevant questions for this continuing literature review include: What other dimensions of time have been identified and what is their significance? Are there instances in which time interferes with, or at least does not facilitate, the development of a trusting relationship? For instance, in Pask's (1994) "philosophical analysis of trust" she identifies another sub-dimension of *time* (amount). In the following quote, time (long-term relationship) is seen as possibly being a detrimental or undermining condition rather than a facilitating one.

(For) . . . those who are nursed over long periods of time. Such experience may lead clients to entrust more than competence to their nurse. For such instances, what set out as a contractual relationship between client and nurse, may develop into a relationship of greater significance, particularly from the point of view of the client. (p. 192)

This example introduces the possibility that amount of time consists of a range that includes "too much time" as well as too little time. Thus amount of time, as a range, becomes a condition for the ability to use time effectively, for multiple purposes. At this point, time can be sub-dimensionalized by amount, uses, meanings, and purposes. The above quote also illustrates how long-term relationships are seen to contribute to a shift in the relationship between nurses and clients that is (implicitly) not useful or desirable. Additional dimensions of trust, "competence," and "more than competence" are also found in this quote. Left unexamined is the relationship between amount of time (sub-dimension) and trust, and between competence and trust. How much time is too much or too little for the development of trust? (How) do conditions interact with amount, duration, and uses of time? What is the client's perspective on each of these? The nurse's? When are they shared or discrepant and what difference does shared or discrepant perspective make?

Another dimension of a trusting nurse/client relationship is having a shared goal. All three articles (Pask, 1994; Repper et al., 1994; Trojan & Yonge, 1993) implied that "sharing the same goal" is one dimension of a trusting nurse/client relationship. For instance, in the article by Trojan and Yonge (1993), nurses assume that the primary goal for elderly people is the desire to stay home and to be independent as long as possible. A trusting relationship is, consequently, assumed to be a relationship in which both parties are working to promote the shared goal of independence. Using dimensional analysis, the researcher would ask the following questions to guide further analysis of the literature:

- How important is a shared goal to developing trust?
- How is the goal shared?
- What if there are additional, competing, or more salient goals for one or the other?
- What are the consequences for trust if "independence" is not perceived equally important by both the nurse and the elderly client as a goal to reach?
- Do goals have to be consistent?
- Does the client also perceive the relationship as an instrument?
- Is sharing a goal the basis of developing trust or is it a consequence of trust?

Attempting to define the relationship of goal sharing to trusting would raise the above questions. Although not stated explicitly, this suggests that nurses and elderly individuals (clients) must share the same goal (e.g., independence) if they wish the outcomes of the care to be "effective." It implies that if clients do not share this goal (independence) with the nurse, they cannot develop a trusting relationship. A dimensional analysis that examines the relationships among dimensions would raise theoretical and practical questions about the coupling of effective nurse/client relationships and shared goals. It would also inquire into the differences between effective and trusting relationships. Furthermore, the researcher would want to understand how nurses and clients come to "share the same goal," who defines the goal(s), and how this process of defining goals influences trusting relationships.

Authors who publish in this body of literature refer frequently to the nurse/client relationships as an instrument, a nursing intervention, with a specific goal in mind that is thought to be shared between nurses and clients. For instance, Repper, Ford, and Cooke (1994) state that " . . . developing and maintaining the client-case manager relationship was *the central vehicle through which* the needs of service users were assessed, direct care delivered, and the necessary service coordinated" (p. 1103; italics added). This also introduces a new sub-dimension, that is, using the relationship as an instrument to achieve a goal.

A dimensional analysis would explore the inclusion of the client perspective and evidence for it, whether that perspective is discovered or attributed and what happens when the goal is not shared, addressing whether the clients' perspective is grounded in the study or is an assumed and attributed perspective. This could lead the researcher to important empirical questions.

Repper, Ford, and Cooke (1994) also describe "sharing the same goal" as a condition for developing trusting relationships, but it is conceptualized differently than in the Trojan and Yonge (1993) article. Specifically, sharing the same goal, and hence, "being realistic" about the outcome of the care becomes the condition for developing a trusting relationship. The authors report:

> The first guiding principle for constructing a working relationship was realism. Several case managers explained the importance of realistic expectations as a strategy to overcome possible frustration (p. 1099).

Repper, Ford, and Cooke suggest that one of the consequences of being realistic is to avoid disappointment in regard to the outcome of care. The link between "being realistic" and time (as a condition for becoming realistic) is reflected in the recognition that time may pass before change (becoming realistic) occurs. Thus, time may be required before becoming realistic and "sharing the same goal" is actually achieved. Sub-dimensionalizing time also leads to the conclusion that time must be used to allow clients to go at their own pace. It is important to remind the reader that dimensions and the relationships among them are gathered from multiple conceptualizations, across multiple sources. No single author will have presented all the relationships included in the analysis of how the concept is constructed and used.

In sharing this goal, that is being realistic, both the nurse and the client avoid frustration. In conducting a dimensional analysis, the researcher would want to know how "realistic" expectations are defined and who defines them. The authors (Repper et al., 1994) present the following quote from a case manager interviewed in their study, which demonstrates how a client's goal is assessed as "realistic" from the case manager's perspective.

> He [the client] does want to move out into the community. He's going at a very slow pace, on his terms. I see it as a valid relationship with prospects of success, but very long term. If nothing happens before Christmas [6 months] I shouldn't be surprised. I hope something does. (p. 1099)

No data are provided in this particular article reflecting the client perspective on "being realistic." This would be important for a dimensional analysis, which would inquire into how "realistic" is defined by nurses as well as by clients. What happens when nurses and clients disagree about whether or not a goal is realistic, and how does this relate to them developing a trusting relationship? Finally, being realistic appears to be linked to "recognition of their long-term involvement with the client, which enables them to find a way of persevering with the same clients in a flexible way over time" (p. 1099). In other words, a long-term perspective creates a context for the nurse and the client to be realistic with regard to the outcomes of the care, which in turn offers flexibility for the client to achieve their own goals. The nature of realistic goals remains undefined.

Repper, Ford, and Cooke (1994) state that the purpose of their study is "to identify, describe, and provide an understanding of case managers' relationships and interventions with and for clients" (p. 1098). A dimensional analysis would explore the nature of the link between nurse/client relationships and interventions, as conceptualized here and in other texts. These two concepts are often linked, although the nature of that link is generally assumed rather than examined. This would include an investigation of how and in what context relationships and interventions are or are not related to each other and to developing a trusting relationship. It is worth mentioning that these authors use "trusting relationship" and "working relationship" interchangeably. A dimensional analysis would require an analysis of how a trusting relationship and a working relationship (as well as an effective relationship) are similar to or different from each other, how they each develop, and whether there is a link among them. Are they equivalent? In what way are they equivalent? Can you have one without the other?

Repper, Ford, and Cooke (1994) also refer to working with clients. Is "working with" similar to having a working relationship, having an effective relationship, intervening? In another section of the article, they write that "from the outset of the project, the relationship was recognized as central to the work of the case manager" (p. 1098). The researcher conducting a dimensional analysis would ask how the relationship is central—central to what? process, outcomes, purpose?—and what happens when the relationship is not central? Is this a suggestion that the relationship is a strategy for accomplishing work or a condition facilitating work? In either case, a dimensional analysis would explore how each is conceptualized, the dimensions included, and how the dimensions relate to each other. The stated centrality of both trust and relationship for getting the work done is illustrated in this quote:

> Case managers' descriptions of their relationship with clients were marked by frequent references to trust. . . . The importance of trust appeared to lie in its utility. . . . (Repper et al., 1994; p. 1101)

In the literature reviewed, many assumptions remain unexplained or implicit. Inconsistencies discovered either within or across articles provide new possibilities for comparative analysis. Exploring the perspectives and contexts associated with these apparent inconsistencies adds elaboration to the dimensional analysis and increases the richness, complexity, and usefulness of the analysis. Most significantly, such an analysis becomes important in identifying fruitful areas for research.

The use of a dimensional matrix is essential in the process of dimensional analysis. Figure 15-1 presents an integrative matrix illustrating the results of a beginning dimensional analysis, conducted on selected sections of the three articles, on nurse/client relationships. This dimensional matrix reflects one of the dimensions (trust) found in the discussion of nurse/client relationships. It helps the researcher to visually represent and to understand how a given concept is conceptualized in the literature. The same type of matrix could be used with other sources (such as interviews). The purpose of a dimensional matrix is to represent (visually) what dimensions are used to describe a concept and to illustrate the relationships among the dimensions (and sub-dimensions). As an example, the dimensional matrix in Figure 15-1 includes various properties of trusting relationships and is organized as follows: (1) *conditions* (dimensions of the context that influence how the concept is framed/constructed, or affect the constructing); (2) *dimension* (aspects, components, characteristics, attributes, descriptors of the concept, that is, nurse/client relationships—in this case "trust" is the central dimension of nurse/client relationships); (3) *sub-dimensions* (dimensions of trusting relationships); and (4) *consequences* (the consequences of holding and using a particular meaning).

A look at the dimensional matrix reveals that conditions (for the development of trusting nurse/client relationships) tend to be the focus of discussions about nurse/client relationships (effective or working relationships). These conditions are primarily related to time (and its sub-dimensions). Other conditions identified in the dimensional analysis so far include client and nurse characteristics that are seen as necessary to facilitate a trusting or effective relationship. The dimensional matrix would assist the researcher to examine how these conditions are seen

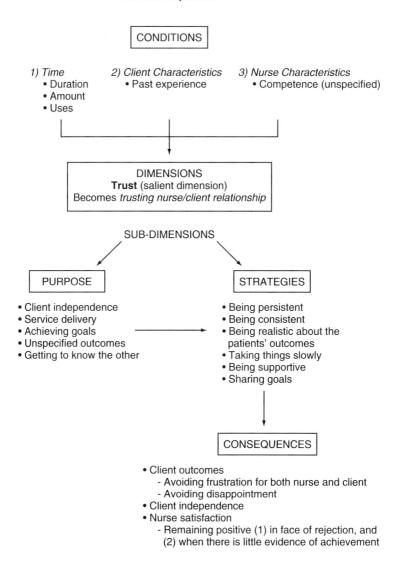

NURSE/CLIENT RELATIONSHIPS
Nurse Perspective

CONDITIONS

1) Time
  • Duration
  • Amount
  • Uses

2) Client Characteristics
  • Past experience

3) Nurse Characteristics
  • Competence (unspecified)

DIMENSIONS
Trust (salient dimension)
Becomes *trusting nurse/client relationship*

SUB-DIMENSIONS

PURPOSE

  • Client independence
  • Service delivery
  • Achieving goals
  • Unspecified outcomes
  • Getting to know the other

STRATEGIES

  • Being persistent
  • Being consistent
  • Being realistic about the
    patients' outcomes
  • Taking things slowly
  • Being supportive
  • Sharing goals

CONSEQUENCES

  • Client outcomes
      - Avoiding frustration for both nurse and client
      - Avoiding disappointment
  • Client independence
  • Nurse satisfaction
      - Remaining positive (1) in face of rejection, and
        (2) when there is little evidence of achievement

Figure 15–1   Dimensional Matrix: Conceptualization in selected nursing literature on nurse/client relationships, from nurses' perspectives.

to be related to the development of a trusting nurse/client relationship. For example, how client past experience, as well as sub-dimensions of past experience, influences the development of nurse/client relationships is not clear. This lack of clarity could direct the researcher to seek more details on this particular condition (past experience) and how it is related to nurse/client relationships. The same could be said for nurse characteristics. Additionally, the matrix suggests (through its underdevelopment of conditions) that the meaning of competence needs to be clarified. It is unclear what competence is, how it varies by context or perspective, and the nature of its influence on developing a trusting relationship. Time and its sub-dimensions have been consistently identified as an important condition for developing a trusting (effective/ working) nurse/client relationship. Hence, the dimensional matrix helps clarify the absence of conceptualization about nurse/client relationships that are not long term. It is unclear how lack of time (duration/long-term) is related to the development of trusting or effective nurse/ client relationship. This observation would be important in guiding the researcher to search for discussions related to this shorter time and the development of nurse/client relationships.

As represented in Figure 15-1, trust is the most salient dimension (thus far identified) of nurse/client relationships. It should be noted that the dimensional matrix is a working tool that would be altered in response to further analysis (of additional texts) that do not specify trust as central to nurse/client relationships. At this point, trust has been found to be central to the texts reviewed (either explicitly or implicitly). Therefore, as conceptualized in reviews done *to this point*, nurse/client relationships seem to be equivalent to trusting nurse/client relationships (as well as to effective and working nurse/client relationships). However, because "working" and "effective" relationships both seem to assume trust, trust becomes the central dimension. Focusing now on trusting nurse/client relationships as the concept to be analyzed, the researcher examines how trusting nurse/client relationships are conceptualized.

The dimensional matrix suggests that trusting a nurse/client relationship is generally described using the dimensions (1) purpose and (2) strategies. That is, discussion of trusting nurse/client relationships focuses on the purpose of the relationship and the strategies used to achieve it. In addition, the sections of texts selected for the analysis reflect the assumption that strategies identified will lead to certain consequences (also found in the dimensional matrix). Furthermore, the dimensional matrix clarifies the absence of specific links between purpose and consequences, and between strategies and consequences. These become important issues in directing the researchers' continuing selection and analysis of texts. An additional consideration represented in the dimensional matrix is the general absence of any (sub) sub-dimensions of purposes, strategies, and consequences. In other words, these concepts are left fairly vague and undefined. One explanation for this is that the concepts are so familiar as to not be seen to require specification, suggesting the possibility that recognition-recall is truncating the analytic processes involved in understanding and describing these phenomena. It is also clear from the dimensional matrix (as representing the dimensional analysis so far) that the influence of perspective and/or context on conceptualization of (effective, working) trusting nurse/client relationships is not integrated into this analysis. An important step at this point would be to return to the texts reviewed and to seek further literature, to clarify how/whether a change in perspective or context alters the dimensional matrix found in Figure 15-1.

A Short Note on Perspectives

We have mentioned throughout this chapter that "perspectives" are central to dimensionalizing. One of the strategies to accomplish this is to pay attention to how the voices of subjects are integrated into the analysis. A good example of how this would be done is found in the study conducted by Trojan and Yonge (1993) that looked at developing trusting relationships between home care nurses and elderly clients. The authors present a quote from one subject of their study (nurse): "I think it is more that I want them to trust me. They let me into their home as a guest. I'm just a stranger in their home. . . . " (p. 1905). Although not highlighted in Trojan and Yonge's analysis, this statement suggests that the nurse takes the role of guest and as stranger. A dimensional analysis is useful to pursue such analogies. If these analogies are used in the nurses' understanding of the relationship, how do they relate to the purpose and conditions identified? What are the dimensions of "being a guest?" This might indicate a look at how guest relationships are described elsewhere (comparative analysis). Does the analogy work for a nurse/client relationship? If it is contradictory, what is the significance of this contradiction? For example, if a home nurse defines herself as a "guest," what does she mean by that and is this image inconsistent with her actions? What does it mean to see oneself as stranger?

Dimensionalizing this analogy raises many questions: What purpose does a guest come with? How do guests relate to and interact with hosts? Is there a goal, an outcome to coming into your home as a guest? Does a guest (P) go into someone's home (O) in possession of confidential information about the host? Does the host O have similar confidential information about the guest P? What is the consequence of continuing to see herself as a guest? What are the consequences for the relationship of understanding this as a guest/host relationship? How does this understanding relate to other dimensions and conditions? There is a danger of perpetuating roles that contradict the nurse's purpose or the client's understandings. That certainly has implications for trust. What is the nurse's understanding of "self as a nurse," as part of the relationship? Does this influence how they act and interact, and the language they use to describe their relationships with their clients? Seeing oneself as a guest suggests equal power with the host, an assumption that must also be questioned. This example illustrates an incongruity between how some nurses see themselves and how they act. Continuing to see oneself as a guest (inconsistency with the way she acts) allows the nurse to sidestep important questions. In other words, this sort of analogy allows nurses to maintain an image of themselves that in fact is very inaccurate.

A dimensional analysis would use comparisons to other types of relationships in order to make the dimensions of "being a guest" more visible. This is a good strategy to demonstrate which dimensions of "being a guest" apply to the nurse/client relationships and which do not apply. Then the next step in the analysis will be to bring the analysis of this analogy to the concept of trust and ask: When nurses act in ways that are contradictory with the ways that they perceive themselves, what are the consequences for the relationship they develop and maintain with the client—and, how does this affect the trust that exists between the two of them?

CONCLUSION—HOW CAN DIMENSIONAL ANALYSIS CONTRIBUTE TO KNOWLEDGE DEVELOPMENT?

This chapter is a first attempt to introduce dimensional analysis as a method to conduct concept analysis in nursing. This particular analytic approach is proposed to researchers who want to understand how concepts are socially constructed and the implications of that for research, theory development, and practice. Dimensional analysis can be most effectively used when the purpose of the analysis is:

1. To describe how a concept is socially constructed.
2. To describe how social constructions vary by perspectives.
3. To uncover assumptions underlying the logic of a concept—i.e., how concepts are used and the consequences of particular uses.
4. To explicate contextual dimensions (conditions) that can account for variations in uses and meanings of a concept.
5. To identify inconsistencies, contradictions, and gaps in the construction and use of concepts.
6. To identify inconsistencies between empirical and theoretical work on a concept.

Thus, to describe how a concept is socially constructed using the dimensional analysis approach as an analytic method, the researcher must demonstrate the links among the perspective presented in the literature pertaining to the concept, the assumptions found in this literature with regard to the concept, the significant conditions influencing the use of the concept, and the consequences for practice and implementation. Dimensionalizing is an effective way to render visible processes by which concepts are constructed and used in the nursing culture.

In summary, a dimensional analysis examines many unquestioned (sometimes cherished) assumptions about the nature of phenomena and relationships among them. A dimensional analysis will raise questions about scientific and practical knowledge, as well as common sense; concepts that experts may agree on but that are not defined precisely because it seems irrelevant or foolish to ask the question—"what does that mean?" (why is trust important, what is a trusting relationship); and commonly accepted, but sometimes poorly understood assumptions that researchers may overlook. Dimensional analysis explores how the concept is organized; its logic; its contextual variation; the consequence of various meanings and uses; and how these elements of the analysis relate to each other. The content of this chapter reflects only a few aspects of a more global schema. We are well aware that many other dimensions of nurse/client relationships are included in the three articles (Pask, 1994; Repper et al., 1994; Trojan, & Yonge, 1993) selected to illustrate the methods of dimensional analysis. The application section serves to assist the reader in conducting the procedures necessary to use dimensional analysis for a given concept. The reader is invited to read the work of Bowers (1984), Canales (1998), Jayne (1993), McCarthy (1992), and Poulin (1994) for examples of completed dimensional analyses of the literature, and Schatzman (1991) for more in-depth explication of dimensional analysis.

It is our belief that dimensional analysis can contribute in a powerful manner to concept and knowledge development in nursing, and can raise important empirical questions relevant to both research and practice. In this chapter, we have tried to highlight some of the strengths of dimensionalizing the literature; that is, (1) to uncover unquestioned assumptions about a given concept that are built into theory, research, and practice, and (2) to identify important questions and inconsistencies that need to be addressed. The centrality and meanings of trust in nurse/client relationships is one example of this. Indeed, we have raised many questions about trust and its relevance to nurse/client relationships. We hope that we have identified, through a partial dimensional analysis, some questions about nurse/client relationships that could guide future research. We believe at least some of these questions would not have been raised through other methods of concept analysis, hopefully illustrating the unique contribution dimensional analysis can make.

We have raised many more questions in this chapter than we have answered. The reader will certainly be aware that these are empirical questions that have important implications. What would one do with all these questions? The questions raised uncover areas in which the concept of trust remains unexplored or poorly understood. Therefore, another strength of dimensional analysis is to identify areas for further fruitful research about concepts. In the case of nurse/client relationships, these areas include the relevance of trust, as well as other dimensions including the significance of trust, and variations across perspectives and contexts. Thus, the numerous questions raised in the previous section of this chapter identify areas in which we need more knowledge related to the concept of trust in nurse/client relationships.

A unique and important contribution of dimensional analysis for concept analysis is the significance of perspectives. For example, while many authors claim to present clients' perspectives in their studies, it is more accurate to say that the clients' perspectives are suggested, created, constructed, attributed, and thus conceptualized by nurse professionals (with the exception of Thorne & Robinson, 1988a, 1988b). This also has implication for nursing education. The client perspective is constructed; it represents shared understandings of clients' perspectives that come from the nurse experts. The assumption that relationships between nurses and clients are directly related to the outcomes of care was also discovered by inquiring into the relationship among dimensions. The nature of the relationship that allows this to occur is largely unarticulated (i.e., words like efficient, effective). Further, the discussion uses mostly instrumental terms rather than relationship terms—for example, they are about outcomes of relationships, not relationships themselves. Questions left unproblematic and unexplored include: What is the nature of a trusting relationship—how do I know this is a relationship I want? Dimensional analysis explores these assumed relationships, examines our taken-for-granted notions (recognition-recall) that are rarely examined. Furthermore, many articles related to trusting relationships between nurses and clients refer to trust; sometimes in the title of their article and sometimes in the discussion, but without much attention to trust beyond passing mention (despite its centrality). Trust and its significance are simply assumed, but the nature and logic of that assumption remain unexamined.

When should a dimensional analysis be conducted? We suggest that researchers select dimensional analysis when the purpose of the analysis is to understand how a concept is constructed and used in the nursing culture. Dimensional analysis is a particularly useful approach to concept analysis when multiple perspectives have to be taken into account in developing knowledge around a nursing concept. We have also found dimensional analysis to be a powerful way to identify inconsistencies in the use or meaning of concepts when the concept is familiar and when its nature and significance appear obvious or taken for granted. Finally, the centrality of context in dimensional analysis makes this approach quite fruitful in understanding how meaning and uses of concepts shift across contexts.

REFERENCES

Bowers, B. J. (1984). Intergenerational caretaking: Processes and consequences of creating knowledge. (Doctoral dissertation, University of California, San Francisco, 1984). *Dissertation Abstracts International, A45*(02), 663.

Blumer, H. (1969). *Symbolic interactionism. Perspective and method*, Berkeley, California: University of California Press.

Canales, M. K. (1998). Changing perceptions of the other: Teaching practices of doctorally-prepared Latina nursing faculty; A grounded theory study. Unpublished doctoral dissertation, University of Wisconsin, Madison.

Charon, J. M. (1997). *Symbolic interactionism: An introduction, an interpretation, an integration*. (5th ed.). Englewood Cliffs, NJ: Prentice-Hall.

Dewey, J. (1938). *Logic: The theory of inquiry*. New York: Henry Holt & Co.

Jayne, R. L. (1993). Self-regulation: Negotiating treatment regimens in insulin-dependent diabetes (diabetes mellitus) (Doctoral dissertation, University of California, San Francisco, 1993). *Dissertation Abstracts International, B54*(03), 1334.

Poulin, K. L. (1994). Toward a grounded pedagogy of practice: A dimensional analysis of counseling supervision (Doctoral dissertation, University of Oregon, 1993). *Dissertation Abstracts International, B54*(09), 4931.

Repper, J., Ford, R., & Cooke, A. (1994). How can nurses build trusting relationships with people who have severe and long-term mental health problems? Experiences of case managers and their clients. *Journal of Advanced Nursing, 19*(6), 1096–1104.

Rodgers, B. L. (1993). Concept analysis: An evolutionary view. In B. L. Rodgers & K. A. Knafl (Eds.), *Concept development in nursing* (pp. 73–92). Philadelphia: W. B. Saunders.

Schatzman, L. (1980). (1999). *Dimensional analysis: Outline in precis form.* Unpublished manuscript.

Schatzman, L. (1991). Dimensional analysis: Notes on an alternative approach to the grounding of theory in qualitative research. In K. R. Maines (Ed.), *Social organization and social process essays in honor of Anselm Strauss* (pp. 303–314). New York: Aldine De Gruyter.

Schatzman, L., & Bowers, B. J. (1999). Dimensional analysis as research method. Unpublished manuscript.

Shalin, D. N. (1986). Pragmatism and social interactionism. *American Sociological Review, 51*(Feb.), 2–29.

Snelson, C. (1992). Trust as a caring construct with the critically ill: a beginning exploration. *National League for Nursing Publications, 2465*, 157–166.

Strauss, A. L. (1978). *Negotiations: Varieties, contexts, processes and social order.* San Francisco: Jossey-Bass.

Strauss, A. L. (1987). *Qualitative analysis for social scientists.* Cambridge: Cambridge University Press.

Stryker, S. (1980). *Symbolic interactionism. A social structured version*. Menlo Park, CA: Benjamin/Cummings.

Thorne, S. E., & Robinson, C. A. (1988a). Health care relationships: The chronic illness perspective. *Research in Nursing & Health, 11*, 293-300.

Thorne, S. E., & Robinson, C. A. (1988b). Reciprocal trust in health care relationships. *Journal of Advanced Nursing, 13*, 782-789.

Trojan, L., & Yonge, O. (1993). Developing trusting, caring relationships: Home care nurses and elderly clients. *Journal of Advanced Nursing, 18*, 1903-1910.

Washington, G. T. (1990). Trust: a critical element in critical care nursing. *Focus on Critical Care, 17*, 418-421.

Wendt, D. (1996). Building trust during the initial home visit. *Home Healthcare Nurse, 14*(2), 92-98.

16

Beyond Analysis: Further Adventures in Concept Development

Beth L. Rodgers

The history of concept development in nursing, as in other disciplines whose members have addressed this form of inquiry, demonstrates an overwhelming emphasis on the *analysis* of concepts. The literature in this area has progressed from basic exploration of the conceptual foundations of the discipline (Hardy, 1974; Johnson, 1959; Kim, 1987; Meleis, 1997), to methods and methodologies of analysis (Chinn & Jacobs, 1983; Chinn & Kramer, 1991; Rodgers, 1989; Rodgers & Knafl, 1993; Sartori, 1984) and, finally, to a substantial number of published reports of completed analyses (see Bibliography for this text). This attention to concept analysis has made numerous contributions to nursing, particularly by pointing out areas of vagueness and ambiguity and through the efforts of researchers to resolve some of the pressing conceptual problems in the discipline.

A negative outcome of this effort, however, is that the overemphasis on concept *analysis* can detract from a broader focus of inquiry on concept *development*. Concept analysis is merely one approach to confronting conceptual problems in the discipline. Recognition of an emerging shift in emphasis to *development* is evident in the fact that critiques are beginning to appear in which authors have questioned the validity and usefulness of existing approaches and have begun to suggest alternatives for advancing the knowledge base (Morse et al., 1996; Paley, 1996; Rodgers, 1989; Rodgers & Knafl, 1993; Schwartz-Barcott & Kim, 1986; Wuest, 1994).

There is no sound reason to abandon analysis of concepts as an approach to concept development. What is needed, however, is recognition of the role of analysis in concept development and use of results in practice and subsequent investigations; use of appropriate methodologies to enhance existing definitions by clarifying certain aspects of a concept, including individual and contextual variations; and inquiry to identify new concepts evident in situations relevant to nursing (see Chapters 2 and 6).

For these activities to make sense and be justifiable within the realm of nursing research, such efforts must be derived from a sound philosophical foundation concerning concepts and concept development. The cycle of concept development (Rodgers, 1989; Rodgers & Knafl, 1993) provides a basis for understanding the nature and fit of inquiry to develop concepts, as discussed elsewhere. Significant aspects of this philosophical foundation that provide direction for future concept development activities include (1) application and "testing" of concepts; (2) the discovery of new concepts and interrelationships among concepts; (3) contextual variations and the construction of concepts, which points to the need for discovery, critique, and deconstruction; (4) alternate forms of expression, communication, and adoption of concepts; and (5) methodological advances consistent with these foci. The following discussion demonstrates how each of these activities of concept development can be accomplished to enhance the conceptual repertoire of the discipline.

BEYOND ANALYSIS: APPLICATION AND TESTING OF CONCEPTS

As noted in previous discussion of the analysis of concepts (see Chapter 6), one of the primary roles of concept analysis is associated with its heuristic function. Concept analysis is not an end point in concept development; instead, the major focus is to provide a clear and rational starting point for further inquiry. Consequently, one reasonable step to take after an analysis is completed is to apply, or test, and evaluate the concept to determine its usefulness. A concept is only of utility and value to the extent that it serves its intended purpose. This utility, therefore, must be evaluated through practical application and testing.

The concept of grief provides a significant example of the need for application and testing of results of analysis. Analysis of appropriate literature had revealed a strong cultural and normative component of the concept, with authors implying frequently that grief varied across cultural contexts (Rodgers & Cowles, 1991). However, there was little research to support this idea other than descriptions of rituals associated with the death of a loved one. These rituals do not necessarily reflect an individual's experience of grief itself, however. Further, for the results of the analysis to be useful, it was necessary to examine the "fit" of the definition derived from the literature-based analysis with members of varying cultural groups. Cowles (1996) subsequently conducted a series of focus groups to evaluate and expand the definition derived through the initial analysis.

Another form of "testing" involves the actual application of results of analysis to different situations and contexts. Through application, the strengths and limitations of the concept are identified, and suggestions for improvement of the usefulness of the concept, or the generation of related concepts, can be accomplished. It is difficult to find actual examples where this has occurred, however. Indeed, a primary reason that the usefulness of concept analysis may be questioned is the fact that results rarely are used in practical situations or, if they are being used, this use, along with evaluation and refinement, is seldom documented or shared in the professional literature. Investigators who have done analyses of concepts are somewhat responsible for this situation when they present their results as "absolutes"—the definitive definition of the concept under investigation—and argue in their discussions of findings that the concept should now be "used" in practice, typically with no discussion of what "use" might entail. From another viewpoint, the lack of application of results of analyses shares similarities with problems concerning research utilization in general and the lack of practical application of findings from any study.

As with any form of research, results of analyses must be applied to determine their effectiveness in capturing relevant situations and phenomena and in communicating about significant interests in nursing. Evaluation should be conducted and results of evaluation, along with refinements, need to be presented to ensure a continuing process of concept development and the existence of a useful conceptual repertoire in the discipline. The concept of suffering, for example, needs to be applied and tested, and ultimately refined and improved, as nurses encounter people who they presume to be, or who are likely to be (based on the context and the definition of the concept) suffering.

Other contextual variations also can be explored through a process of application and testing. Interdisciplinary variations may be worth studying to determine if, and how, the use of a concept varies across disciplines. If this focus is not included in the initial literature-based analysis, then examining such potential variation as evident in the writings of authors of different disciplines is an appropriate first step in discovering such variation. Interviews may provide interesting insights as well and could be used to explore perspectives among different types of practitioners within a discipline. Kersbergen (1997) used this approach to uncover differences and similarities in the concept of *managed care* held by administrators and actual "case managers" as a means to expand and clarify the definition derived from a review of the literature. Investigation of such "use" of a concept provides "real-world" examples of the application of the concept and can reveal important areas for further development.

Another obvious example of this importance of applying and testing the results of analysis is the development of taxonomies. Persons involved in the development of nursing diagnoses, particularly, have used analysis procedures to identify the defining attributes of the concepts that constitute the diagnostic statements and categories. At present, developers of diagnoses generally devote considerable effort to testing, evaluating, and subsequently refining diagnostic categories to improve their usefulness in nursing practice. It has not always been the case, however, that testing and evaluation occurred with the regularity and rigor that are evident with current research efforts. Performing these activities and forms of inquiry can only expedite and improve the effectiveness of categories as they are developed. Examining the usefulness of the conceptual category in actual practice situations provides a necessary basis for refining the concept to ensure its continuing practical utility.

Evaluation and testing cannot be considered "one-time" activities, however. As the situations in which nurses practice and the problems they face continue to change and evolve, the conceptual repertoire must be evaluated continually to ensure that the primary concepts in nursing continue to be useful and relevant. Application needs to be evaluated continually to avoid perpetuating the use of concepts that become archaic over time or that lack relevance in new contexts.

BEYOND ANALYSIS: DISCOVERY OF NEW CONCEPTS AND INTERRELATIONSHIPS

The discovery (or construction) of new concepts actually may be one of the most enduring methods of concept development. Often, however, researchers conducting inquiry that leads to such discovery do not seem to think of their work as concept development research. Qualitative research provides many examples where new concepts have been discovered and relationships explored or enhanced. In many types of qualitative research, the investigation results in the delineation of new concepts through the researcher's discovery of themes or patterns in the data. The work of Knafl and Deatrick (1990) provides a prominent example with their development of *family management style* as a concept to capture families' means to deal with the chronic illness of a child in the family. Cowles and Rodgers (1997), as another example, studied the experiences of significant others of PLWAs (persons living with acquired immunodeficiency syndrome [AIDS]) and discovered the concept of *character portrayal*. This concept concerned the participants' manner for depicting the basic character of the PLWAs and presented stark contrasts in comparison to the concept of *haloing,* which is documented widely in the literature of grief and bereavement. This discovery contributed both a new concept to the field of grief and bereavement and illustrated the relationship of this concept to one established previously.

Because of the emphasis on discovery in most qualitative research, this form of inquiry is particularly appropriate and valuable in the discovery of new concepts. Interviews and observations can provide new insights into situations and phenomena and new ways of conceptualizing experiences. Exploring phenomena among different populations or across settings can help to clarify relationships among concepts as well. Although concept development may not be the primary focus of researchers in the conduct of such studies, recognition of the contributions of such work to concept development will help to expand the conceptual repertoire of the discipline.

Quantitative studies also can contribute to concept development. Although discovery is not a common purpose of quantitative research, some types of designs and analyses still may render new ideas or concepts. One obvious example concerns studies in which factor analysis is used to analyze data. The individual factors identified through the analysis easily can result in the construction of new concepts. It is common, for example, for a researcher using factor analysis in regard to determining the psychometric properties of a new research instrument to deal with an important phenomenon to identify concepts or, on occasion, constructs, and relationships among these concepts as they are associated with the phenomenon of interest. Often, this result is dependent on the nature of the study and the creativity of the researcher in developing language that captures the sense of a factor.

BEYOND ANALYSIS: CRITIQUE AND DECONSTRUCTION

Some philosophical consensus, supported by empirical studies, exists in support of the idea that concepts are constructed and socially or contextually bound. This philosophical foundation supports the need to identify contextual variations, as described previously, to explore how a concept is used in different contexts (such as by members of different disciplines or cultural groups) as well as used in different temporal and situational contexts (such as *grief* associated with a death and with job loss, relocation, etc.). But another important point for consideration of concepts stems from this philosophical foundation as well. the existence of variation on the part of people who use a particular concept points out the fact that social, cultural, and disciplinary factors have a role in the formation or construction of concepts. An important and valuable focus for inquiry, therefore, is the deconstruction of concepts to identify how they have been constructed in different contexts and critique to determine how the values and norms of that context have influenced the formation and use of the concept.

There are relatively few examples in the literature of this form of inquiry for concept development. However, there are authors who have invoked critical theory or techniques of deconstruction to explore the implications of important ideas in nursing (Irvine & Graham, 1994; Phillips, 1993; Wuest, 1994), and some new techniques have been applied recently to accomplish this purpose (Caron & Bowers, see Chapter 15). However, there is a need for more work in this area as a part of the development of concepts that will be of significant use in nursing and elsewhere.

Standard techniques of analysis typically address what the concept *is*—its attributes and other defining characteristics. Although approaches and interpretations vary in regard to the degree of certainty or absoluteness associated with the nature of the concept (see Chapter 2). But the general purpose is similar in the focus on defining characteristics. A complete understanding of a concept, however, is possible only with a thorough exploration of its origins, contextual relevance, and implications, in other words, how and why the concept developed and the possible effects of the conceptualization on segments of society and, for nursing's purposes, recipients of health care. Deconstruction and critical analysis can help to ensure that nurses are aware of the implications of the use of particular concepts as they are applied in various situations.

BEYOND ANALYSIS: ALTERNATE FORMS OF EXPRESSION

Investigators working on concept development, to date, have relied almost exclusively upon written or spoken language. For analysis purposes, the investigator typically reviews published literature to explore ideas associated with a concept and thus arrives at a definition of the concept. Occasionally the literature review is supplemented with interviews and observations; but these also rely on a discursive language, obviously in the case of interviews, but also in the documentation and communication of observations. The tremendous potential that exists for examination of nondiscursive forms of presentation, such as music and dance, has not been explored adequately in "scientific" inquiry. The distinction between verbal and written and nondiscursive forms of communication could be considered a remnant of the logical positivist view of science. In this view, there was a clear separation between art and science; science was defined very narrowly and with an emphasis on higher order math (calculus) as the language of science (Ayer, 1959; Carnap, 1956; Schlick, 1959). Wittgenstein (1921/1981) initially argued for a discursive language that "mirrored" the natural world, and only later saw language as less ordered or structured and as a tool for expression and the sharing of ideas. This emphasis on written or spoken language as the source of data is reasonable, to a great extent, due to the primary role of language in learning, socialization, enculturation, and communication. The fundamental importance of language, however, does not preclude attention to other forms of communication and conceptualization. At present, nondiscursive forms of communication continue to be relegated to aesthetics rather than "science."

Some forms that immediately come to mind are the media of art and music, as well as other performing arts. A recent example of the way that concepts can be shared through the performing arts is the multimedia dance performance *Still/Here*, created by noted choreographer Bill T. Jones. Jones wanted to create a dance that would convey the experience of terminal illness. To create this work, he invited people with life-threatening conditions to express their experience through dance and other forms. The expressions of these people were then used as a basis for the choreography of *Still/Here* and the multimedia aspects of this performance (including videotape of these participants). The individuals faced with life-threatening conditions were highly diverse in all sociodemographic and health-related characteristics. Despite the fact that none had professional dance experience, they had no difficulty expressing their experiences through movement This particular work has generated both controversy and critical acclaim (Croce, 1994-1995; Gates, 1994; Teachout, 1995). Nonetheless, it is clear that the power and potential value of communication other than through words can have significant implications for concept development.

Music is another form of expression, going far beyond merely having a good "beat" or a pleasing melody. Instead, it serves as a medium for expression of the ideas and experiences of the creator, and is valued for the variety of responses it invokes in the listener. Visual arts are a similar form of expression and communication. In fact, some things cannot be expressed easily through discursive language, yet may be communicated quite effectively through the arts. All the thoughts, emotions, and perceptions that are not easily "put into words" might be expressed through other forms. Similarly, a focus on alternate forms of expression can shed light on definitions and meanings that are otherwise obscured by language.

The frequent use of metaphor and simile in language offers some testimony to the difficulty faced in attempts to "put into words" some ideas, emotions, or experiences. Simile and metaphor allow the speaker to use language to express ideas, yet in an attempt to convey something other than what the words alone would accomplish. The speaker (or writer) can say that something is *like* something else, without having to say what the something *is*. Although simile and metaphor involve language, the "meaning" of such expressions lies beyond the actual words. As an example, consider the words of a participant in a study of significant others of PLWAs as she described her experience upon hearing of her brother's diagnosis: "It's like someone took their fist and just hit me as hard as he could right here [placing fist over middle of chest]." The interviewer/listener most likely will have a vivid sense of what a part of the grief experience was for that person, perhaps even more clearly than if the respondent had described or defined it in specific terms. Although respondents in this, and other studies have had considerable difficulty in their attempts to describe what grief *is*, rarely have they had difficulty in expressing their experience in other ways, such as through simile, metaphor, or through their actions and movements.

Discursive language serves us well. But it also limits and constrains the sharing of ideas or concepts. Language actually may veil the definition of concepts; the concept of *grief* does not involve being hit in the chest as an attribute, and a researcher who fails to look beyond the surface of language may miss some very important cues regarding the definition of a concept. Equally important to remember is that discursive language is not the only way in which concepts are shared. Language is, essentially, one type of sign; other signs and symbols may be of tremendous value in our attempts to understand concepts.

Methodological Approaches

Methodological improvements, innovations, and advances also are needed to further concept development in nursing. A vast array of methodologies and procedures is available for use in nursing inquiry. Researchers have made significant contributions to the discipline, employing various methods to address significant problems in the discipline. However, diverse methods are not discussed or used often specifically for purposes of concept development.

The need at present is for methodological advances consistent with nondiscursive forms of expression. Examination of works *about* art can be supplemented by interviews with those who experience art as well as the creators of art to determine the ways in which concepts are communicated through such media. In a related area, some work has been done regarding art as a teaching-learning tool. Cowles (1997, personal communication), for example, has for some time had students in a class on death and dying use various forms of media, including collage and crayons, to present their views on death and dying.

Inquiry of this type can provide important information about concepts of interest and forms of expression other than language. Such information ultimately may be of use also in developing nursing interventions to promote expression and understanding. Such forms of expression often are more valuable than words and typically provide an important means to capture things that are not easily articulated using a common language.

Some of the methodologic developments needed were described in previous sections. In addition to these implications for methodology, however, researchers can consider new approaches specific for concept development. In 1986, Schwartz-Barcott & Kim presented their "Hybrid Model," a significant methodological advance developed specifically for concept development. Rather than merely applying existing methods to resolve conceptual problems and develop or clarify concepts, researchers need to consider the current state of the concepts of interest and formulate approaches that will solve the identified problems best.

In a sense, the call for new methodologies for concept development represents a tautology. All research, to some extent, contributes to the development of concepts. When a researcher uses biophysiologic instruments to measure pain response in association with different pain management interventions, the researcher is contributing to the development of the concept of pain. By recognizing specifically how research can contribute to conceptual aspects of the discipline using different methodologies, nurse scholars can enhance the likelihood that conceptual progress continues in the knowledge base of nursing.

CONCLUSION

Nurse researchers have made important contributions to concept development over the past several decades. Throughout this activity, however, the emphasis has been primarily on the *analysis* of concepts. Significant accomplishments can be made in nursing if researchers and scholars recognize the potential for concept development that goes "beyond analysis." Continuing progress will be enhanced if researchers develop studies to apply and test results of analysis, to discover new concepts and relationships, to expand existing concepts by studying contextual constructions, and to explore alternate forms of expression and new methodologies for concept development.

REFERENCES

Ayer, A. J. (Ed.). (1959). *Logical positivism*. Glencoe, IL: Free Press.

Carnap, R. (1956). *Meaning and necessity*. Chicago: University of Chicago Press.

Chinn, P. L., & Jacobs, M. K. (1983). *Theory and nursing: A systematic approach*. St. Louis: Mosby.

Chinn, P. L., & Kramer, M. (1991). *Theory and nursing: A systematic approach.* (3rd ed.). St. Louis: Mosby.

Cowles, K. V. (1996). Cultural perspectives of grief: An expanded concept analysis. *Journal of Advanced Nursing, 23,* 287–294.

Cowles, K. V., & Rodgers, B. L. (1997). Struggling to keep on top: Meeting the everyday challenges of AIDS. *Qualitative Health Research, 7,* 98–120.

Croce, A. (1994, December 26; 1995, January 2). Still/here [dance review]. *The New Yorker, 70,* 54–56.

Gates, H. L. (1994, November 28). The body politic. *The New Yorker, 70,* 112–118.

Hardy, M. E. (1974). Theories: Components, development, evaluation. *Nursing Research, 23,* 100–107.

Irvine, R., & Graham, J. (1994). Deconstructing the concept of profession: A prerequisite to carving a niche in a changing world. *Australian Occupational Therapy Journal, 41*(1), 9–18.

Johnson, D. E. (1959). The nature of a science of nursing. *Nursing Outlook, 7*(5), 291–294.

Kersbergen, A. L. (1997). Defining managed care in an evolving health care environment. (Doctoral dissertation, University of Wisconsin-Milwaukee, 1996). *Dissertation Abstracts International, B 57/12,* 7450. (AAC#9717140)

Kim, H. S. (1987). Structuring the nursing knowledge system: A typology of four domains. *Scholarly Inquiry for Nursing Practice, 1*(2), 111–114.

Knafl, K. A., & Deatrick, J. A. (1990). Family management style: Concept analysis and development. *Journal of Pediatric Nursing, 5*(1), 4–14.

Meleis, A. I. (1997). *Theoretical nursing* (3rd ed.). Philadelphia: J. B. Lippincott.

Morse, J. M., Hupcey, J. E., Mitcham, C., & Lenz, E. R. (1996). Concept analysis in nursing research: A critical appraisal. *Scholarly Inquiry for Nursing Practice, 10,* 253–277.

Paley, J. (1996). How not to clarify concepts in nursing. *Journal of Advanced Nursing, 24,* 572–578.

Phillips, P. (1993). A deconstruction of caring. *Journal of Advanced Nursing, 18,* 1554–1558.

Rodgers, B. L. (1989). Concepts, analysis and the development of nursing knowledge: The evolutionary cycle. *Journal of Advanced Nursing, 14,* 330–335.

Rodgers, B. L., & Cowles, K. V. (1991). The concept of grief: An analysis of classical and contemporary thought. *Death Studies, 15,* 443–458.

Rodgers, B. L., & Knafl, K. A. (Eds.). (1993). *Concept development in nursing: Foundations, techniques, and applications.* Philadelphia: W. B. Saunders.

Sartori, G. (1984). *Social science concepts: A systematic analysis.* Beverly Hills, CA: Sage.

Schlick, M. (1959). The turning point in philosophy. In A. J. Ayer (Ed.), *Logical positivism* (pp. 53–59). Glencoe, IL: Free Press.

Schwartz-Barcott, D., & Kim, H. S. (1986). A hybrid model for concept development. In P. L. Chinn (Ed.), *Nursing research methodology: Issues and implementation* (pp. 91–101). Rockville, MD: Aspen.

Teachout, T. (1995). Victim art. *Commentary, 99,* 58–61.

Walker, L. O., & Avant, K. C. (1983). *Strategies for theory construction in nursing.* Norwalk, CT: Appleton-Century-Crofts.

Wittgenstein, L. (1981). *Tractatus Logico-philosophicus* (D. F. Pears and B. F.

McGuiness, Trans.). Great Britain: Whitstable Litho. (Original work published 1921)

Wuest, J. (1994). A feminist approach to concept analysis. *Western Journal of Nursing Research, 16*, 577–586.

Exploring Pragmatic Utility: Concept Analysis by Critically Appraising the Literature

Janice M. Morse*

Exploring the pragmatic utility of the concept(s) involved is the foundation of any social science research program. The pragmatic principle of concept evaluation includes determining the "applicability of concepts to the world" or the degree to which they are "operationalized" (Morse, Hupcey, Mitcham, & Lenz, 1996). Although determining pragmatic utility somewhat overlaps with the other principles of concept evaluation (i.e., the epistemological, logical, and linguistic principles) and in turn also contributes to the researcher's appreciation of the level of maturity of the concept (see Morse, Hupcey, Mitcham, & Lenz, 1996; Morse, Mitcham, Hupcey, & Tason, 1996), it is a task that contributes to understanding the function of the concept or the role it plays in research.

Pragmatic utility is determined by critically appraising the literature, but it is a procedure that differs from other types of literature summaries. A critical appraisal of the literature differs from a *literature review,* in which all of the research pertaining to a particular topic is summarized. It differs from a *critical analysis,* in which the researcher criticizes or challenges the *ideas* of other authors. It differs from a *review article,* in which the researcher summarizes the major contributions to research in a particular area, and it differs from a *research review,* in

*Acknowledgements: The author thanks Janice Penrod, M.S., and Judy Norris, Ph.D., for their comments during the development of this chapter. This research is supported by NIH, NINR, 2R01 NR02130-08, and AHFMR #57 61032.

which the researcher attempts to identify what is known and where the gaps in the research are or to identify the next logical step, hypotheses, or research questions to be tackled in order to continue inquiry. Rather, a *critical appraisal of the literature* contributes to a research program in another significant way: the exploration and development of the concepts themselves and the role they play in inquiry.

A critical appraisal of the literature is conducted in order to explore the pragmatic utility of concepts embedded in or emerging from a research program. It provides information about the *usefulness of the concept* to science, which in turn provides guidance about what research approaches should be used to further the research program and in what aspect of the concept—or in what area or dimension—concept development needs to occur. A critical appraisal of the literature provides information about various conceptualizations of the concept (whether overt or covert) and ways the concept is being used by other researchers in their models and in theory. Finally, it provides information about implicit and explicit assumptions and contributes to the evaluation of the logical coherence of the concept.

Thus, exploring the pragmatic utility of a concept is a way to evaluate the "state of the art" of the concept's application and utilization. Inquiry using critical appraisal of the literature is more than synthesizing and summarizing the literature—it is a process of active inquiry *using the literature as data*. The end result pushes knowledge beyond what is presently known about the concept and reveals new insights, poses significant questions, and provides direction about which level of inquiry and which methods should be used in the next phase of the research program.

The purpose of this chapter is to introduce methods of concept analysis that use the literature as data,* but before these methods are outlined, I will clarify what is meant by a concept and describe how one determines sampling adequacy and appropriateness for the selection of the literature.

THE ANATOMY OF A CONCEPT

Concepts are conceptual representations of phenomena, or in this context where the focus is on behavioral concepts, they are names given to clusters of behaviors that together form some function or purpose. The components of concepts are attributes or characteristics that distinguish one concept from another. Concepts have boundaries that delimit cases, showing what is and what is not an instance of that

---

*These methods differ dramatically from those described by Walker and Avant (1995), who recommend *review* of the literature and the creation of fictitious cases to illustrate the identification of conceptual attributes.

particular concept. Attributes are characteristics of the concept, and all of the identified attributes must be present in every case for the case to be considered an example of that particular concept. The pattern in which these attributes appear in the concept are context-bound, and it is this feature that gives rise to different manifestations of the concept.*

TYPES OF CONCEPTS

The types of concepts that are of primary interest to nurse researchers are *behavioral concepts,* or labels given to clusters of behaviors. Examples of behavioral concepts important to nursing are empathy, caring, hope, trust, social support, and so forth. These differ from concrete phenomena, such as incontinence, fatigue, or stress, which are more amenable to direct measurement. Because concrete entities can be measured directly, it is absurd and very clumsy to examine them using the indirect methods used for examining concepts described in this volume.

Behavioral concepts may be described as everyday concepts or scientific concepts. *Everyday concepts* are those used in ordinary language, are usually defined in the dictionary and, because they are abstract, are associated with many contexts (i.e., broad), do not have particular definitions, and are not narrowly confined to specific situations. Everyday concepts function to facilitate communication by providing labels for abstract ideas or clusters of behaviors. They enable shared meanings to be communicated when the object or representation cannot be clearly observed or directly measured.

Scientific concepts, on the other hand, are developed by researchers to refer to particular behaviors or entities. They are carefully defined as *operational definitions*, and it is this definition that gives the concept its particular scientific meaning, often relating to a specific context. In this sense scientific concepts are created by the researcher, their attributes are assigned or designated by the researcher (usually as variables, or indirectly as indices), and they are particular to the situation ascribed by the researcher (i.e., they are context-bound). Definitions of scientific concepts are therefore considered *narrow.* Confusion occurs when the concept label is used by many researchers who are unaware that they are assigning slightly different meanings to the same concept label (Tatje, 1970). In addition, researchers may use the same formal definition of the concept but, in practice, ascribe different attributes to the concept.

The dynamic nature of language results in the shift of concepts to or from the realm of scientific language to everyday language or vice versa.

---

*For example, consider patterns of hope (Morse & Doberneck, 1995).

Concepts may be developed by the scientific community that have appeal to the nonscientist, and eventually these concepts are adopted into everyday language, removed from the specific scientific context, and earn their place in the dictionary. An example of one that is making such as transition is the concept *empathy*, which was claimed as a scientific term from the lay lexicon in the 1950s through the work of Carl Rogers, was used in clinical psychology and the caring profession (including nursing) for several decades, and is presently being returned to the public. *Social support* is also of interest at this time, as I feel it is presently undergoing a transition. It was introduced as a scientific concept by Kaplan in 1974, and social support, although now used in everyday language, has not yet appeared in the dictionary (Hupcey, 1998). Other concepts that are a part of everyday language and are attracting the interest of researchers (and may therefore be considered to be in transition, being investigated and incorporated into scientific theory) are *hope* and *trust*.*

Serious problems occur when the researcher does not examine the concept as it is used and unquestioningly adopts it. First, such practices add to the confusion in science. An excellent example of such confusion was the concept of *caring*, which was used unquestioningly in nursing. As we will discuss later, concept analysis for pragmatic utility revealed that caring was used in the research literature with many different assumptions and purposes and in many different forms (Morse, 1986), with the result that several meanings of caring implicitly developed. Second, because relatively little interaction occurs among the social science disciplines, because of the slight differences in focus of these disciplines (and therefore differences in the application of the concepts), and because these disciplines rarely share literatures, a concept may develop slightly different definitions and meanings in two or more disciplines. An example of such variation is the concept of *trust*. It is important that such variation be explicated. Third, parallel concepts, which refer to the same or very similar phenomena, may develop in different disciplines: for example, *perception* (from nursing), *social construction of reality* (from sociology), and *cultural perspectives* (from anthropology).

From the above it should be evident that in the behavioral sciences nurse researchers frequently use and develop everyday concepts as *scientific concepts* or adopt concepts developed in another discipline for use in nursing in the context of patient care. Movement of concepts from scientific to everyday language also occurs—and vice versa. Thus, examining concepts, both everyday and scientific concepts, that appear

---

*Incidentally, qualitative research plays an important role in the development and the adoption of such concepts into nursing science because qualitative methods provide the means to explore the lay meaning of the term.

in the scientific literature in order to establish pragmatic utility is an important task. Not only does this analysis clarify the research literature but it also guides the course along which inquiry should proceed. That is, it provides important insights into the type of research that can and should be conducted.

PRINCIPLES OF ASSESSING PRAGMATIC UTILITY

The recent trend in nursing research has been to guide researchers by presenting a series of steps that can be systematically followed. The intent of this procedural approach is to clearly state *how* to use this method correctly, reliably, and validly. However, it simplifies the procedure and does not do justice to the cognitive work inherent in inquiry. Nor does this procedural approach allow for the nuances that emerge with each new topic and context. There is a tendency, particularly in concept development research, for researchers to follow these instructions superficially, and as a consequence, the results are often trivial. Writing stepwise instructions does not allow for an appreciation of the depth of inquiry, nor paradoxically does it ensure *rigor*. I have, therefore, written the following *guiding principles*. While some direct instructions cannot be avoided, the intent is that these instructions be used with wisdom, thoughtfulness, and, if necessary, cautiously added to or deviated from. The reader will note, however, that in this method all of the principles of rigorous research continue to have pertinence and relevance.

Principle 1: Be Clear About the Purpose of the Inquiry

Although the exact question may be modified during the course of inquiry, the researcher must have at least a research focus (identified as the concept or phenomenon to be investigated) and have a preliminary question to guide the initial work in the library.

Phenomenon Versus Concept

The first step is to clearly delimit the concept being explored. Occasionally a phenomenon may have several concepts that refer to it, and as previously stated, these concepts may have the same or slightly different meanings. Therefore, it is important to identify *all* of the terms used. Prepare a list of search terms by concept, subject word, or term. If using a concept, be certain to identify the allied concepts. Also add the converse: For example, if searching for trust, also search for mistrust or distrust; if searching for hope, also search for hopeless and even for despair. This will ensure that your search is comprehensive and complete.

A word of warning: Note we are delimiting by *topic*. That is, we are selecting a word and similar terms to use as our search terms. If a word is ambiguous, we do not search the alternative meanings of the word. Walker and Avant (1995, p. 41) use the example of *coping*. In addition to coping as a behavior, they include the copings on buildings, coping saws, coping as a method of trimming a falcon's beak, and coping as an ecclesiastical garment. Alternative meanings do *not* help us with the search for pragmatic utility, and alternative meanings are ignored.

Principle 2: Ensure Validity

To ensure that the sample of literature is adequate and appropriate, it is imperative that all relevant data bases are searched. Unless your research question is specific to nursing, data bases of all relevant disciplines should be searched. Ignoring a particular data base may leave a gap that will threaten validity.

It is most important to become familiar with the literature; therefore, *obtain all references*, both articles and books. Copy all articles, and read the literature carefully. I cannot emphasize enough that this research cannot be conducted using only the abstracts obtained from the indexing service—the entire article is needed. As you are reading each article, pay particular attention to (and highlight) any definitions of the term (and any attribution for the term), the study's research question, and any assumptions listed. Consider exploration of the concept within a "school of thought," and if possible, begin to organize the articles into stacks according to underlying assumptions or how similar concept definitions are used.

A problem may develop if the researcher adheres to only one bibliographic data base (no matter how "comprehensive") because of the danger of disciplinary bias. Sometimes, allied concepts may share attributes, and in this case, it will be necessary to search both concepts and compare and contrast the two. In order for analysis to proceed, there must be enough literature available that uses the selected concept, thereby ensuring that the criterion of sampling adequacy will be met (see Morse, 1986). If there is only scant literature available, that is an indicator that the concept is immature, and a qualitative study must be conducted to develop the concept (see Morse, Hupcey, Mitcham, & Lenz, 1996).

Develop a System for Maintaining Bibliographic Records

The amount of literature identified—as a simple count of the number of articles—should be large, and it needs to be large if you are using this method of concept analysis. If you have identified only a few articles, unless those few articles are rich and theoretically comprehensive, your sample will be inadequate.

Because you are using a large and comprehensive literature as data, a system for bibliographic retrieval must be organized and used. Catalogue all articles into a computerized system such as *Procite.**

Principle 3: Identify Significant Analytical Questions

Attain Comprehension with the Topic

It is imperative that the researcher become familiar with all the pertinent literature, copy it, and read it all. Highlight (emphasize) definitions and variables used because these are indicators of the concept's attributes or characteristics.

Seek out, identify, and record assumptions used in the articles. The assumptions or author's perspective may be clearly stated. Alternatively, assumptions may be inferred from: (1) the research question(s) asked in the study; (2) the researcher's focus or "bias," or (3) the general content of the article, such as by making inferences from the variables used in the article or the items listed in the instruments used. Recall that research is not value free, and the author's bias, perspective, or theories used provide, albeit indirectly, a means to infer the researcher's perspective on the concepts. As the reading progresses, it may be possible to sort the literature into piles according to the major (or most interesting) assumptions identified. By this stage, you should be able to talk about the literature with confidence and describe and categorize various approaches.

Refine the Research Question

The continuous reading, sorting, cataloguing and thinking about the articles assists with the refinement of the research question. Inasmuch as the research question *determines the purpose of the analysis* and the approach used, this is a critical step. The research question will arise from your open and querying reading about the concept: Think—is there consensus within the literature about the definition of the concept? Do definitions vary from article to article? Are definitions missing or not stated? Is the concept used in the same way, and is it used consistently from study to study? Is the concept used consistently among different disciplines?

The research question is important because it determines the purpose of the analysis and the principles and mechanism for comparing and sorting the literature. Reevaluate your overall question in light of what

---

*Procite is available from Research Information Systems, Carlsbad, California.

has been learned about the topic: Is your question the result of a need to clarify the concept? To compare or to contrast disciplinary perspectives? To determine adequacy by contrasting competing concepts? To identify conceptual gaps/boundaries when explaining phenomena? To identify conceptual adequacy?

Note that the research question need not arise from a curiosity present at the beginning of the study, but it may be reconceptualized in the process of reading the copious literature. Indeed, you may not have been aware of the problems or strengths in the concept before delving into the literature.

The Nature of the Overall Question Dictates the Design of the Remainder of the Study; the Research Question Dictates the Organization of Data for Comparison

Researchers must always be aware of their rationale for asking research questions, and they should be aware of the type of results that they intend to obtain. The rationale for conducting the study remains a constant reminder of the overall desired goals. For instance, you may be interested in different *disciplinary perspectives* on the concept. Because each discipline provides a different context in which to use the concept, while the conceptual attributes remain the same, the various disciplinary contexts emphasize different attributes, resulting in different conceptual forms. Similarly, as authors or major "schools of inquiry" tend to cluster in disciplines (or even within disciplines, institutions, or geographic areas), the analysis may cluster by major contributors or researchers who tend to use the same conceptual definitions. Occasionally, one or two authors will have made significant contributions, and therefore, it may be pertinent to the research goals to sort the concept by definition: for example, to sort stress by articles using Selye's definition versus "others."

Another design that may be of interest to researchers is by method. By *method* I do not mean research method, but rather how the concept is researched and described, for this provides insight into how the concept or phenomenon has been perceived. For example, the phenomenon of nurses' ability to assess the patient's condition without the patient verbalizing complaints has been accounted for by the concepts of inference, sublimation, empathy, and insight. Consider how this phenomenon was researched: Did the researcher interview nurses or *observe* nurses assessing patients to describe the concepts used? Did the researcher interview nurses about unsuccessful as well as successful incidents? As discussed later, these concepts all have distinct attributes, and using different methods to examine the same phenomenon sheds light on how the concepts were perceived.

Researchers may find it more convenient to sort literature by time periods. Such an approach provides information on the changing use of the concept and even on the profession's value of the concept. For instance, when studying comfort, McIlveen and Morse (1995) sorted the literature by decades, comparing and contrasting the changing role of comfort in the literature. Other researchers may elect to use historical events: for instance, sorting the literature by such milestones as the First and Second World Wars, the Depression, the post–World War II boom years, and so forth.

Alternatively, the researcher may elect to sort the literature by quality-(ies) or perspectives of the concept. This is the most difficult type of analysis because the qualities are not always immediately obvious. An example of one such study is an examination of the conceptualizations of caring, which will be discussed later.

Unfortunately, it is not possible to combine too many of these purposes. Each time the data are "split," the amount of data in each category is further reduced and introduces a problem of thin data or an inadequate number of articles (data) available for analysis in each category.

The Research Question Aids in the Identification of the Analytical Questions

The analytical questions (i.e., the questions actually asked of the data) are the essence of the analysis—the most important part of the analysis—for it is these questions that enable the process of comparison; and it is the comparison that determines the parameters (boundaries) of the concept or the differences between the perception of the concept or differences in the attributes when comparing concepts. I cannot emphasize enough that these questions, which come from a profound understanding of the literature, are the most significant contribution to the analysis and the strength of the study.

The analytical questions can only be identified once the researcher is familiar with the literature. Until the researcher has an excellent grasp on the concept and its components and has looked at the literature critically, she or he will not be able to identify questions that may be asked of all conceptual dimensions. Analytical questions may be discussed within the literature, or may arise within some of the literature, or may be developed from dimensions regarding assumption about the preconditions or the outcomes, that is, the *use* of the concept. This point will be more easily understood by examining the analytical questions used in the examples later in this chapter.

Principle 4: Synthesize Results

Set the Stage So You Can See the Whole: The Key to Developing an Adequate Means and Appreciating the Dimensions of Difference

Seeing the whole matrix allows the researcher to ask analytical questions across dimensions and identify commonalities and differences. Prepare a worksheet by taping large sheets of paper together so they cover a tabletop. Construct a matrix, with the analytical questions in the left column and the selected dimensions across the top. Draw in the columns and complete the matrix. Questions answered appropriately may have "Yes," "No" or "Exceptions," the names of the first author, and the bibliographic number of the article written in the cells. Occasionally the best quotation—or most represented summary—may be written in the cell for future reference. Or the analytical question may demand that the description be listed in the cell—again with the citation number of the article.

There is a distinct *dis*advantage to using a computer for recording responses to comparative analytical questions because one cannot view the whole matrix at once on the screen. Even if the matrix is relatively complete, it will require much printing and taping pages together to form the complete sheet. My recommendation for this task is to use a pencil and paper; more specifically, obtain a very large sheet of paper and draw multiple columns and cells.

One word of warning: It is important not to consider the categories within the cells as rigid or inflexible, and do not make value judgments about the appropriateness or inappropriateness of the derivations of the conceptualization. Using cells to identify dimensions is merely an analytical tool, and the process of abbreviating and separating necessarily simplifies, perhaps unfairly separating the statements from the context of the article as a whole. But it is a technique that enables the identification of differences and makes the process of analysis exciting, interesting, and possible.

If working as a team, *divide the task into cohesive areas and allocate tasks accordingly.* Making a team member responsible for distinct areas enables analytical questions to be asked within the context of team meetings. The adage "many heads are better than one" is true in this context, especially if you are working with a multidisciplinary team. The different theoretical bases of each team member stimulate a greater variety of questions, which, in turn, moves the analysis along more quickly and results in a richer, more comprehensive product. Initially, the answers to questions may be abbreviated on the chart, with the chart completed at a later time.

Compilation of "Results"

Once the analysis has been completed, the researchers must then prepare an article that accurately reports the results. The first step, always, is to outline the article and prepare the tables or figures. One needs to be creative about the best way to present many authors on a single table or figure, giving consideration to the format of the journal to which the completed article will be submitted. Occasionally, the journal editor will not permit a full bibliographic list to be included with the article, allowing only major references. In this case, include a footnote so that interested readers may write to the senior author for the complete bibliographic list. If it is essential for attribution, a coding system may be developed to identify the primary author for each citation (see Figure 17-1). The referencing style of the American Psychological Association (APA) is often too cumbersome for use on complex tables. In this case, consider using a number-citation style, such as University of Chicago.

When writing the article, it is important to maintain a balanced perspective. Be certain to point out new findings and points that reinforce the status quo. Above all, be clear; contrast and explain facts in detail so that your reader is not struggling to follow you or to seek out your point.

To reiterate, the type of approach to the literature will depend on the level of development of the concept and, consequently, the researcher's purpose in conducting the analysis, from which, of course, the research question is derived. Only those concepts that are reasonably well developed may be analyzed using these methods. Principles of sampling dictate there must be adequate literature available in order to conduct this type of analysis. When asking analytical, comparative questions of the data (literature), the researcher must have an adequate base to answer the questions. If there are too few articles, or the articles do not contain adequate information (that is, the data base is inadequate), then the concept is immature, and a qualitative study must be conducted. *This is a basic principle of sampling that holds true for all research methods.* The main purpose for conducting this analysis is to ensure pragmatic utility: to clarify concepts, to compare and contrast the use of concepts in particular disciplines, to compare conceptual adequacy with competing concepts, to identify conceptual gaps and boundaries, and to identify conceptual inconsistencies within a concept.

ESTABLISHING PRAGMATIC UTILITY

Example One: Clarifying Concepts; Clarifying Caring

Occasionally concepts are widely used, and there is an extraordinarily large volume of literature available. But despite the "popularity" of the concept and its extensive use and broad application, much about the concept probably remains implicit. The researcher may sense that despite superficial cohesion or unity of perspectives, there are important differences that have remained unexplicated, and it is these differences that are leading to conceptual confusion and different research agendas. It becomes important to identify implicit values/assumptions underlying the concepts and to make the different theoretical perspectives explicit.

Such was the case of caring in the late 1980s. Caring was generally considered to be a very important concept to nursing, and several major theorists considered it to be the keystone of nursing. Such theorists as Leininger, Watson, Roach, and Ray considered caring to be the "essence" or the "core" of nursing. Despite this apparent unified focus among these researchers, I was disconcerted that there were important differences in perspective that remained submerged, and a clarification of the concept was needed.

The huge volume of caring literature revealed that the concept was amenable to concept analysis; dozens of articles were retrieved from nursing alone. From this large number, seminal articles by authors who were considered to be major contributors were selected for analysis. These articles contained a definition of caring, or if an explicit definition was not contained in the article, it was possible to classify the theoretical perspective of the author from an examination of the research approach, research questions, and underlying assumptions. For instance, Stevenson (1990) examined all the quantitative literature on care, selecting her sample by searching the titles of articles for the word *care*, documenting the procedural aspects of care. Aamodt (1989), on the other hand, explored the patient's perspective as a recipient of care, implying that the concept is reflected in nursing behaviors and is recognizable by the patient. If care was described as a *process*, the author usually depicted relationships in a diagram containing arrows illustrating the implied or explicit connections; others did not consider care as a process or the outcomes of care in their conceptualization of care.

Thus, an examination of the definitions of care and the models of care in each article identified care as a static concept or as a process and revealed the philosophical or definitional commonalities. These articles were placed in piles according to their commonalities and were labeled accordingly.

Five conceptualizations of care were identified, and it was noted that some authors linked two or more conceptualizations in their models. These conceptualizations were as follows: caring as a human trait, caring as a moral imperative, caring as an affect, caring as an interpersonal relationship, and caring as a therapeutic intervention. In addition, two outcomes were identified, as some researchers noted one or both of

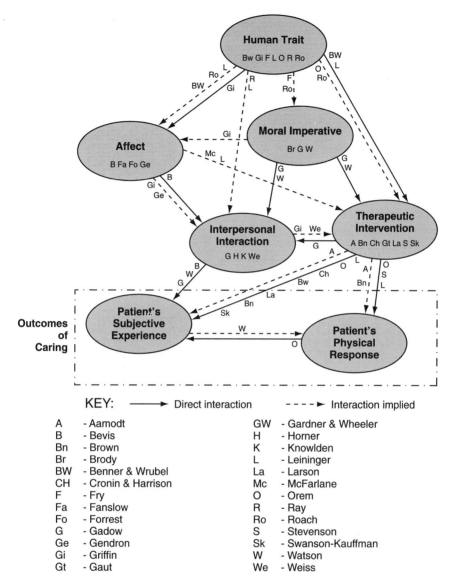

KEY: ——————► Direct interaction   - - - - ► Interaction implied

A	- Aamodt	GW	- Gardner & Wheeler
B	- Bevis	H	- Horner
Bn	- Brown	K	- Knowlden
Br	- Brody	L	- Leininger
BW	- Benner & Wrubel	La	- Larson
CH	- Cronin & Harrison	Mc	- McFarlane
F	- Fry	O	- Orem
Fa	- Fanslow	R	- Ray
Fo	- Forrest	Ro	- Roach
G	- Gadow	S	- Stevenson
Ge	- Gendron	Sk	- Swanson-Kauffman
Gi	- Griffin	W	- Watson
Gt	- Gaut	We	- Weiss

Figure 17–1 The interrelationship of five perspectives of caring.

these: caring as the subjective experience of the patient and caring as the physical response of the patient (Figure 17–1). From this literature sort, the main characteristics of each perspective were then described.

A second publication was built on this initial categorization, comparing the linkages between categories and the purposes and the outcomes of each author's perspective (Morse, Bottorff, Neander, & Solberg, 1991) (Table 17–1). This analysis provided further detail on the implications

Table 17–1 The Major Components of Five Perspectives on Caring

Human Trait	Moral Imperative	Affect	Interpersonal Interaction	Therapeutic Intervention
Essential for being human	Foundational basis—Nurse virtue	Empathy, feeling and concern for, another	An exchange characterized by respect and trust	Nursing actions that meet patient's needs
Universal	Nurse-centered	Nurse-centered	Mutual involvement	Patient-centered
Necessary for survival	Maintain dignity of patients	Nurse must feel compassion to be able to nurse	Develop a type of intimate relationship	Implementation meets patient's goals
Essential way of being	Guides decision making, provides the "oughts" behind the "shoulds"	Feeling motivates the nurse; nurse feels better when able to "really nurse"	Process that can enhance growth of both patient and nurse	If actions are appropriate, the patient improves regardless of how nurse feels
Constant, long-lasting	Constant concern for patient	Nursing is defined in relation to affect. However, affect may vary with kind of patient, stage of relationship, and/or situational demands	Is likely to vary with ability or desire of patient to be involved with nurse and situational demands	Varies with situational demands and in relation to knowledge and skill of nurse

of the diverse conceptualizations of caring for nursing practice and the strengths and weaknesses of these conceptualizations. Analytical questions were developed, such as: Is caring unique to nursing? Does the caring intent of nursing vary between patients? Can caring be reduced to behavioral tasks? and Does the outcome of caring affect the patient? The nurse? Or both the patient and the nurse? The sorting of authors according to these questions further pushed the analysis (Table 17-2). Finally, we asked: Does caring take place with individuals or with groups? It was noted that caring between individuals was clearly described, but the caring process for families or communities (at the institutional or societal level) was poorly described and needed further development.

These two articles exploring caring clearly revealed that *if* caring is the "essence of nursing," then which theoretical perspective (or all) constitutes this essence? The pragmatic utility of caring as a concept is poorly developed, and this analysis revealed previously unrecognized gaps, inadequacies, and areas that needed further qualitative work.

Example Two: Determining Adequacy by Contrasting Competing Concepts; Accounting for Inference and Insight in Nursing Assessment

Recall that behavioral concepts represent a phenomenon or collections of behavioral actions that have some meaning and have been given a name. The abstract nature of these concepts means that not only are they difficult to measure directly, but several concepts may emerge that account for the same phenomenon. This is an awkward situation because these concepts then compete with varying degrees of acceptance, according to the discipline of origin, amount of conviction or adequacy of explanation, faddishness, and even practical concerns, such as ease of operationalism and measurement. Of importance, however, is that the concepts, while accounting for the same phenomenon, may contain different sets of behaviors and be at different levels of maturity. When the investigator is interested in a particular phenomenon, it is important to compare and contrast the conceptual adequacy of these competing concepts rather than simply accept them as different disciplines' labels for the same concept. It is worse still to choose one and ignore the other concept labels and their accompanying literatures, writing them off as "different concepts" altogether and therefore concepts that are irrelevant to the present phenomenon.

Early in the 1990s I was interested in expert nurses' insight into a patient's condition or state, that is, the documented ability of nurses to predict an impending crisis and deterioration in the patient's condition without the patient explicitly reporting his or her symptoms, feelings,

Table 17–2 Authors' Perceptions of Selected Characteristics of Caring

Is Caring Unique in Nursing?

Yes		No	
Brody	Roach	Benner & Wrubel	Horner
Knowlden	Watson	Bevis	Ray
Leininger		Fry	
McFarlane		Griffin	

Does the Caring Intent of Nursing Vary Between Patients?

Yes	No	
Griffin	Brody	Gendron
Horner	Fanslow	Leininger
Ray	Fry	Watson

Can Caring Be Reduced to Behavioral Tasks?

Yes	No	
Brown	Benner & Wrubel	Gadow
Gaut	Bevis	Griffin
Larson	Brody	Horner
Leininger	Fanslow	Knowlden
McFarlane	Fry	Roach
Orem	Forrest	Watson
Swanson-Kauffman		
Weiss		
Wolf		

Does the Outcome of the Caring Affect:

The Patient?	The Nurse?	Both the Patient and the Nurse?
Brown	Brody	Benner & Wrubel
Gaut	Fanslow	Bevis
Gendron	Forrest	Gadow
Larson	Fry	Griffin
Leininger	Roach	Horner
Orem		Watson
Swanson-Kauffman		
Wolf		

or needs. With this ability, clinicians have the ability to assess patient cues and the insight to comprehend their meaning and to respond with the appropriate clinical intervention and, therefore, provide comfort.

Despite the importance of this ability to "sense patient needs," use "inference and insight," or to "read the patient," it is poorly understood, and seven concepts compete to explain the phenomenon: intuition, inference, "knowing the patient," countertransference, empathy, compathy, and embodiment (Morse, Miles, Clark, & Doberneck, 1994). Initially, the definitions, mechanisms, and application of the seven concepts were compared. However, adequate literature was available for only three of them (i.e., intuition, emotional empathy, and inference), and therefore, these three competing concepts were compared for pragmatic utility. Significant analytical questions were identified, and wherever possible, authors were sorted into cells on a large template. The following questions were asked of the concepts:

1. Were these abilities something common to all humans as a part of "human nature," a characteristic—a "quality"—of most nurses, or alternatively, as Benner and Tanner (1987) suggest, a quality of an excellent nurse acquired in the process of becoming expert?
2. Were the concepts perceived to be a special gift, ability, or talent?
3. Was the degree of ability to use the concepts influenced or enhanced by the nurse's personal past? For example, are nurses more empathetic if they themselves have personally experienced illness or bereavement prior to commencing their nursing careers?
4. Is a relationship with the patient a precondition for the phenomenon to occur?
5. Can the concept be taught or enhanced in the classroom or at work?

Analytical questions were asked about the characteristics of or assumptions about the *processing* of the information when the nurses were assessing patient cues:

1. Was the nurse's response emotional, cognitive, or physical?
2. At what level of awareness does the concept occur (i.e., conscious, subconscious, or unconscious)?
3. Did the nurses experience identification with the patient? If so, was this identification psychosocial, physical, or both?

Finally, we examined the *outcome* or the reported results of the nurse's use of the concept:

1. Was the concept considered a complex process and/or a product (such as a feeling or a therapeutic intervention)?
2. Was the concept accurate in predicting or judging the patient's condition or state?
3. Was the experience described by the concept positive or beneficial to patient care, negative or potentially harmful, or could it be either positive or negative?

From the above analysis, it was concluded that these three competing concepts had much in common (depicted by overlapping characteristics). However, there were also distinct differences, which related to the epistemological origins and/or nursing interpretation, translation, adoption, and utilization of the concepts. Problems arose both from misinterpretation and from the borrowing of concept, resulting in two authors using the same concept name but implicitly using different meanings. Often there were problems with the research design, such as *intuition* being investigated by interview (rather than observational methods), despite the fact that it was described as "a look that patients get" and nurses repeatedly being unable to describe the "look." Furthermore, only reports of *successful* intuits were considered in the analysis (see Benner & Tanner, 1987). Both of these problems do not assist with the application of the concept; in fact, it demonstrates an important pragmatic mismatch between the concept and the research conducted.

In conclusion, the lack of fit between the complex behaviors inherent in "reading the patient," the research, and clinical application may be because none of the concepts considered met the pragmatic principle for concept evaluation. It is possible that the appropriate concept had not yet been considered in nursing research (such as sublimation) or that the appropriate concept had not yet been developed. Nevertheless, a critical analysis of the literature assessing the pragmatic utility of the competing concepts was a simpler, less costly (both in research dollars and time) way to arrive at this conclusion than approaching the problem in the traditional way of systematically experimenting with these concepts.

DISCUSSION

Several factors are most important in the pragmatic assessment of concepts. For example, it cannot be stressed enough that *all* the literature must be pulled, read, and carefully considered. This means that the researcher must be very careful not to "drown" in the volume of data, become overwhelmed, and lose control of the material, for when this happens ideas are lost and inquiry comes to standstill. It is important to maintain control of the literature with a data base, develop a system to record ideas and attribution of those ideas, develop a system of bibliographic retrieval, and learn that not all articles should be prioritized equally (or even incorporated) into the analysis. Some articles are "key" references; they are theoretically rich, and should be prioritized and referred to frequently, with the researcher paying more attention to them in the analysis than to others. Articles that add little information may be excluded from the analysis. Unfortunately, until the researcher has read all of these articles, it is not possible to sort the "wheat from the chaff."

It is the identification of analytical questions that guides the research forward and enables the research process itself to make a unique and creative contribution to the literature. Much thought must go into the identification of these questions because the study will be only as strong as the analytical questions asked. The analytical questions provide the dimensions by which the researcher actually explores the concept and subsequently redefines the concept itself. For this reason, this method can only be used with relatively mature concepts, once again using *adequate literature* as data.

Although the researcher develops creative insights, these insights are not coming, as with qualitative meta-analysis, from the qualitative data presented in each study, but from the operational definitions, conceptual descriptions, assumptions, and even from the questions asked in each study. The literature used may be qualitative or quantitative research, or it may be theoretical or philosophical essays. It is unrealistic to assume that the answers to each analytical question are clearly evident in every article—often these answers must be inferred, and sometimes creatively. For instance, it is possible to derive answers from such sources as the items of Likert Scales or by using inference when the author asserted the converse. Clearly, researchers making such inferences must do so with caution, discussion, agreement within the team, and with the appropriate use of footnotes anchoring their data collection matrix to the original source.

This method of concept analysis to establish pragmatic utility and using the literature as data has developed over a period of time and as a result of conducting analysis on concepts that were perceived to be significant to nursing and inherent in the construct of comfort. Results from these studies reveal that the method enables new insights to be developed about the concept, and by using the literature as data, the research may proceed without the collection of raw data. Pragmatic assessment of concepts is an important tool in commencing a research program because it provides information about the adequacy and appropriateness of concepts for research or for clinical application.

REFERENCES

Aamodt, A. (1989). Ethnography and epistemology: Generating nursing knowledge. In J. M. Morse (Ed.), *Qualitative nursing research: A contemporary dialogue*. Rockville, MD: Aspen.

Benner, P., & Tanner, C. (1987). Clinical judgment: How expert nurses use intuition. *American Journal of Nursing, 87*, 23-31.

Hupcey, J. E., Penrod, J., Morse, J. M., & Mitcham, C. (in review). A multidisciplinary analysis of the concept of trust.

Hupcey, J. E. (1998). Social support: Assessing conceptual coherence. *Qualitative Health Research, 8*(3), 304-318.

McIlveen, K. M., & Morse, J. M. (1995) The role of comfort in nursing care: 1900-1980. *Clinical Nursing Research, 4*(2), 127-148.

Morse, J. M. (1986). Qualitative and quantitative methods: Issues in sampling.

In P. Chinn (Ed.), *Nursing research methodology: Issues and implementation* (pp. 181–193). Rockville, MD: Aspen.

Morse, J. M., Anderson, G., Bottorff, J., Yonge, O., O'Brien, B., Solberg, S., & McIlveen, K. (1992). Exploring empathy: A conceptual fit for nursing practice? *Image: Journal of Nursing Scholarship, 24*(4), 274-280.

Morse, J. M., Bottorff, J., Anderson, G., O'Brien, B., & Solberg, S. (1992). Beyond empathy: Expanding expressions of caring. *Journal of Advanced Nursing, 17*, 809-821.

Morse, J. M., Bottorff, J., Neander, W., & Solberg, S. (1991). Comparative analysis of the conceptualizations and theories of caring. *Image: Journal of Nursing Scholarship, 23*(2), 119-126.

Morse, J. M., & Doberneck, B. M. (1995). Delineating the concept of hope. *Image: Journal of Nursing Scholarship, 27*(4), 277-285.

Morse, J. M., Hupcey, J., Mitcham, C., & Lenz, E. (1996). Concept analysis in nursing research: A critical appraisal. *Scholarly Inquiry for Nursing Practice, 10*(3), 253-277.

Morse, J. M., Miles, M. W., Clark, D. A., & Doberneck, B. M. (1994). "Sensing" patient needs: Exploring concepts of nursing insight and receptivity used in nursing assessment. *Scholarly Inquiry for Nursing Practice, 8*(3), 233-254.

Morse, J. M., Mitcham, C., Hupcey, J., & Tason, M. (1996). Criteria for concept evaluation. *Journal of Advanced Nursing, 24*(2), 385-390.

Morse, J. M., Solberg, S. M., Neander, W. L., Bottorff, J. L., & Johnson, J. L. (1990). Concepts of caring and caring as a concept. *Advances in Nursing Science, 13*, 1-14.

Stevenson, J. (1990) A review of the quantitative literature on care. In J. Stevenson & T. Tripp-Reimer (Eds.), *Knowledge about care and caring: State of the art and future development.* Kansas City, KS: American Academy of Nursing.

Tatje, T. A. (1970). Problems of concept definition for comparative studies. In R. Naroll & R. Cohen (Eds.), *A handbook of method in cultural anthropology* (pp. 689-696). Garden City, NY: Natural History Press.

Van der Steen, W. J. (1993). *A practical philosophy for the life sciences.* Albany, NY: State University of New York Press.

Walker, L. O., & Avant, K. C. (1995). *Strategies for theory construction in nursing* (3rd ed.). Norwalk, CT: Appleton & Lange.

CHAPTER

18

Research Careers and Concept Development: The Case of Normalization

Kathleen A. Knafl and Janet A. Deatrick

A variety of disciplines and philosophical perspectives are evident in the concept development literature. These include wide-ranging discussions about the nature of concepts and human cognition, methodological guidelines for carrying out analyses of specific concepts, and scholarly debates about the merits of different concept development activities (McCloskey & Glucksberg, 1978; Medin, 1989; Morse, Hupcey, Mitcham, & Lenz, 1996; Paley, 1996). In nursing, much attention has been directed to the analysis of specific concepts using one of several analytical protocols advocated by nurse authors (Chinn & Kramer, 1991; Rodgers, 1989; Walker & Avant, 1988). Although there has also been considerable debate on the relative merits of these approaches to concept analysis, a common underlying goal is the synthesis of knowledge regarding a particular concept, typically with an eye to identifying defining attributes or criteria (Knafl & Deatrick, 1993). Recently, a number of authors have advocated the use of qualitative research methods to advance concept development (Morse, Mitcham, Hupcey, & Tason, 1996; Schwartz-Barcott & Kim, 1993). In contrast to the concept analysis literature that focuses on taking stock of what is known about a particular concept, this recent literature emphasizes the further refinement and development of concepts through systematic data collection and analysis. Relatively little attention has been directed to the interplay of analytical and empirical approaches to concept development. Our intent in this chapter is to explore that interplay as it has evolved in our own research.

Over the past 15 years we have sustained an enduring interest in normalization, a concept that has proven useful in understanding and explaining family response to childhood illness and disability. Our interest in normalization has led us in a variety of directions including formal concept analyses and multiple empirical studies (Deatrick, Knafl, & Murphy-Moore, in press; Knafl & Deatrick, 1986; Knafl, Deatrick, & Kirby, in press). We have learned a great deal about normalization; we also have learned a great deal about the process of concept development and the ways in which both analytical and empirical endeavors can contribute to that development. Much of our learning has been trial and error. Conceptual angst and methodological uncertainty have been interspersed with moments of insight and intellectual satisfaction. In retrospect, we have been on an extended scholarly adventure. We undertook our first concept analysis prior to much of the more sophisticated debate on the topic; our early qualitative studies were launched prior to general acceptance of qualitative methods in nursing. Although we have learned a great deal along the way, many of our hard-earned lessons and insights were not appropriate for inclusion in a typical research report or theoretical presentation. Although they were shared with colleagues and students in seminars and informal discussion, they did not make their way into the formal literature. The writing of this chapter has provided us with an opportunity to systematically reflect on the various processes that have contributed to the development of the concept of normalization. As such, it includes the official history of the concept as reported in the published literature and the personal story of our particular adventure in concept development. Following brief discussions of the history of concept development in nursing and the evolution of the concept of normalization, our focus will turn to the inside story of our work on normalization and the conceptual and methodological struggles and insights that accompanied our contributions to its development. Our hope is that these insights will prove useful to readers who, like us, are committed to advancing the conceptual underpinnings of nursing science and practice.

THE GROWTH AND DEVELOPMENT OF NURSING CONCEPTS

Concepts, like people, have developmental histories. Following an initial act of creation, some are carefully nurtured and thrive while others are neglected or fall into disuse, contributing relatively little to the advance of science. Contemporary thinking on the nature of concepts emphasizes their developmental qualities and directs our attention to how they are used and change over time. Within nursing, Rodgers (1993) argued in favor of an evolutionary view of concepts that builds on contemporary philosophical views. She suggests viewing concepts as dynamic and states:

> this notion of development and refinement reveals the emphasis placed on conceptual change . . . I do not consider the attributes of a concept to be a fixed set of necessary conditions, or an essence. Consequently, according to this view, this cluster of attributes may change, by convention or by purposeful redefinition over time to maintain a useful, applicable, and effective concept. (p. 75)

She developed an approach to concept analysis that took into account their evolving nature.

As discussed in Chapter 3 of this volume, nurse theorists have had a long-standing interest in concept development and this interest gave rise to the delineation of a variety of approaches to concept analysis. These approaches, though varied, are directed to synthesizing the literature on a particular concept. They contribute to concept development by integrating current knowledge and providing direction for subsequent research and theory development.

Qualitative research also has a long history of contributing to concept development in nursing. In particular, grounded theory and phenomenological approaches have been used to both identify and develop concepts. As early as 1967, Quint advocated the use of empirical approaches to concept development, and Chenitz and Swanson (1986) noted that "a grounded theory is done to produce abstract concepts and propositions about the relationships between them." Examples of concepts that have been identified and developed in grounded theory studies include: responsible subversion (Hutchinson, 1990); negotiated partnerships (Powell-Cope, 1994); and transformed parenting (Seideman & Kleine, 1995). Whereas grounded theorists emphasize linkages among an array of concepts that comprise an empirically based theory, phenomenologists have focused on identifying the underlying structure of a given concept. For example, Jacobson (1994) identified three underlying dimensions of children's stressful life experiences and Swanson (1990) described the essential components of caring in neonatal intensive care. Both grounded theorists and phenomenologists have directed their attention to the discovery and description of concepts that are relevant for understanding a wide spectrum of health- and illness-related experiences.

Until Schwartz-Barcott and Kim (1986) developed the hybrid approach of concept development, little was acknowledged about the interplay between the empirical concept development approaches of qualitative researchers and the analytical approaches described in texts on theory development. Schwartz-Barcott and Kim made a notable contribution to the discipline when they discussed the advantages of combining analytical and empirical approaches to concept development. Their presentation of the hybrid approach described how one first reviews the literature with the intent of developing a working definition of a concept and then further develops the concept through qualitative data collection. They described how to use participant observation to further develop a concept of interest and reported that between 1980 and 1993 they and their students examined over 70 concepts using the hybrid approach (Schwartz-Barcott & Kim, 1993).

Jan Morse's (1995) recent work on advanced techniques of concept development also advocated incorporating analytical and empirical approaches to concept development. Morse differentiated a variety of concept development activities (delineation, comparison, clarification, correction, identification), all of which were grounded in a thorough review of the literature that set the stage for subsequent data collection activities using qualitative methods. This interplay of analytical and empirical activities is reflected in the development of the concept of normalization.

ORIGIN AND HISTORY OF NORMALIZATION

The concept of normalization had its origins in the work of sociologists interested in deviance and identity. In 1957, Schwartz published an article entitled "Perspectives on Deviance—Wives' Definitions of Their Husbands' Mental Illness," in which she described how women used what she termed a normalcy framework to explain their husband's increasingly bizarre behavior. By defining the behavior as accidental, temporary, or linked to unusual circumstances, women in this study sustained a definition of their husbands as mentally normal. Building on Schwartz's work, Davis (1963) used the term *normalization* to describe how some, though not all, families in which there was a child with polio defined and managed their situation. In addition to exploring how these families regained their view of their family as normal, Davis also described the kinds of behaviors families engaged in to sustain what they viewed as a normal family life. In these sociological studies, the concept of normalization contributed to the explanation of deviance disavowal or the individual's or family's ability to reject threats to a valued identity—in these studies, the view of oneself and one's family as normal. Subsequent studies (Birenbaum, 1971; Darling, 1979; Roskies, 1972; Voysey, 1975) pointed to the importance of external validation, including that from health care professionals, in supporting individuals' and families' normalization efforts. In particular, insights from these early authors linking normalization to external validation pointed to the potential clinical significance of the concept for practice disciplines.

Health care providers not only could support the family's claim to a normal identity, they could contribute to developing strategies that sustained normal family roles and routines. The results of these early studies were synthesized in our first analysis of the concept (Knafl & Deatrick, 1986). The analysis was based on the assumption that normalization was a clinically and theoretically relevant concept and used Chinn and Jacobs's (1983) approach to concept analysis. It resulted in the identification of four defining criteria: (1) acknowledge existence of impairment; (2) define family life as normal; (3) define social consequences of impairment as minimal; (4) engage in behaviors to demonstrate normalcy.

A subsequent analysis (Deatrick, Knafl, & Murphy-Moore, in press) that was based on Rodgers' approach to concept analysis identified 34 additional publications reporting work on the concept, 19 of which explicitly contributed to its continued development. This second analysis led to our further refinement of the original four defining attributes of normalization and the addition of a new attribute. Table 18–1 compares the original and revised attributes of normalization and points to the continuing evolution of the concept as a result of ongoing empirical and analytical activities.

In particular, studies completed between our first and second analysis of the concept have provided insights into the origins of families' normalization efforts (Robinson, 1993) and the development of management behaviors and routines that sustain a normalized family life (Bossert et al., 1990; Dashiff, 1993; Deatrick, Knafl, & Guyer, 1993; Hatton et al., 1995). They also have revealed how the defining attributes of normalization vary across illness and family contexts. For example, in families where members agree on the desirability of adopting a normalcy lens for viewing their situation, they are likely to support one

Table 18–1   Defining Attributes of Normalization in 1986 and 1998

1986	1998
1. Acknowledges existence of condition	1. Acknowledges existence of condition and its potential to threaten lifestyle
2. Defines family life as normal	2. Adapts normalcy lens for defining child and family
3. Engages in behaviors to demonstrate the normalcy of their family life	3. Engages in parenting behaviors and family routines that are consistent with normalcy lens
4. _____	4. Develops a treatment regimen that is consistent with normalcy lens
5. Defines social consequences of condition as minimal	5. Interacts with others based on view of child and family as normal

another's normalizing behaviors. In contrast, when family members disagree on the desirability of adopting a normalcy lens, normalizing efforts by one member are likely to be a source of conflict in the family (Knafl et al., 1996).

The most recent analysis of the concept also indicated that, in contrast to early studies that had been conducted primarily by sociologists interested in theoretical questions regarding deviance and identity, more recent studies were conducted exclusively by nurse researchers interested in family response to illness and the role of nurses in supporting family adaptation. Our two analyses of the concept also pointed to the contribution of qualitative methods to concept development. Our search of the literature, which was rigorous and designed to be exhaustive, revealed that, with one exception, all studies were based on qualitative approaches.

This brief overview of the development of the concept of normalization points to the interplay of empirical and analytical approaches to concept development. The analytical review of these studies revealed the overarching, defining attributes of normalization and provided direction for future studies. For example, in our most recent analysis, we (Deatrick, Knafl, & Murphy-Moore, in press) recommended that subsequent research pay greater attention to contextual variation in how normalization is manifested and to the varying outcomes of normalization for the family and individual family members. Despite their usefulness, however, analytical efforts are limited in the extent to which they can further the development of a particular concept. Ongoing development depends on further research, ideally research that explicitly builds on the insights and recommendations of prior analyses.

In the next section, we take a closer look at how we have alternated analytical and empirical activities in our own efforts to develop the concept of normalization. Our intent is to demonstrate how these two domains of activity mutually inform one another by providing an "insider" view of our collaborative and individual work.

OUR PERSONAL ADVENTURES IN CONCEPT DEVELOPMENT

Our concept analysis activities evolved in three overlapping phases as we moved from discovery of concept analysis as a useful analytical tool to recognition of the benefits of alternating analytical and empirical approaches to knowledge development. These phases, though not recognized as such as we moved through them, became apparent to us as we reflected on our work in preparing this chapter. We have labeled them *Exploring New Territory, Parallel Play,* and *Making Connections.* Each was characterized by different dominant activities and different major insights and lessons regarding the process of concept development.

EXPLORING NEW TERRITORY

Although we have been working on developing the concept of normalization for over 15 years, we began our work by accident when Janet Deatrick was working as Director of Nursing Research at Shriners Hospital in Chicago. The year was 1980 and we had teamed up to explore "The Impact of Osteogenesis Imperfecta on the Family." We have since abandoned our focus on impact, which suggests that families are passive in the face of chronic illnesses, in favor of studying how families actively manage illness challenges, but this was early in our research careers and we were studying impact. We were focusing on osteogenesis imperfecta (OI) because of the unique challenges it presented to families and because it was one of the major patient groups served by the hospital.

In discussing our proposed research with nursing and medical staff, we were both perplexed and intrigued when they expressed concern about families who reported minimal impact of their child's OI on the family or the child. Staff were concerned that these families were denying the seriousness of their child's condition and feared that a consequence of this denial would be failure to attend to the child's special needs. However, our subsequent interviews with some of these families revealed that parents fully understood the seriousness of the child's illness, but also felt that in many important ways their child and family were normal. Moreover, they readily shared with us examples of typical childhood and family activities as well as the strategies they had developed to create and sustain what they defined as a normal family life. Their accounts were similar to those reported by Davis (1963) in his study of families in which a child had polio. He had conceptualized this kind of response as a process of normalization; staff viewed it as denial.

Based on these experiences, we felt that we wanted to explore more systematically the differences between the concepts of normalization and denial. In addition to being of theoretical interest, we recognized the profound clinical significance of interpreting a parent's response to childhood illness as denial versus normalization. Whereas denial was likely to be viewed as cause for concern and to motivate interventions directed to helping parents have a more accurate understanding of their situation, we believed that if staff understood the concept of normalization, they would interpret the same family behaviors very differently. Responses that were seen as inappropriate when viewed through a denial lens would be seen as healthy and appropriate when understood as normalization.

Although we knew that we wanted to do something to explore the differences between denial and normalization, we were unsure what approach to take. At this time Knafl also was teaching a master's level course in nursing theory and was exploring possible texts for an upcoming offering of the course. The year was 1983 and a colleague recommended a new book by Chinn and Jacobs on theory development. Within minutes of reviewing the section describing concept analysis, she was on the phone to Deatrick. As luck would have it, we had found an approach that would help us conceptually delineate normalization from denial. Soon thereafter we launched our first formal analysis of the concept of normalization. We decided to focus on normalization rather than denial both because it was a relatively unexplored concept in nursing and because we believed it had potential clinical usefulness. Moreover, we were able to use concept analysis techniques to explore the difference between normalization and denial by developing denial as a case example of a related concept. Although we did not develop all the kinds of case examples suggested by Chinn and Jacobs, we followed their guidelines for identifying defining criteria for normalization as closely as we could. We didn't explore other approaches to concept analysis and certainly did not fully understand that there were philosophical issues associated with doing a concept analysis. We were pleased with the manuscript we developed and submitted to *Research in Nursing and Health* (RINAH), but were entirely unsure how the reviewers would evaluate it. Concept analysis was a new area of endeavor for us and, in contrast to our sense of competence as qualitative researchers, we were relatively unschooled and unsure of our abilities in what for us was virgin territory. To our delight the reviewers for RINAH liked the manuscript, although one questioned whether a concept analysis was appropriate for publication in a research journal. Margaret Grier, the editor at that time, thought that it was appropriate, and the manuscript was published (Knafl & Deatrick, 1986).

We learned several important lessons as a result of that first analysis. The experience with staff that triggered our search for a strategy to compare normalization and denial was an important lesson in the real world significance of concepts. In subsequent conversations with staff, they were quick to recognize the clinical implications of defining family behavior as normalization rather than denial. They also appreciated the usefulness of an approach to reviewing the literature that resulted in a set of defining criteria that could be used to determine whether one's clinical assessment was valid. Rodgers (1991) has discussed the clinical usefulness of concept analysis. She argued that "concept analysis helps the nurse identify and assess complex patient care situations, communicate patient needs, develop nursing diagnoses, and select nursing interventions" (p. 33).

In addition, the responses to the first publication also contributed to our growing recognition of the complexities of concept analysis. We were intrigued with concept analysis and continued to read on the topic and discuss our efforts with colleagues. In particular, a series of conversations with Dr. Beth Rodgers sensitized us to some of the philosophical issues surrounding concept analysis. Not only were we convinced that concept analysis was a useful endeavor, we knew that if we ever did another analysis, we would need to consider a wider array of analytical options and articulate our position on the nature and purpose of concept analysis. However, in 1987 we had growing research involvements and no particular plans to undertake another concept analysis.

Following submission of the proposal, Knafl had time for more thoughtful consideration of the possible link between concept analysis and the proposed study. Until then, she had viewed them as relatively separate spheres of endeavor. Although both the concept analysis of normalization and the planned study "How Families Define and Manage Childhood Chronic Illness" (DMCI) addressed a common subject matter, they did not build directly on one another. However, the concept analysis of normalization had revealed how useful analytical techniques could be for clarifying the attributes of a concept, and Knafl was beginning to think about how a formal concept analysis of family management style (FMS) would contribute to the conceptual underpinnings of the DMCI project even while the proposal was being reviewed. She contacted Deatrick to discuss the possibility of another concept analysis. We discussed our interest in doing a concept analysis on management behaviors, one component of the FMS model, as well as developing a special issue of *The Journal of Pediatric Nursing* to highlight research consistent with the model.

In the end, we decided to undertake a formal analysis of the concept of FMS as well as review the literature about management behaviors. Because we both were continuing to do research related to family response to chronic illness, we thought formal analyses would serve to clarify our conceptualization of how the family as a unit responds to illness and disability. The analysis of FMS presented us with some challenges we had not faced in the analysis of normalization. Unlike normalization, the term *family management style* was not routinely used in the literature. Although researchers (Anderson, 1981, 1986; Benoliel, 1970; Darling, 1979; Davis, 1963; Krulik, 1980) had described how the family unit responded to the challenges of childhood illness, there was no generally accepted terminology for referring to family unit response. We were planning the analysis of a concept that had not been "officially" named and thus would not have been referenced as a key term for searching the literature. Moreover, because we were more knowledgeable of the various approaches to concept analysis than we had been when we undertook our analysis of normalization, we knew it was important to consider a variety of analytical options. We wanted to make sure that our approach was consistent with both our purpose and our view of concepts. In the end, we chose an approach described by Sartori (1984). Although not well known in nursing, Sartori's method was uniquely suited to the exploration of a relatively unformed concept such as FMS. The method allowed us both to reconstruct the concept of FMS based on the literature and offer a tentative reconceptualization to guide further research and theory development. Using Sartori's method, we completed an analysis of the modest literature on family unit response to childhood illness and disability and developed a working model (as opposed to a set of defining criteria) of FMS (Deatrick & Knafl, 1990). The model conceptualized FMS as the configuration formed by the individual family members' definition of their situation and their illness management behaviors.

For Knafl, the concept analysis of FMS, which was completed following the submission of the DMCI proposal, in conjunction with her discovery of Schwartz-Barcott and Kim's (1986) hybrid model, led to some subtle, but nonetheless important changes in how she viewed the intent of the DMCI study and how it eventually was carried out. What had been initiated as a grounded theory study aimed at conceptualizing family response to chronic illness was implemented as a concept development project guided by the principles underlying the hybrid model of concept development.

For Deatrick, further understanding about management behaviors advanced her evolving work regarding pediatric advanced practice nursing (PAPN). A series of empirical projects and papers resulted concerning PAPNs facilitating children with chronic conditions and their families based on the FMS model and the management behaviors used by family members (Deatrick & Knafl, 1990; Deatrick, Faux, & Moore, 1993; Deatrick, Feetham, Hayman, & Perkins, 1993; Deatrick, Knafl, & Guyer, 1993).

Although parallel play with regard to our empirical and analytical endeavors had characterized our efforts during much of this phase of our work, the eventual lesson we learned had to do with the ways in which these activities could inform one another. In retrospect the lesson seems obvious—something we should have recognized all along. However, it wasn't until we explicitly linked the analytical and empirical aspects of our work that we fully appreciated how concept analysis and qualitative research could be used in concert to develop nursing concepts. This recognition has since helped us to bring these activities into closer, more deliberate alignment. We now see our knowledge synthesis efforts as well as our ongoing research on family response to illness as part of a single, more encompassing endeavor: the development of a scientific basis for the nursing care of children and families.

CONTINUING CONNECTIONS

There continues to be an ebb and flow in our engagement in analytical and empirical endeavors. Sometimes one is the major focus of our work, sometimes the other. However, we have learned how useful it can be to engage in major knowledge synthesis activities in conjunction with ongoing research. Our continuing work on the concept of normalization provides a good example of the benefits of interspersing knowledge synthesis and creation.

Knafl's DMCI study revealed some interesting findings regarding how normalization is variously manifested in families in which there is a child with a chronic illness. In that study, data had been collected at two points in time from roughly 200 family members in 60 families. Thematic analysis of that large qualitative data set led to the identification of five distinct family management styles (Knafl et al., 1996). Normalization themes were evident across all five styles, but were revealed in different ways. In the Thriving and Accommodating Styles, normalization was an overarching theme that characterized the family's definition of the situation and the focus of their management behaviors. In contrast, normalization in the Enduring Style was seen as a desirable, but unreachable goal. In the Struggling Style it was a source of bitter family conflicts when parents held different ideas about its appropriateness as a goal for their child or family. Parents in the Floundering Style described normalization as a fluctuating goal or discussed management behaviors that were inconsistent with normalization. These findings stimulated our thinking about the continuing development of the concept of normalization. Based on our past experiences, we believed that another formal analysis of the concept of normalization would both situate our own work in the broader literature and clarify the current usage of the concept.

Deatrick's research and that of her students also had continued to explore families' normalization efforts, especially the management behaviors that supported normalization. For instance, Susan Sullivan-Bolyai (in progress) is investigating the experience of parenting infants with insulin-dependent diabetes mellitus. Like other students with whom Deatrick is working, she is exploring the range of management behaviors used by parents and how these behaviors vary with regard to their goal, underlying conceptual dimension, implementor, and foci (Deatrick & Knafl, 1990).

At this point, it had been 10 years since the publication of our first analysis of the concept of normalization. During that time, we, as well as other authors, had continued to apply and develop the concept, indicating to us that it would be useful to undertake a second, formal analysis. Moreover, during that same time span there had been notable advances related to concept analysis. New approaches such as Rodgers' evolutionary model had been published (1989), and Morse (1995, 1996) had begun writing on the contribution of qualitative research to concept development. Both of these authors had emphasized the importance of considering how the defining attributes of a concept are manifested across different situational contexts, something we had not taken into account in our initial analysis.

Although we had read and discussed individual articles on normalization as they were published between 1986 and 1996, we had not reviewed the body of literature as a whole. Once again we decided to undertake a formal concept analysis. Our intent was to identify how the defining attributes of the concept might have changed over time as well as to provide direction for our own work. Unlike our prior analytical efforts, this was seen from the outset as an essential step for advancing the science as well as our own programs of research. Because of our interest in how the concept of normalization had changed over time, we selected Rodgers' approach to concept analysis because it views concepts as ever-changing and evolving (1989, 1993). The results of this second analysis are summarized in Table 18–1.

The analysis revealed that the concept has continued to evolve. Although it is a relatively well developed concept as evidenced by considerable research and multiple synthesis attempts, it was also clear to us, based on our most recent analysis, that there are multiple opportunities for even further development. For example, relatively little effort has been directed to bridging work done at the micro and macro levels. To date, research has focused on internal family management. With the exception of Anderson's work (1981, 1986), little effort has been directed to the relationship between the cultural value attached to normalcy and the family's subjective experience of illness. Also, relatively little work has been done to develop nursing interventions directed to initiate or support a family's normalization efforts, even though normalization promotion is an intervention listed in the Nursing Intervention Classification system (NIC) (Knafl, Deatrick, & Kirby, in press; McCloskey & Bulechek, 1996). The NIC framework lists 22 nursing activities directed to helping families achieve successful normalization, all of which merit further refinement and testing. We have also been challenged to consider ethical dimensions of this concept (Tishelman & Sachs, 1998).

As expected, this most recent analysis of normalization has provided direction for our research, which focuses on looking at normalization in the context of computer-assisted illness management and developing and testing interventions aimed at normalization promotion.

FINAL THOUGHTS

On occasion, one has the good fortune to be asked to write a chapter that triggers serious reflection on especially intriguing issues and processes. This chapter provided us with such an opportunity. In writing it, we were pushed to take stock of our own programs of research with an eye to identifying some of the important lessons we had learned along the way. It is clear to us that concepts thrive when their developers use both analytical and empirical approaches. Formal concept analysis forces us to situate our work in that of the larger scientific community. Our most recent review of the concept of normalization revealed that nurse researchers do not always pay sufficient attention to building on the work of others. In spite of the considerable body of research related to normalization, most authors cited two or fewer articles on normalization in support of their own work. In our eagerness to develop our own programs of research, we must take care to acknowledge and explicitly build on prior work. As nursing science matures, it becomes increasingly important to hone and develop our abilities both to synthesize and expand on current knowledge in the field. Knowledge synthesis when combined with further empirical study of a concept of interest is the most effective and efficient approach to concept development in nursing. Much of our own research to date has been based on qualitative methods. However, we do not see an inherent link between concept development and a particular method. Although certain qualitative approaches such as grounded theory and phenomenology are well suited to the identification and early development of concepts, other methodologies are likely to be more appropriate for exploring the various manifestations of a given concept or testing interventions related to the concept. Finally, we would argue that time spent in concept development is time well spent both in terms of advancing nursing science and clinical practice. Concepts shape how we think about the patients, families, and communities with whom we work. They direct our observations and our actions based on those observations. Important in their own right and as the building blocks of theory, they merit our careful attention and nurturance.

REFERENCES

Anderson, J. M. (1981). The social construction of illness experience: families with a chronically ill child. *Journal of Advanced Nursing, 6,* 427–434.

Anderson, J. M. (1986). Ethnicity and illness experience: ideological structure and the health care delivery system. *Social Science Medicine, 22*(11), 1277–1283.

Benoliel, J. (1970). The developing diabetic identity: A study of family influence. In M. Batey (Ed.), *Community nursing research: Methodological issues in research* (pp. 14–32). Boulder, CO: Western Interstate Commission on Higher Education.

Birenbaum, A. (1971). The mentally retarded child in the home and the family life cycle. *Journal of Health and Social Behavior, 12,* 55–65.

Bossert, E., Holaday, B., Harkins, A., & Turner-Henson, A. (1990). Strategies of normalization used by parents of chronically ill school age children. *Journal of Child Psychiatric Nursing, 3*(2), 57–61.

Chenitz, C., & Swanson, J. (1986). *From practice to grounded theory: Qualitative research in nursing.* Menlo Park, CA: Addison-Wesley.

Chinn, P., & Jacobs, M. (1983). *Theory and nursing: A systematic approach.* St. Louis: Mosby.

Chinn, P. L., & Kramer, M. (1991). *Theory in nursing: A systematic approach* (3rd ed.). St. Louis: Mosby.

Darling, R. (1979). *Families against society: A study of reactions to children with birth defects.* Beverly Hills: Sage Publications.

Dashiff, C. J. (1993). Parents' perceptions of diabetes in adolescent daughters and its impact on the family. *Journal of Pediatric Nursing, 8*(6), 361–369.

Davis, F. (1963). *Passage through crisis: Polio victims and their families.* Indianapolis: Bobbs-Merrill.

Deatrick, J. A., & Knafl, K. A. (1990). Management behaviors: Day-to-day adjustments to childhood chronic conditions. *Journal of Pediatric Nursing, 5*(1), 15–22.

Deatrick, J. A., Faux, S. A., & Moore, C. (1993). The contribution of qualitative research to the study of families' experiences with childhood illness. In S. Feetham, S. Meister, J. Bell, & C. Gillis (Eds.), *The nursing of families* (pp. 61–69). Newbury Park, CA: Sage.

Deatrick, J. A., Feetham, S., Hayman, L., & Perkins, M. (1993). Development of a model to guide advanced practice in family nursing. In S. Feetham, S. Meister, J. Bell, & C. Gilliss (Eds.), *The nursing of families* (pp. 147–154). Newbury Park, CA: Sage.

Deatrick, J. A., Knafl, K., & Guyer, K. (1993). The meaning of caregiving behaviors: Inductive approaches to family theory development. In S. Feetham, S. Meister, J. Bell, & C. Gilliss (Eds.), *The nursing of families* (pp. 38–45). Newbury Park, CA: Sage Publications.

Deatrick, J. A., Knafl, K. A., & Murphy-Moore, C. (in press). Reanalysis and further development of the concept of normalization. *Image: Journal of Nursing Scholarship.*

Hatton, D., Canam, C., Thorne, S., & Hughes, A.-M. (1995). Parents' perceptions of caring for an infant or toddler with diabetes. *Journal of Advanced Nursing, 22,* 569–577.

Hutchinson, S. A. (1990). Responsible subversion: A study of rule-bending among nurses. *Scholarly Inquiry for Nursing Practice: An International Journal, 4*(1), 3–17.

Jacobson, G. (1994). The meaning of stressful life experiences in nine-to-eleven-year-old children: A phenomenological study. *Nursing Research, 43,* 95–99.

Knafl, K., Breitmayer, B., Gallo, A., & Zoeller, L. (1987). How families define and manage a child's chronic illness. Funded by the National Center for Nursing Research, Public Health Service (Grant #NR01594).

Knafl, K., Breitmayer, B., Gallo, A., & Zoeller, L. (1996). Family response to childhood chronic illness: Description of management styles. *Journal of Pediatric Nursing, 11*(5), 315–326.

Knafl, K. A., & Deatrick, J. A. (1986). How families manage chronic conditions:

An analysis of the concept of normalization. *Research in Nursing & Health, 9,* 215-222.

Knafl, K., & Deatrick, J. (1990). Family management style: Concept analysis and development. *Journal of Pediatric Nursing, 5,* 4-14.

Knafl, K. A., & Deatrick, J. A. (1993). Knowledge synthesis and concept development in nursing. In B. L. Rodgers & K. A. Knafl (Eds.), *Concept development in nursing: Foundations, techniques, and applications* (pp. 35-50). Philadelphia: W. B. Saunders.

Knafl, K., Deatrick, J., & Kirby, A. (in press). Normalization promotion. In M. Craft-Rosenberg & J. Denehy (Eds.), *Nursing interventions for the childbearing and childrearing family.* Newbury Park, CA: Sage.

Krulik, T. (1980). Successful "normalizing" tactics of parents of chronically ill children. *Journal of Advanced Nursing, 5,* 573-578.

McCloskey, J. C., & Bulechek, G. M. (1996). *Nursing Intervention Classification (NIC).* St. Louis: Mosby.

McCloskey, M., & Glucksberg, S. (1978). Natural categories: Well defined or fuzzy-sets? *Memory and Cognition, 6,* 465-472.

Medin, D. L. (1989). Concepts and conceptual structure. *American Psychologist, 44,* 1469-1481.

Morse, J. M. (1995). Exploring the theoretical basis of nursing using advanced techniques of concept analysis. *Advances in Nursing Science, 17*(3), 31-46.

Morse, J. M., Hupcey, J. E., Mitcham, C., & Lenz, E. R. (1996). Concept analysis in nursing research: A critical appraisal. *Scholarly Inquiry for Nursing Practice: An International Journal, 10*(3), 253-277.

Morse, J. M., Mitcham, C., Hupcey, J. E., & Tason, M. C. (1996). Criteria for concept evaluation. *Journal of Advanced Nursing, 24,* 385-390.

Paley, J. (1996). How not to clarify concepts in nursing. *Journal of Advanced Nursing, 24,* 572-578.

Powell-Cope, G. (1994). The experience of gay couples affected by HIV infection. *Qualitative Health Research, 5,* 36-62.

Quint, J. C. (1967). The case for theories generated from empirical data. *Nursing Research, 16,* 109-114.

Robinson, C. A. (1993). Managing life with a chronic condition: The story of normalization. *Qualitative Health Research, 3*(1), 6-28.

Rodgers, B. L. (1989). Concepts, analysis and the development of nursing knowledge: The evolutionary cycle. *Journal of Advanced Nursing, 14,* 330-335.

Rodgers, B. L. (1991). Using concept analysis to enhance clinical practice and research. *Dimensions of Critical Care Nursing, 10,* 28-34.

Rodgers, B. (1993). Concept analysis: An evolutionary view. In B. Rodgers & K. Knafl (Eds.), *Concept development in nursing: Foundations, techniques, and applications* (pp. 73-92). Philadelphia: W. B. Saunders.

Roskies, E. (1972). *Abnormality and normality: The mothering of thalidomide children.* Ithaca, NY: Cornell University Press.

Sartori, G. (1984). *Social science concepts: A systematic analysis.* Beverly Hills, CA: Sage.

Schwartz-Barcott, D., & Kim, H. (1986). A hybrid model for concept development. In P. L. Chinn (Ed.), *Nursing research methodology: Issues and implementation* (pp. 91-101). Rockville, MD: Aspen.

Schwartz-Barcott, D., & Kim, H. (1993). An expansion and elaboration of the hybrid model of concept development. In B. L. Rodgers & K. A. Knafl (Eds.), *Concept development in nursing: Foundations, techniques, and applications* (pp. 107-134). Philadelphia: W. B. Saunders.

Seideman, R., & Kleine, P. (1995). Theory of transformed parenting: Parenting a child with developmental delay/mental retardation. *Nursing Research, 44,* 38-44.

Sullivan-Bolyai, S. *The experience of parenting young children with IDDM.* Unpublished doctoral dissertation, Yale University.

Swanson, K. M. (1990). Providing care in the NICU: Sometimes an act of love. *Advanced Nursing Science, 13*(1), 60-73.

Tishelman, C., & Sachs, L. (1998). The diagnostic process and boundaries of normality. *Qualitative Health Research, 8*(1), 48-60.

Voysey, M. (1975). *A constant burden: The reconstruction of family life.* London: Routledge and Kegan Paul.

Walker, L. O., & Avant, K. C. (1988). *Strategies for theory construction in nursing* (2nd ed.). Norwalk, CT: Appleton & Lange.

Concept Development Situated in the Critical Paradigm

Judith Wuest

A pproaches to concept development in nursing rely upon synthesis and analysis of existing knowledge, and qualitative exploration of subjective experience. The outcome of such approaches is a conceptual definition or understanding that corresponds with the dominant meanings and beliefs in the discipline and in society. These dominant views are normally those of the most powerful. The mandate of nursing is to attend to health of all people; therefore, knowledge that is useful for nursing practice also must reflect views from the margins and the influence of domination on those views. One strategy for ensuring that nursing knowledge does not promote marginalization is to augment concept development with concept critique. Without such critique, concept development in nursing may be a process of perpetuating *what is* rather than introducing *what could be*. Concept development within a critical paradigm, that is, concept critique, differs markedly from traditional approaches discussed because it is based on distinctly different ontological, epistemological, and methodological assumptions (Guba & Lincoln, 1994). In the following discussion, I will discuss paradigm differences, put forward a case for the critical approach, and suggest some approaches to concept critique. The intent is to foster further debate and dialogue about the place of the critical perspective in knowledge development in nursing. This chapter extends my earlier thinking, which focused on feminist concept analysis (Wuest, 1994).

PARADIGM DIFFERENCES IN CONCEPT DEVELOPMENT

In nursing, concept development has been addressed primarily through Wilson-derived methods of concept analysis (Morse, 1995). Such approaches, Morse argued, often result in trivial and insignificant contributions to nursing's theoretical base. Hupcey, Morse, Lenz, and Tasón (1996) recently observed that nurse researchers, preoccupied with these methods of concept analysis, have failed to ask such fundamental questions as "What do I want to find out? Why do I want to know? And for what purpose?" (p. 207). Such questions lead to a consideration of the paradigm that guides the inquiry. Emphasis in Wilsonian-based concept analysis has been on clarification of the empirical referents of particular concepts as a first step in theory development. Such approaches (Chinn & Kramer, 1991; Walker & Avant, 1995) are based on positivist assumptions that there exists a singular objective reality that can be known only by reductionism and control of contextual influences and that knowledge of this reality allows for prediction and control of phenomena (Guba & Lincoln, 1994; Rodgers, 1989, 1993). If there is one reality or truth, then it follows that each concept will have a set of empirical referents that will be universally applicable.

Rodgers (1989, 1993) put forward an evolutionary approach to concept analysis that replaced this positivist static definition with a more fluid interpretation. The assumptions in this approach are more consistent with the naturalistic paradigm in which multiple context-dependent realities exist and are understood in a hermeneutical/dialectical process (Guba & Lincoln, 1994). Rather than seeking the essential attributes of a concept, the goal in the evolutionary approach is to uncover the dynamic nature of concepts, dynamic in the sense that concepts change with both time and context. Because the underlying premise is that concepts and their meanings are formed through social interaction, emphasis is placed on exploring the ways that the concept has evolved. By exploring usage and application in specific contexts, the range, scope, and limitations of the concept are evident. Concept analysis is ongoing and contextually specific.

The goal of concept development within the critical paradigm is neither prediction and control, as in the positivist paradigm, nor understanding, as in the naturalistic paradigm. The goals of the inquiry in the critical paradigm are critique and transformation (Guba & Lincoln, 1994). Within this paradigm, reality is virtual and shaped by social, political, economic, cultural, and gender values. This virtual reality consists of "historically situated structures that are, in the absence of insight, as limiting and confining as if they were real" (Guba & Lincoln, 1994, p. 111). Personal meanings then are "shaped by societal structures and communication processes and are therefore all too often ideologic, historically bound, and distorted" (Campbell & Bunting, 1991, p. 5). In order to achieve the goals of critique and transformation, the central activities of concept development in this view are examination of the ways that concepts have been shaped by historical structures, exploration of the overt and hidden meanings of the concept, and dialogue and reflection about the potential within these meanings for injustice, exploitation, or constraint. This reflective process is the antithesis of positivist approaches and results in knowledge that is inherently emancipatory (Eastland, 1994).

Concept development in this paradigm then is a dialogic process of concept critique, a questioning and reexamining that heightens consciousness and transforms awareness of concept meaning. This process is grounded in critical hermeneutics, a branch of interpretive theory based not only on the assumption that meanings are constituted over time but also that many meanings are socially oppressive, representing the interests of the few (Thompson, 1990). The focus of the critical dialogue moves beyond subjective meaning to consideration of ideological forces. This process is not one of essentializing, that is "the reduction of concepts to an essence" (Miller, 1997, p. 147); nor does it result in substituting one definition of a concept with another, but rather in revealing a plurality of definitions (Allen, 1987). Within nursing, knowledge development based on the critique of domination within social structure is in its infancy (Stevens, 1989), and race, class, and gender bias have yet to be questioned in any systematic way (DeMarco et al., 1994). A critical nursing science has the potential to uncover the ways that social, political, economic, gender, and cultural factors interact to influence health or illness experiences (Ford-Gilboe et al., 1995).

The Critical Tradition

Critical traditions in inquiry are rooted in critical social theory, feminist theory, critical postmodernism, and poststructuralism (McCormick & Roussy, 1997). Although each of these viewpoints has unique features, Kincheloe and McLaren (1994) identified the following common broad assumptions that underpin social and cultural criticism within the critical tradition: "thought is fundamentally mediated by power relations that are socially and historically constituted" (p. 139); facts are influenced by ideology or values; "the relationship between concept and object . . . is never stable or fixed and is often mediated by the social relations of capitalist production and consumption" (p. 140); language is central to conscious and unconscious awareness; some groups are marginalized in society and oppression is enhanced when these groups accept their social status as natural; there are many forms of oppression (race, class, gender, etc.) and focusing on one form ignores the interconnections;

and "mainstream research practices are generally . . . implicated in the reproduction of systems of class, race, and gender oppression" (p. 140). My discussion of concept development in the critical tradition will be informed by these assumptions.

WHY IS A CRITICAL VIEWPOINT SIGNIFICANT IN CONCEPT DEVELOPMENT?

Within nursing, concepts are foundational as the building blocks of theory, the foci of research, and the phenomena of practice (Wuest, 1994). Dorothy Smith (1990), a sociologist, offered some insights regarding the significance of concepts to a discipline:

> We begin with and return to the conceptual structure. . . . The actualities of living people become a resource to be made over into the image of the concept. The work becomes that of transposing the paramount reality into the conceptual currency in which it is governed. (Smith, 1990, p. 53)

The dominant ideology of a discipline is embedded in the conceptual language, creating a "conceptual imperialism" in that this accepted conceptual language controls the ways that practice is interpreted or experienced (Smith, p. 115). When nursing concepts are analyzed by examining current and past usage, and synthesizing and reducing this existing knowledge, conceptual imperialism is bolstered and never challenged. Wilsonian approaches to concept analysis produce "ideas that we think are new and yet only contain and restrict us . . ." (Brennan, 1997, p. 483).

Dominant concepts and the conceptual frameworks or theories in which they are located guide practice and knowledge development. Evaluation of approaches to concept development and the products of this work is commonly achieved by post-positivist standards that include congruence with existing knowledge and peer review according to Guba and Lincoln (1994). Collins (1991) argued that black women's standpoints remained unacknowledged because the community of experts called upon to validate developing knowledge largely consists of white men who maintain their expertise by not challenging the basic beliefs of the larger culture. Within nursing, perspectives from the margins may also be suppressed because the dominant views of the most powerful nursing leaders, editors, investigators, and academics provide the standard against which new meanings and interpretations are measured. McCormick and Roussy (1997) observed that the metanarratives of nursing theories reflect the cultural assumptions of Western, privileged, white, middle-class women and called for examination of the assumptions that underlie the central concepts to reveal the role of power and the issues of marginality in the health and illness experience. A particular concern is the perpetuation of patriarchal perspectives within nursing knowledge development, perspectives that ignore or discount race, class, or gender (Wilson-Thomas, 1995). Assumptions of normality and homogeneity that underpin traditional knowledge development in nursing obscure the diversity of human experience (Hall et al., 1994). For example, the practice of identifying universal critical attributes in traditional concept analysis obscures the influence of race, gender, and class on conceptual meaning.

If concepts are to be developed in such a way that they do not perpetuate the viewpoints of the most powerful nursing voices, more emancipatory approaches must be considered. Allen (1992) argued that no singular set of criteria or kind of evidence is sufficient for the development of emancipatory knowledge. Although objective observation has limitations, so do the subjective perspectives of particular groups. The key elements of emancipatory science lie in what Allen called "situated" discourse that addresses the underlying social conditions and assumptions that inform the dialogue. "Whatever 'the real' is, it is discursive" (Lather, 1991, p. 25). Concepts that are of any interest are inherently subjects of dispute (Paley, 1996). "Every truth is incomplete, partial, and culture bound" (Miller, 1997, p. 153).

LANGUAGE AND THE CRITICAL TRADITION

Concepts are neither an independent objective reality nor a mental structure expressed in words; "they are enmeshed in language" (Paley, 1996, p. 576). Language is pivotal within the critical paradigm. In traditional science, concepts are mirrors of reality; in hermeneutic philosophy, concepts are a way of fixing our beliefs in language that both opens up new understandings and puts limits on what can be known (Thompson, 1990). Thompson noted, ". . . concepts are not just value neutral, ahistorical entities that more or less accurately mirror our worlds. Rather, concepts are conditioned by our historical era and by our social interests" (p. 241).

Reality then is shaped and constructed by language that is bound to the social and ideological (Lather, 1991; Miller, 1997). "This moves social inquiry to new grounds, the grounds of 'discourse' where the ways we talk or write are situated within social practices, the historical conditions of meanings, the positions from which texts are both produced and received" (Lather, p. 89). Thus, the meanings of words or concepts are determined by the theoretical structures in which they are positioned (Paley, 1996). An underlying assumption of critical hermeneutics is that language has multiple meanings according to the position of the social actor, not all interpretations are equally heard or seen as legitimate, and "it is important to demystify socially oppressive meanings that may be unnoticed by participants themselves" (Thompson, 1990, p. 258). When dominant social forces express concepts in the language of the majority, the voices of those on the margins are silenced (Hall et al., 1994). Some fundamental ideologies that are entrenched in social structures and contribute to inequity are racism, sexism, classism, ageism, and heterosexism (Stevens, 1989).

Conceptual Language and Nursing

Concepts are fundamental to the development of nursing theories that inform practice and research. The challenge in theory development is in using conceptual language that is abstract but inclusive of the variation of human experience, particularly the experiences of the marginalized (Hall et al., 1994; Wuest, 1997). But words selected to name nursing concepts are often chosen for their congruence with the dominant, accepted language of the discipline or because research related to such named concepts is more likely to be funded or published (Müller & Dzurec, 1993). Because maternal-fetal relationships were named *maternal-fetal attachment*, subsequent research has focused on attachment rather than alternative possibilities such as adaptation (Müller & Dzurec, 1993). Nurse researchers frequently ignore the nuance that accompanies words selected to name phenomena. Such nuances include "the various meanings of any one word, the images that are peculiar to that word at a given point in history, the theories that have incorporated that word as a name or adjective, and the emotional or political contexts of the word" (Müller & Dzurec, 1993, p. 16). By failing to consider these dimensions, nursing concepts may represent only dominant perspectives. Hall, Stevens, and Meleis (1994) asked "How might problems be renamed and reconceptualized according to the experiences of those who reside far from societal center?" (p. 35). This question is fundamental to ensuring that knowledge development in nursing has relevance to diverse populations.

CRITICAL APPROACHES

The foregoing discussion provides ample rationale for the inclusion of concept critique in the process of knowledge development in nursing. This raises questions related to the process and conditions of such critique. The literature offers some direction in terms of both critical methods and exemplars.

Critical Methods

The critique of accepted and institutionalized meanings is vital to social transformation (Thompson, 1990).

The "suspicion" behind critical hermeneutics then is intended to go behind "commonsense," socially acceptable meanings, and to uncover hidden meanings that may be unnoticed by the social actors themselves but that, nevertheless, function to sustain and reproduce social inequities and injustices. (p. 265)

Definition frequently rests on the negation of something that is in opposition and meaning is derived from the contrast, for example, male/female, presence/absence, employment/motherhood, family leave/child care (Miller, 1997; Scott, 1990). The meaning of a word, then, is determined "as much by what it is not as by what it is" (Miller, p. 145). Meaning is discovered by taking apart those oppositions, examining their interdependence, and considering the social and historical influences.

Stevens (1989) suggested that critique is a process that takes place in the following ways: oppositional thinking to uncover oppressive ideology in the rules and assumptions underlying historical, cultural, and political structures; reflection on the structural changes to make uncoerced knowledge and action possible; analysis of the barriers to communication and action; dialogue that raises consciousness of social, political, and economic contradictions; and action that is "informed, deliberate behavior and verbalization by those experiencing oppression that seeks to bring about social change" (p. 60). A critical theory approach then enables nurses to "challenge traditional norms, in order to uncover hidden meanings and constraining sociopolitical barriers to optional health for all" (Wilson-Thomas, 1995, p. 574).

Collins (1991) offered additional insights related to knowledge, social relations, and domination. She argued that it is necessary to understand oppression in terms of one overarching theoretical system of interlocking race, class, and gender oppression that stimulates the rethinking of basic social science concepts. This stance allows for considering other oppressions such as age, sexual orientation, religion, and ethnicity. According to Collins,

> Placing African-American women and other excluded groups in the center of analysis opens up possibilities for a both/and [sic] conceptual stance, one in which all groups possess varying amounts of penalty and privilege in one historically created system. In this system, for example, white women are penalized by their gender, but privileged by their race. Depending on the context, an individual may be an oppressor, a member of an oppressed group, or simultaneously oppressor and oppressed. (p. 225)

Such a position suggests each person's knowledge is partial and situated; by sharing such partial knowledge through dialogue, difference can be transcended.

DeMarco, Campbell, and Wuest (1993) in their discussion of feminist critique provided some direction for a critical approach to concept analysis. In particular, conceptual meanings need to be examined for overt bias and also for exclusion of meanings that may be significant. A critical consideration is the way that concepts are operationalized in research that tests theory. Frequently instruments are developed using homogeneous, accessible populations with the outcome that they are meaningless in diverse populations. There is little point in instruments being reliable and valid if they are not adequate; that is, if they are not relevant or grounded in diverse experience (Hall & Stevens, 1991). Thus, it is important that the process of concept development include looking for meaning "beyond and behind what one has been socialized to believe is there" (p. 26).

In an earlier paper, I suggested feminist concept analysis as a means of uncovering racial, class, and gender bias inherent in concepts (Wuest, 1994). Although this approach began to address the use of conceptual definitions that may have been meaningless in the contexts of people's lives, it still relied heavily on traditional approaches to concept analysis, albeit with consideration of subjective experiences, contextual dependency, and multiple definitions. From a critical viewpoint, it failed to address the limited contribution of subjective perspectives, if the participants accept historical tradition as truth. A critical approach to concept development moves beyond subjective understanding of conceptual meaning to reflective exploration of the assumptions and social conditions that inform such understandings.

Exemplars in Nursing Literature

Critical approaches to understanding specific concepts are visible in the nursing literature. Allen (1987) used a critical approach in the definition of *family*, noting the variation in the definition related to historical periods and the influence of powerful social influences. He cautioned against a rigid definition of family noting the implications for women in terms of potentially limiting work outside the home, perpetuating constricting gender identity, and contributing to a sense of entrapment. Chopoorian (1986) and Stevens (1989) have critically examined the concept of *environment*. Although Chopoorian did not allude to critical social theory, she offered a solid critique of nursing's interpretation of environment as "society or setting to which people adapt or conform" (p. 40), arguing that this conceptualization excludes persons who "reject accommodation to environments that present intolerable or unacceptable social, political, or economic circumstances" (p. 40). She contended that such a conceptualization results in nursing failing to examine "the dominant social, political, and economic structures that produce behaviors associated with class relationships, power relations, political interests, economic policies, and ideologies such as sexism, racism, ageism, classism that influence persons in their worlds—behaviors that interfere with health and that eventually cause illness" (p. 41). This, in turn, results in practice focusing on individual adaptation rather than strategies to change the environment. Based on the premise that concepts include an organization of sub-concepts, Chopoorian argued for nursing consciousness of three sub-categories of environment: social, economic, and political structures; human and social relations; and everyday life. Examination of each of these sub-concepts was conducted to reveal the influence of structural processes on health.

Stevens (1989) expanded Chopoorian's critique and explicitly put forward critical social theory as a means of not only critiquing the concept of *environment* but also as action "to transform the environmental conditions that constrain health and human potential" (p. 56). Rather than examining the concept of environment in isolation, Stevens used a critical social theory approach to examine the impact of an expanded conceptualization of environment on the issues arising from the use of an acne medication that causes severe birth defects. Specifically she examined the oppressive structures that constrain health, limit life possibilities, and restrict equal and fully conscious participation in society. This analysis becomes a base for nursing action at both individual and community levels, and for nursing research.

Some authors have included elements of critique in their analyses of concepts. Müller and Dzurec (1993, p. 20), discussing the example of maternal-fetal *attachment* versus *binding-in,* argued for maximizing the power of the name of a concept by considering "the political, historic, social, biologic, environment, and psychologic contexts in which a phenomenon is found *before* the name is imposed" and by choosing a name that best reflects the investigators' understanding of the contextualized phenomenon. Thus, their position was that a critical approach should be taken prior to assignment of a name to a phenomenon. Once the name is selected, a contextualized concept analysis is recommended. Messias (1996), in an examination of *undocumentedness,* proposed a feminist process of concept exploration for identifying and situating concepts relevant to nursing. Concept exploration includes identifying the disciplinary perspective of the investigator, reflexivity, and examining the historical, social, political, and legislative contexts of the concept. Although this process does not specifically critique the influences of historical shaping, the consideration of the historical, social, political, and legislative context initiates questioning of diverse influences.

METHODS FOR CONCEPT CRITIQUE

A critical method of concept development involves ongoing critique of the meanings of concepts through exploration of ideological forces and contextual relevance. The goal of such critique would not be a singular definition. The goal would be to transform awareness with regard to the ideological influences that shape the meanings of concepts and to apply this more complete knowledge to research and practice such that oppression is reduced. Concept critique could be enacted in various ways. I propose three possible approaches: a participatory research project, a critical review of existing knowledge, and a critical perspective brought to bear on a concept analysis.

Participatory Research

Ideally the process of concept critique would be a collaborative, dialogic process played out in a participatory research project with stakeholders being partners in the exploration. Participatory research is a complex and difficult process (Wuest & Merritt-Gray, 1997). Unless the initiative for such a process comes from a community or special interest group, it is likely that the investigator will be making decisions about the relevancy of particular stakeholders, and the ways to engage them in such a project. Because the explicit goal of a critical approach is emancipation and change, participants, normally referred to as agents, are not being asked to merely share their views but also to engage in dialogue that explores the ways the way their subjective views have been influenced by dominant ideologies, and to take action to address power imbalances and legitimize diverse perspectives. A fundamental assumption here is that the knowledge gained will be partial, in that it is situated in this specific context. But at the same time, the knowledge gained has potential to add to a more complete understanding by challenging or adding to the dominant view. The investigator would link with those for whom the concept has sufficient relevance that agents would be willing to invest their time and energy. For example, if the concept of interest is *noncompliance*, the investigator might engage the interest of families, individuals, or health professionals who deal with a specific chronic illness. Alternatively a particular marginalized group such as low-income people who encounter structural constraints in managing their health might be interested in examining this concept.

Assuming agents are willing to participate, agreement could be made for regular discussions over several weeks. Discussions would include sharing personal meanings and discussing the diversity in those meanings; exploring the underlying assumptions of personal meanings; considering the social, political, economic, and cultural forces that influence those assumptions; examining the potential for discrimination, marginalization or social injustice in those meanings; and finally deciding upon and planning particular actions. The dialogue could begin with talk about the personal meanings of *compliance* and *noncompliance*. Such discussion would begin to tease out and challenge the underlying assumptions of the concept, such as "health care professionals know best" or "compliance with medical regimens results in better health" or "individuals can control their own behavior." Such assumptions might raise questions of professional versus personal knowledge, the legitimacy of professional power, and victim blaming. Dialogue could further illuminate such contradictions or barriers such as how someone earning minimum wage can afford to buy a healthy diet or take time off work to attend clinic appointments.

Although it is impossible to know how the dialogue might actually evolve, the role of the investigator would be to facilitate dialogue to uncover hidden social, economic, political, and cultural assumptions related to the concept, and to look at the barriers or conditions that reinforce those assumptions and constrain other action. The facilitator would need to introduce issues related to public policy that might influence meanings of compliance. For example, when exploring the notion that compliance is aligned with the assumption that people can exert control over their own health by doing what they are told, it would be important to examine whether individuals do have control. Structural barriers such as drug patent legislation, health insurance legislation, availability and cost of public transportation, employment policies regarding sick time, and cost of wholesome food could be introduced for discussion. Although personal meanings would inform the dialogue, new constructions or understandings would emerge as agents raised new perspectives and issues.

The facilitator could also have the group consider the ways that their evolving understanding of *noncompliance* might be received by persons marginalized by gender, ability, race, age, etc. The goal here would relate to raising collective consciousness of how structures influence the meanings held to be true, and how those dominant meanings are in themselves barriers and constraints. The assumption of participatory research is that change occurs as part of the research process. Through dialogue about the meaning of a concept, change occurs as agents develop wider understanding of sites of social, economic, and political oppression related to a particular concept and are better able to evaluate their personal situations. Agents may choose as a result of this transformation to plan strategies to address issues uncovered.

At this level critical concept development is a full-fledged participatory research project with a goal of both emancipatory action and knowledge development. Thus, to engage in concept development of this nature commits the investigator to partnership and participatory work with the group until the agents reach their goal. One obvious limitation is that it may be difficult to find and engage agents in such work. If agents are willing to meet with the investigator individually but are reluctant to commit to meeting over time with a group, another strategy might be to have a single dialogue with each interested individual, summarize key issues raised, and use this as a base for one group discussion. This limited commitment might be more appealing and if the discussion is useful and interesting, the group may consider meeting again. A final challenge is that the investigator will need to reach agreement with the agents regarding the ownership of conceptual knowledge that emerges from the project. In participatory projects, the goals of the agents and academic investigators are often different and issues such as authorship and content of final reports and publications need to be addressed. Despite these constraints, the conceptual knowledge that emerges from such a project is likely to challenge dominant views and raise exciting issues for nursing.

Critical Review

Campbell and Bunting (1991) noted that the most frequent method employed by critical theorists for knowledge development has been the critical review. The goal in critical review is to "decipher the ideology or determine the 'social illusion' " (p. 6) in the ways that the concept is presented in the literature used by nursing. Concept critique as a critical review can be a solitary strategy in which the meanings of a specific concept in text resources are identified with attention to historical and contextual evolution. The intent is not to arrive at a singular meaning, as in concept analysis, but to uncover the range and scope of conceptual meaning. The investigator would at the same time explore the ways that the social, cultural, or political structures influenced the development of the meaning and the use of the concept in the discipline. A starting point could be determining historically when the concept emerged within the discipline, followed by an exploration of the social and disciplinary circumstances that contributed to its emergence. For example, *noncompliance* became a focus for nursing in 1970 when Marston reported that most research in the area was conducted by physicians and behavioral scientists and posited that encouraging people to follow physician orders was a concern of nurses. Because this occurred at a time when nursing was attempting to build a scientific knowledge base to gain credibility as a profession, it is not surprising that nurses gravitated to a domain already legitimized by the powerful profession of medicine (Wuest, 1993).

By situating the textual meanings in the existing sociopolitical structures of the particular historical time, it becomes possible to illuminate the ideological influences and the ways that the discipline has come to accept dominant meanings as truth. In the case of *compliance/*

noncompliance, another dominant historical influence was sociological sick-role theory in which the patient is obligated to seek medical attention and cooperate with a physician (Parsons, 1951). The underlying assumption was that following physician directions will result in cure. This theoretical perspective also gave legitimacy to the concept, particularly for nurse researchers who were obtaining their doctoral education in disciplines such as sociology.

The evolution of the concept over time is also a focus of the critical review. In the case of *compliance,* definitions changed from the initial "doing what one is told by professionals" to choosing to participate in a regimen mutually developed between the professional and the client (Dracup & Meleis, 1982). This evolution is reflective of the movement in nursing theory toward mutual goal setting and client participation. The inclusion of *noncompliance* in the taxonomy of nursing diagnoses (Kim, 1986) was another significant step in embedding the concept in nursing's textual reality. Consideration of the factors that have influenced the development of such a taxonomy is critical in understanding the structural pressures that influence the adoption and usage of this concept. Factors outside of nursing also need to be considered such as the structure of health care systems, health care insurance, or payment of health professionals for they may contribute to the meanings of central concepts. Another strategy for uncovering the dominant ideology is examining the debate and dialogue in the literature. In the case of *compliance,* it is necessary to explore discussion that has challenged the prevailing viewpoint (Burckhardt, 1986; Edel, 1985; Erlen, 1997; Thorne, 1990; Wuest, 1993).

A final strategy is to systematically question or examine the literature for sites of exclusion or bias. Have the theoretical frameworks, instruments, and studies relevant to compliance considered issues of race, gender, age, education, culture, or class? Has the emphasis been on the individual or has the larger system been considered in the debate? Considering possible sites of oppression explicitly helps to uncover the ways that the meanings of a concept are or are not appropriately reflecting diversity.

The outcome of this critical review will be a new conceptual understanding illuminated by historical assumptions that have been made explicit. Such a review challenges dominant perspectives and provides important groundwork for nurses to expand their vision of particular concepts such that they are applicable to more diverse populations in both research and practice. The transformation that takes place with such a critical review is within the professional who conducts this internal dialogue. The extent to which others are influenced depends on the availability of such critique through literature or public presentation.

Concept Analysis with a Critical Perspective

The final way of enacting the critical viewpoint in concept development is the application of a critical perspective to existing methods of concept analysis. This strategy is less powerful but may be acceptable to investigators who otherwise do not consider the critical approaches possible or feasible. It may be argued applying a critical perspective to concept analysis crosses paradigm boundaries in that the epistemological, ontological, or methodological assumptions may be incongruent. However, there is increasing recognition of the value that other paradigm perspectives or insights bring to particular investigations (Denzin & Lincoln, 1994; Ford-Gilboe et al., 1996; Reinharz, 1992), especially if usefulness is one of the evaluation criteria. A critical perspective raises fundamental questions about both the adequacy of the conceptualization and the potential for injustice, marginalization, or discrimination of specific groups particularly if practice or research is grounded in the outcome of the analysis.

This strategy would involve completing the concept analysis by whatever means chosen and then critically examining the outcome for exclusionary bias, and potential for power imbalance. Investigators could conduct this examination on concept analyses that they themselves carried out or on ones found in the literature. Within this strategy, the goal of transformation would be met only to the extent that the investigator became aware of the discriminatory nature of the meaning given to the concept. A beginning point would be to explore the applicability of the defining attributes to diverse groups such as those identified by age, race, gender, culture, socioeconomic status, etc. Investigator ability to answer such a query may be limited by personal understanding of such diverse groups. Consulting literature specific to selected marginalized groups or obtaining subjective views of diverse people would help to sensitize the investigator to particular limitations of the concept analysis. The latter approach is essential for the meanings attributed to concepts to be significant in people's lives.

Collins (1991) cautioned that oppression can occur at personal, community, and institutional levels. This highlights the importance of considering the meanings at each of these levels. One needs to consider the ways that the designated conceptual meanings may contribute to power imbalances. This question demands identification of the assumptions that underlie each defining attribute as well as consideration of the political, cultural, social, and economic influences that inform such assumptions. Such questions will help the investigator consider potential sources of social injustice that are not visible to people themselves.

Concept critique at this level is limited in that the approach begins with a more traditional analysis that is not aimed at emancipation or change. However, the strength of such exploration is that it may be considered feasible by those who would not consider a critical review or a participatory project. It is important that the critical perspective be brought to bear on concept analysis because many nursing studies are conducted based on definitions that do not reflect either the realities of participants' lives. Moreover, many conceptual meanings are limited by consideration only of individual factors and failure to include the influence of systemic factors. A critical perspective added to concept analysis is a vital first step in expanding the relevance and usefulness of concept development techniques.

CONCLUSIONS

The major reason for initiating concept development is normally to clarify meaning such that a body of knowledge can be developed related to the concept. A risk in any attempt to discover universal meanings is that such meanings will ignore the voices of those on the margins and only resonate with perspectives of the dominant culture. It is clear from the foregoing analysis that a critical approach to concept development uses debate, dialogue, and critical review to produce new, partial, and time-limited meanings that are bound to the sociostructural conditions or theoretical positions that inform them. It would seem that with such situated meanings, knowledge accumulation is difficult.

Guba and Lincoln (1994) suggested that within the critical paradigm, knowledge "grows and changes through a dialectic process of historical revision that continuously erodes ignorance and misapprehension and enlarges more informed insights" (p. 114). Because all knowledge is situated in a particular context, it is partial and unfinished, not universal (Collins, 1991). Knowledge evolves through communication and dialogue whereby dominant perspectives are decentered, and diverse viewpoints are heard and neither suppressed nor given primacy. The outcome is a more complete understanding, but one that is always modifiable in response to new perspectives.

It is important that our quest for knowledge development does not reproduce or sustain oppression. In our efforts to develop common reference points for practice and research in nursing, we can deny neither the subjective diversity of meaning nor the social or historical construction of the concept. By using methods of concept critique, we move beyond exploration and synthesis of currently accepted meanings and produce new understandings that are partial, situated, and evolving. At first glance, this seems to doom nursing to uncertain knowledge of our basic phenomena. Upon reflection, there is a realization that by avoiding universals, we can begin to uncover the ways that social injustice and power imbalances influence the health of all.

REFERENCES

Allen, D. (1987). Critical social theory as a model for analyzing ethical issues in family and community health. *Family & Community Health, 10*(1), 63-72.

Allen, D. (1992). Feminism, relativism, and the philosophy of science. In J. Thompson, D. Allen, & L. Rodrigues-Fisher (Eds.), *Critique, resistance, and action: Working papers on the politics of nursing* (pp. 1-20). New York: National League for Nursing.

Brennan, M. (1997). A concept analysis of consent. *Journal of Advanced Nursing, 25,* 477-484.

Burckhardt, C. (1986). Ethical issues in compliance. *Topics in Clinical Nursing, 7*(4), 9-13.

Campbell, J., & Bunting, S. (1991). Voices and paradigms: Perspectives on critical and feminist theory in nursing. *Advances in Nursing Science, 13*(3), 1-15.

Chinn, P., & Kramer, M. (1991). *Theory and nursing: A systematic approach* (3rd ed.). St. Louis: Mosby.

Chopoorian, T. (1986). Reconceptualizing the environment. In P. Moccia (Ed.), *New approaches to theory development* (pp. 39-54). New York: National League for Nursing.

Collins, P. (1991). *Black feminist thought: Knowledge, consciousness, and the politics of empowerment.* New York: Routledge.

DeMarco, R., Campbell, J., & Wuest, J. (1993). Feminist critique: Searching for meaning in research. *Advances in Nursing Science, 16*(2), 26-38.

Denzin, N., & Lincoln, Y. (1994). Introduction. In N. Denzin & Y. Lincoln (Eds.), *Handbook of qualitative research* (pp. 1-17). Thousand Oaks, CA: Sage.

Dracup, K., & Meleis, A. (1982). Compliance: An interactionist approach. *Nursing Research, 31,* 31-36.

Eastland, L. (1994). Habermas, emancipation, and relationship change: An exploration of recovery processes as a model for social transformation. *Journal of Applied Communication Research, 22,* 162-176.

Edel, M. (1985). Noncompliance: An appropriate nursing diagnosis. *Nursing Outlook, 33,* 183-185.

Erlen, J. (1997). Ethical questions inherent in compliance. *Orthopaedic Nursing, 16*(2), 7780.

Ford-Gilboe, M., Campbell, J., & Berman, H. (1995). Stories and numbers: Coexistence without compromise. *Advances in Nursing Science, 18*(1), 14-26.

Guba, E., & Lincoln, Y. (1994). Competing paradigms in qualitative research. In N. Denzin & Y. Lincoln (Eds.), *Handbook of qualitative research* (pp. 105-117). Thousand Oaks, CA: Sage.

Hall, J., & Stevens, P. (1991). Rigor in feminist research. *Advances in Nursing Science, 13,* 16-27.

Hall, J., Stevens, P., & Meleis, A. (1994). Marginalization: A guiding concept for valuing diversity in nursing knowledge development. *Advances in Nursing Science, 16*(4), 23-41.

Hupcey, J., Morse, J., Lenz, E., & Tasón, M. (1996). Wilsonian methods of concept analysis: A critique. *Scholarly Inquiry for Nursing Practice, 10,* 185-220.

Kim, M. (1986). Nursing diagnosis: A Janus view. In M. Hurley (Ed.), *Classification of nursing diagnoses: Proceedings of the sixth conference* (pp. 1-14). St Louis: Mosby.

Kincheloe, J., & McLaren, P. (1994). Rethinking critical theory and qualitative research. In N. Denzin & Y. Lincoln (Eds.), *Handbook of qualitative research* (pp. 138-157). Thousand Oaks, CA: Sage.

Lather, P. (1991). *Getting smart: Feminist research and pedagogy with/in the postmodern.* New York: Routledge.

Marston, M. (1970). Compliance with medical regimens: a review of the literature. *Nursing Research, 19*, 312-323.

McCormick, J., & Roussy, J. (1997). A feminist poststructuralist orientation to nursing praxis. In S. Thorne & V. Hayes (Eds.), *Nursing praxis: Knowledge and action* (pp. 267-284). Thousand Oaks, CA: Sage.

Messias, D. (1996). Concept development: Exploring undocumentedness. *Scholarly Inquiry for Nursing Practice, 10*(3), 235-252.

Miller, S. (1997). Multiple paradigms for nursing: Post-modern feminisms. In S. Thorne & V. Hayes (Eds.), *Nursing praxis: Knowledge and action.* (pp. 140-156). Thousand Oaks, CA: Sage.

Morse, J. (1995). Exploring the theoretical basis of nursing using advanced techniques of concept analysis. *Advances in Nursing Science, 17*(3), 31-46.

Morse, J. (1996). Concept analysis in nursing research: A critical appraisal. *Scholarly Inquiry for Nursing Practice, 10*, 253-277.

Müller, M., & Dzurec, L. (1993). The power of the name. *Advances in Nursing Science, 15*(3), 15-22.

Paley, J. (1996). How not to clarify concepts in nursing. *Journal of Advanced Nursing, 24*, 572-578.

Parsons, T. (1951). *The social system.* Chicago: The Free Press.

Reinharz, S. (1992). *Feminist methods in social research.* New York: Oxford University Press.

Rodgers, B. L. (1989). Concepts, analysis, and the development of nursing knowledge: The evolutionary cycle. *Journal of Advanced Nursing, 14*, 330-335.

Rodgers, B. L. (1993). Concept analysis: An evolutionary view. In B. L. Rodgers & K. Knafl (Eds.), *Concept development in nursing: Foundations, techniques, and applications* (pp. 73-92). Philadelphia: W.B. Saunders.

Scott, J. (1990). Deconstructing equality-versus-difference: or uses of poststructuralist theory for feminism. In M. Hirsch & E. Fox Keller (Eds.), *Conflicts in feminism* (pp. 134-148). New York: Routledge.

Smith, D. (1990). *The conceptual practices of power: A feminist sociology of knowledge.* Toronto: University of Toronto Press.

Stevens, P. (1989). A critical social reconceptualization of environment in nursing: Implications for methodology. *Advances in Nursing Science, 11*(4), 56-68.

Thompson, J. (1990). Hermeneutic inquiry. In L. E. Moody (Ed.), *Advancing nursing science through research,* Vol. 2 (pp. 223-280). Newbury Park, CA: Sage.

Thorne, S. (1990). Constructive non-compliance in chronic illness. *Holistic Nursing Practice, 5*, 62-69.

Walker, L., & Avant, K. (1995). *Strategies for theory construction in nursing* (3rd ed.). Norwalk, CT: Appleton & Lange.

Wilson-Thomas, L. (1995). Applying critical social theory in nursing education to bridge the gap between theory, research, and practice. *Journal of Advanced Nursing, 21*, 568-575.

Wuest, J. (1993). Removing the shackles: A feminist critique of non-compliance. *Nursing Outlook, 41*, 217–224.

Wuest, J. (1994). A feminist approach to concept analysis. *Western Journal of Nursing Research, 15*, 577–586.

Wuest, J. (1997). Fraying connections of caring women: An exemplar of including difference in the development of explanatory frameworks. *Canadian Journal of Nursing Research, 29*, 99–116.

Wuest, J., & Merritt-Gray, M. (1997). Participatory action research: Practical dilemmas and emancipatory possibilities. In J. Morse (Ed.), *Completing a qualitative research project* (pp. 283–306). Thousand Oaks, CA: Sage.

Concept Development of Nursing-Sensitive Patient Outcomes*

Meridean L. Maas, Sue Moorhead, Janet P. Specht,
Deborah Perry Schoenfelder,
Elizabeth A. Swanson, Marion L. Johnson,
and Bonnie L. Westra

Patient outcomes research has major implications for nursing practice and care delivery, as well as for building theory to develop the science of nursing. Concerns about cost, quality, and distribution of health care drive the need to demonstrate the effectiveness of nursing management and clinical interventions. These forces and the recognized need for standardized nursing languages (Lange & Jacox, 1993; Maas et al., 1996; McCloskey & Bulechek, 1994) highlight the necessity for a classification of nursing-sensitive patient outcomes. The Nursing Outcomes Classification (NOC) (Iowa Outcomes Project, 1997), developed by a research team at the University of Iowa College of Nursing, is a comprehensive classification of patient outcomes influenced by nursing interventions that completes the standardized languages for the three nursing process elements of the Nursing Minimum Data Set (Werley & Lang, 1988). Comprehensive standardized languages for nursing diagnoses (Martin & Scheet, 1992; North American Nursing Diagnosis Association, 1997; Saba et al., 1991) and nursing interventions (Iowa Interventions Project, 1996; Martin & Sheet, 1992; Saba et al., 1991) were previously developed and published.

The ability to assess the efficacy and effectiveness of interventions to

*Research funded by Sigma Theta Tau International and the National Institutes of Health, Institute of Nursing Research R01 NR04347.

treat nursing diagnoses has been hampered by the lack of standardized languages. Standardized languages enable the development of computerized nursing information systems and the building of large local and national clinical data bases. When available, these data bases can be mined to examine the linkages among diagnoses, interventions, and outcomes. Further, knowledge will accumulate more rapidly around standardized languages denoting concepts that describe the phenomena of nursing. Finally, the development of concepts describing and classifying nursing phenomena is first-level theory building that facilitates the linking of concepts in hypotheses to be tested for elaboration of middle-range nursing theories (Blegen & Tripp-Reimer, 1997). This chapter briefly overviews the work of the Iowa Outcomes Project (1997) and describes the use of concept analysis by the research team to develop the outcomes and indicators included in the Nursing Outcomes Classification (NOC).

THE IOWA OUTCOMES PROJECT

The NOC research team, funded by Sigma Theta Tau International and the National Institutes of Health, National Institute of Nursing Research, began work in 1989 to: (1) identify, label, validate, and classify nursing-sensitive patient outcomes and indicators; (2) evaluate the validity and usefulness of the classification in clinical field testing; and (3) define and test measurement procedures for the outcomes and indicators.

Following the clarification and resolution of conceptual and methodological issues, the research team defined *nursing-sensitive patient outcome, indicator,* and *measure* and agreed upon an initial inductive research approach. A *nursing-sensitive patient outcome* is defined as a variable patient or family caregiver state, behavior, or perception that is influenced by nursing intervention and conceptualized at a middle level of abstraction (Erben et al., 1992). A *nursing-sensitive outcome indicator* is a variable patient or family caregiver state, behavior, or perception at a lower level of abstraction than an outcome that is responsive to nursing and used for determining an outcome (Maas et al., 1996). An *outcome measure* is a scale that quantifies the status of a patient or family caregiver outcome or indicator.

To accomplish the study aims, the next step of this first phase of the research was to construct a preliminary list of patient outcomes used in nursing, as evidenced in the nursing literature and clinical nursing information systems. More than 4,000 outcome statements, mostly patient goals, were extracted from 20 nursing textbook, care plan manual, and information system sources, representing all clinical settings, nursing specialties, and patient age groups. The outcome statements were distributed to research team members, 150 to 200 statements each on separate slips of paper. In a series of exercises, the team members clustered the outcome statements, based on similarity-dissimilarity, and developed an outcome label for each cluster. After redundancy was removed, an initial list of more than 300 outcome labels, each with a set of outcome statements (indicators) resulted. The next step was to perform a concept analysis of the initial outcome concepts to further develop and validate each outcome and its indicators based on the relevant literature.

CONCEPT ANALYSIS

Broad outcome categories based on the medical outcomes study (MOS) (Tarlov et al., 1989) and the work of Lang and Marek (1990) were developed to organize and perform a concept analysis of each outcome on the initial list. The eight categories were: physiological status; psychological/cognitive status; social and role status; physical functional status; safety status; family caregiver status; health attitudes/knowledge/behavior; and perceived well-being. Eight work groups were formed with research team members, each chaired by a doctorally prepared investigator. Nurse clinicians representing a variety of clinical settings and specialties were invited to join each of the work groups. More than 25 clinicians responded, increasing the size of the research team to more than 40 members. Each work group included faculty, clinicians, and graduate student members and each group was assigned a research assistant to assist with the concept analyses. Each work group was assigned one of the eight outcome categories. Using a two-round Delphi process, each outcome on the initial list was assigned to one of the eight categories and thus to one of the eight work groups. Organizing the initial outcomes and their associated indicators in the broad categories enabled the work groups to focus the review of literature more than would have been possible if the outcomes had been randomly assigned to the work groups.

Method

An adaptation of the method of concept analysis promulgated by Rodgers (1989a) was used to identify a conceptual definition of each outcome concept. Rodgers' method was chosen because she emphasizes rigorous inductive analysis, systematic description, and comparison of most frequent use by diverse disciplines (Rodgers, 1987, 1989a, 1989b). Bonnie Westra, who studied and published with Rodgers (Westra & Rodgers, 1991) and was a member of the NOC research team, guided the development of the concept analysis procedures and assisted with confirming that each work group chair understood the procedures. The guidelines in Table 20–1 for the analysis of each outcome concept

Table 20–1 Guidelines for Concept Analysis of Outcome Concepts

1. Identify literature related to the concept.
   a. Conduct literature searches across nursing and other relevant disciplines.
   b. Select 5–10 key sources that represent conceptual and research bases.
   c. Review instruments that measure the concept.
2. Review each source for definitions, indicators, linkages with nursing interventions, and patient populations.
   a. Complete the attached forms as completely as possible, e.g., instruments may include only definitions and indicators.
3. Compare indicators derived from the literature with indicators generated in the previous exercises.
4. Develop (or refine) an outcome label, a proposed definition for the outcome label, and a list of indicators that reflect all dimensions of the outcome using information from the literature review and indicator lists generated in the previous exercises.
   a. Development of the conceptual definition (Waltz, Strickland, & Lenz, 1991).
      1) Develop a preliminary definition, i.e., your own definition of the concept.
      2) Critically analyze definitions and use of the concept in the literature.
      3) List all definitions of the concept, synonyms, and their definitions.
      4) Select the critical dimensions of the concept, i.e., the key elements that are consistently present.
      5) Construct an outline, table, or diagram to represent the key dimensions of the concept and their indicators.
      6) Determine if the outcome is too complex, i.e., needs to be divided or if outcomes are missing and need to be added.
      7) Restate the conceptual definition based on the above analysis of dimensions and indicators.
   b. Rules for definitions.
      1) The definition must describe the complete meaning of the outcome concept (Kaplan, 1964).
      2) The definition as a whole must be synonymous with the outcome concept (Kaplan, 1964).
      3) The definition must be clear and simple (Kaplan, 1964; Waltz, Strickland, & Lenz, 1991).
      4) The definition must refer to all indicators included with the concept and describe all dimensions of the concept (Kaplan, 1964; Waltz, Strickland, & Lenz, 1991).

c. Development of indicators.
   1) Combine the lists of indicators generated from Phase I and from the literature review.
   2) Remove redundancy from the lists.
   3) Reduce the list of indicators if too long or too numerous to equal 10–12 key indicators. If more than 20 indicators are needed to represent the outcome concept, consider whether there is more than one outcome concept represented.
   4) Obtain additional sources if the list is too short to determine if it is complete.
d. Rules for indicator statements (Waltz, Strickland, & Lenz, 1991).
   1) Indicator statements must be precise with explicit and specific terms used.
   2) Indicator statements must be congruent with the outcome concept so that the meaning of the concept is adequately represented.
   3) Indicator terms must be used in a consistent manner.
   4) Indicator statements must be inclusive so that all dimensions of the outcome concept are represented.
   5) Indicator statements must be measurable so that empirical measures can be developed.
   6) Indicator statements must be sensitive and useful so that they have utility for nursing.
5. Determine the appropriateness of the outcome label (this is ongoing as the definition is developed).
   a. Recommend a new outcome label if needed.
   b. Add new outcome labels as needed.
   c. If the outcome is not consistent with the outcome category, give the label and any associated information to the appropriate work group chair.
   d. Review each label for consistency with the Rule of Standardization (Table 20–2).
   e. Prepare the Outcome File Form for each completed outcome concept.
   f. The final outcome analysis product is the outcome label, a conceptual definition, a list of specific indicators, and a list of references used for the concept analysis (APA style).
   g. Provide all information to the Co-Principal Investigators for review before presenting to the research team, including a copy of all articles used in the review.

were outlined by Westra, approved by the research team, and distributed to each work group chair. Additional examples of concept analysis to develop NOC outcomes are reported in the literature (Swanson et al., 1997).

Sampling of literature was accomplished by conducting extensive literature searches. Based on the frequency of articles in a discipline, articles in at least two disciplines were selected—nursing and one other. Literature from different disciplines were searched depending on the concept. Only English language publications were sampled for each analysis. MEDLINE and CINAHL were the primary searches used. References of key articles also were searched. Keywords used were the outcome label and any synonyms. Investigators were instructed to restrict searches to the last five years except for purposive sampling of classic literature and if fewer than 30 articles were retrieved.

Statements were extracted consistent with the following categories: definitions and indicators of the outcome concept; synonyms; related concepts; references; antecedents; and consequences. Data were inducted to describe themes for each category and subsequently reviewed to identify indicators and other concept characteristics. Comparisons were made across disciplines to locate any unique discipline conceptualizations.

Findings described the concept definition developed from the data. Other themes were identified from the data to describe the concept, including indicators of the outcome concept; synonyms and related concepts; antecedents; consequences; and references (use of concept in reference to an idea, thing, or event).

Following the refinement of the outcome label (Table 20-2) according to language rules developed by the NOC research team, development of the definition, and selection of indicators and a measurement scale, each outcome is reviewed by the research team with language revisions made if indicated. Four to six content literature references are listed with the outcome. The outcome is next evaluated for content validity by expert survey.

Table 20-2   Rules for Standardization of Outcome Labels

Conceptualized at a middle level of abstraction
Concise; stated in five or fewer words
Stated in nonevaluative terms rather than as decreased, increased, or improved state
Does not describe a nurse behavior or intervention
Not stated as a nursing diagnosis
Describes an individual client state, behavior, or perception that is variable and can be measured and quantified
Colons used to make broad labels more specific with the broad label stated first and the more specific after colon

CONTENT VALIDITY BY EXPERT SURVEY

Surveys of master's-degree nurses representing cross sections of clinical specialties, settings, and client age groups were used to rate which indicators are most important to determine each outcome and to rate which indicators were most sensitive to nursing intervention. A revision of Fehring's methodology (Fehring, 1987) for assessing content validity of nursing diagnoses was used to estimate the outcomes' and indicators' content validity and sensitivity to nursing interventions.

Fehring's method for determining content validity for nursing diagnoses was adapted and tested in the preliminary work to validate the content of outcomes describing satisfaction with nursing. McCloskey and Bulechek (Iowa Interventions Project, 1992) used the method to assess the content validity of nursing interventions and argue that adaptation of Fehring's method is consistent with recommendations of ways to construct taxonomies (Fleishman & Quaintance, 1984). The successful use of Fehring's method to validate nursing interventions and the NOC team's pilot work with patient satisfaction outcomes supported the use of the method to assess the content validity of the NOC outcomes.

Surveys were mailed to 175 to 200 randomly selected experts from the mailing lists of nursing specialty organizations. The nurse experts were asked to review the definitions and to rate each indicator of eight to ten outcomes as to: (a) the extent nursing interventions contribute to achievement (sensitivity) (1 = no contribution; 5 = contribution is mainly nursing), and (b) the importance of the indicator to determining the outcome status (content validity) (1 = never important; 5 = always important). Return rates ranged from 30 percent to 65 percent.

Only a few minor changes to the definitions were suggested on the returned surveys, and in each case the outcome label and definition were reevaluated and a change made, if indicated. In general, the majority of indicators were rated at .60 or more, and many met the .80 criterion. Respondents suggested a few additional indicators, and after review by the research team, a few new indicators were added. The results of the surveys indicated that the selection, development, and refinement of the nursing-sensitive outcomes and indicators, based on the qualitative and concept analyses, were content valid and responsive to nursing interventions.

CONCEPT ANALYSIS OF ANXIETY: AN EXAMPLE

One of the concepts assigned to the Psychological/Cognitive Focus Group in the early stages of developing outcomes for NOC was Anxiety. The members of the focus group considered this to be an important problem that nurses treat, and the group felt outcomes that addressed this nursing diagnosis were important to include in the NOC. The literature identifies that anxiety disorders are the most prevalent mental disorders in the United States (Blair & Ramomes, 1996). A preliminary review of major psychiatric nursing textbooks failed to provide much insight into the desired outcomes of anxiety that were useful for the development of this outcome by the focus group. Textbooks focused on the identification and assessment of the problem and its differentiation from the concept of Fear.

The history of Anxiety as a nursing diagnosis presents a rocky course in the development of standardized language for patient problems treated by nurses. The controversy centers on the differentiation of the defining characteristics of Anxiety from those of Fear by members of North American Nursing Diagnosis Association (NANDA). At one point Anxiety was removed from the list of approved nursing diagnoses (Kim & Moritz, 1982), only to be added back at the following NANDA conference. Despite continued efforts to differentiate Anxiety from Fear, the major difference is definitional based on whether the source of the feelings experienced by the individual is known.

Attempts to find key articles for the development of outcomes for anxiety proved to be a significant hurdle. To be consistent with the problem classification of NANDA, the members of the focus group decided to identify and create separate outcomes for Fear and Anxiety. This was partly due to the tremendous amount of literature available for each problem and the identification of separate measurement tools for Anxiety and Fear. More recent work by Whitley (1989, 1992a, 1992b, 1994) and Whitley and Tousman (1996) support anxiety as a concept separate from fear.

An extensive computerized literature search of the concept anxiety since 1993 identified over 5,000 published articles in English with the word anxiety in the abstract. The download of the sources and abstracts of this search filled 12 high-density disks! It is clear that many professionals are concerned with anxiety experienced by individuals and that nurses, regardless of setting, deal with anxiety as a clinical problem. The literature supports that anxiety is associated with preoperative periods, invasive or health-related tests, aging, retirement, cancer, and family member illness, to name a few.

Assessment of anxiety has commonly focused on trait vs. state. Trait anxiety occurs when the individual's self-concept is challenged or threatened in some way. This type of anxiety tends to be a long-standing personality trait and is communicated by a fairly specific behavior pattern (Spielberger, 1975). Patients with trait anxiety are more likely to be treated by psychiatric and mental health nurses. In contrast, state anxiety occurs in response to a situation. The distinctions made between state and trait anxiety are widely accepted, used across disciplines, and clinically useful. The work group noted state and trait distinctions and incorporate them in the data base of indicators.

A total of 13 measurement tools were identified for Anxiety, and studies using each instrument were found (Moorhead & Brighton, in press). The most commonly used measurement tool is the State-Trait Anxiety Inventory (STAI) by Spielberger, Gorsuch, Lushene, Vagg, and Jacobs (1983). Almost 30 studies, many from nursing, were found that use this instrument to measure anxiety in adult patients. The tools used to measure Anxiety in nursing studies indicated the importance of the problem treated by nurses.

Members of the focus group felt it was important to develop outcomes for Anxiety that measure the effects of interventions by nurses regardless of setting or source of the anxiety. Group members wanted the outcome developed to be useful for mental and physical health as well as illness situations. Initial work on Anxiety focused on identifying indicators that captured the level of anxiety experienced by the individual. This led the group to acknowledge the original levels of Anxiety developed by NANDA (mild, moderate, severe, and panic) (Gebbie & Lavin, 1975). The group concluded that their literature review failed to provide clear directions or insight into the outcome needed for Anxiety because they were examining the problem rather than what would be important to assess responsiveness to nursing interventions. Refocusing on the goals and evaluation of treatment of Anxiety as revealed in the literature, indicators of anxiety reduction and anxiety control were identified.

The group decided that Anxiety Control was the preferred term because Anxiety Reduction was a label used in the Nursing Interventions Classification (NIC) (Iowa Interventions Project, 1996). Reexamination of the literature affirmed indicators and supported development of a definition of Anxiety Control. Anxiety Control was defined as the individual's ability to identify and control anxious feelings (Figure 20-1). Indicators for both state and trait anxiety control were included. Surveys of nurse experts validated the outcome and its content, but some suggested that monitoring the amount of anxiety also would be useful before, throughout, and following nursing intervention. Based on the survey, the work group is reexamining whether an outcome for anxiety level is needed in the NOC.

DISCUSSION OF CURRENT AND FUTURE WORK

The development and testing of NOC outcomes is continuing and will continue. The work groups continue to conduct concept analyses of outcomes that are suggested to be added to the Classification. The research team also has begun work on outcomes that are responsive to

Domain-(3)
Class-Self-Control (O)
Scale-(m)

DEFINITION: Ability to eliminate or reduce feelings of apprehension and tension from an unidentifiable source

TITLE: Anxiety Control	Never Demonstrated 1	Rarely Demonstrated 2	Sometimes Demonstrated 3	Often Demonstrated 4	Consistently Demonstrated 5
140201 Monitors intensity of anxiety	1	2	3	4	5
140202 Eliminates precursors of anxiety	1	2	3	4	5
140203 Decreases environmental stimuli when anxious	1	2	3	4	5
140204 Seeks information to reduce anxiety	1	2	3	4	5
140205 Maintains coping strategies for stressful situations	1	2	3	4	5
140206 Uses effective coping strategies	1	2	3	4	5
140207 Uses relaxation techniques to reduce anxiety	1	2	3	4	5

		1	2	3	4	5
140208	Reports decreased duration of episodes	1	2	3	4	5
140209	Reports increased length of time between episodes	1	2	3	4	5
140210	Maintains role performance	1	2	3	4	5
140211	Maintains social relationships	1	2	3	4	5
140212	Maintains concentration	1	2	3	4	5
140213	Reports absence of sensory perceptual distortions	1	2	3	4	5
140214	Reports adequate sleep	1	2	3	4	5
140215	Reports absence of physical manifestations of anxiety	1	2	3	4	5
140216	Behavioral manifestations of anxiety absent	1	2	3	4	5
140217	Controls anxiety response	1	2	3	4	5
Other	_____ Specify	1	2	3	4	5

Figure 20–1 Anxiety control–1402. (Data from Laraia, M. T., Stuart G. W., & Best, C. L. (1989). Behavioral treatment of panic-related disorders: A review. *Archives of Psychiatric Nursing, 3*(3), 125–133; Stuart, G. W., & Sundeen, S. J. (1995). *Principles and practice of psychiatric nursing (5th ed.).* St. Louis: Mosby; Waddell, K. L., & Demi, A. S. (1993). Effectiveness of an intensive partial hospitalization program for treatment of anxiety disorders. *Archives of Psychiatric Nursing, 7*(1), 2–10.)

nursing that characterized family and community units. Perhaps most importantly, NOC outcomes are being added to nursing care planning and documentation software, nursing information systems in all settings, and to textbooks and other media describing nursing clinical decision making and practice in all settings. Finally, the NOC team is conducting research to evaluate the reliability and validity of the outcome measures with clinical data in multiple sites representing the continuum of health care.

Nurses have been documenting the outcomes of their interventions for decades, but the lack of a common language and associated measures for outcomes has impeded data aggregation, analysis, and synthesis of information about the effects of nursing interventions and practice. Outcome evaluation has expanded to include not only the efficacy of health care interventions, but also the effectiveness of interventions. Identifying outcomes responsive to nursing, rather than depending on the use of interdisciplinary outcomes developed mostly for physician practice, is important for the control of quality patient care and the development of nursing knowledge. Agreement on standardized nursing-sensitive outcomes will allow nurses to study the effects of nursing interventions along a continuum of care and across settings. Standardized outcomes that are responsive to nursing interventions will provide data to advance nursing theory development, science, and practice, and will furnish the data needed to inform and influence health care policy makers, a necessity if nursing is to fulfill its social contract.

REFERENCES

Blair, D. T., & Ramones, V. A. (1996). The undertreatment of anxiety: Overcoming confusion and stigma. *Journal of Psychosocial Nursing, and Health Services, 34*(6), 9–19.

Blegen, M. A., & Tripp-Reimer, T. (1997). Implications of nursing taxonomies for middle-range theory development. *Advances in Nursing Science, 19*(3), 37–49.

Erben, R., Franzkowiak, P., & Wenzel, E. (1992). Assessment of the outcomes of health intervention. *Social Science Medicine, 15*(4), 359–365.

Fehring, R. J. (1987). Methods to validate nursing diagnoses. *Heart & Lung, 16*(6), 625–629.

Fleishman, E. A., & Quaintance, M. K. (1984). *Taxonomies of human performance: A description of human tasks.* Orlando: Academic Press.

Gebbie, K. M., & Lavin, M. E. (1995*). Classification of nursing diagnoses: Proceedings of the first national conference.* St. Louis: Mosby.

Iowa Interventions Project. (1992). *Nursing interventions classification (NIC).* St. Louis: Mosby.

Iowa Interventions Project. (1996). *Nursing interventions classification (NIC).* St. Louis: Mosby.

Iowa Outcomes Project. (1997). *Nursing outcomes classification (NOC).* St. Louis: Mosby.

Johnson, S., Brady-Schluttner, K., Ellenbecker, S., Johnson, M., Lassengard, E.,

Maas, M., Stone, J., & Westra, B. L. (1996). Evaluating physical functional outcomes: One category of the nursing outcomes classification system. *MEDSURG Journal of Nursing, 5*, 157-162.

Kaplan, A. (1964). *The conduct of inquiry.* Scranton, PA: Chandler Publishing Company.

Kim, M. J., & Moritz, D. A. (1982). *Classification of nursing diagnoses: Proceedings of the third and fourth conference.* New York: McGraw-Hill.

Lang, N. M., & Marek, K. D. (1990). The classification of patient outcomes. *Journal of Professional Nursing, 6*, 153-163.

Lange, L. L., & Jacox, A. (1993). Using large data bases in nursing and health policy research. *Journal of Professional Nursing, 9*(4), 204-11.

Maas, M., Johnson, M., & Moorhead, S. (1996). Classifying nursing sensitive patient outcomes. *IMAGE, 28*(4), 295-301.

Martin, K., & Scheet, N. (1992). *The Omaha system: Applications for community health nursing.* Philadelphia: W. B. Saunders.

McCloskey, J. C., & Bulechek, G. M. (1994). Standardizing the language for nursing treatments: An overview of the issues. *Nursing Outlook, 42*(2), 56-63.

Moorhead, S., & Brighton, V. (in press). Anxiety & fear. In M. Maas, K. C. Buckwalter, M. Hardy, T. Tripp-Reimer, & M. Titler (Eds.), *Nursing diagnoses, interventions and outcomes for the elderly* (2nd ed.). St Louis: Mosby.

North American Nursing Diagnosis Association. (1997). *Nursing diagnoses: Definitions and classification.* Philadelphia: NANDA.

Rodgers, B. L. (1987). The use and application of concepts in nursing. Unpublished doctoral dissertation. University of Virginia, Charlottesville.

Rodgers, B. L. (1989a). Concepts, analysis, and the development of nursing knowledge: The evolutionary cycle. *Journal of Advanced Nursing, 14*, 330-335.

Rodgers, B. L. (1989b). Exploring health policy as a concept. *Western Journal of Nursing Research, 11*, 694-702.

Saba, B. K., O'Hare, A., Zuckerman, A. E., Boondasj, J., Levine, E., & Oatway, D. M. (1991). A nursing intervention taxonomy for home health care. *Nursing and Healthcare, 12*(6), 296-299.

Spielberger, C. D. (1975). Stress and anxiety. In I. G. Garason & C. D. Spielberger (Eds.), *Stress and anxiety.* Philadelphia: Hemisphere.

Spielberger, C. D., Gorsuch, R. L., Lushene, P., Vagg, P. R., & Jacobs, G. A. (1983). *Manual for the State-Trait Anxiety Inventory.* Palo Alto, CA: Consulting Psychologists Press.

Swanson, E. A., Jensen, D. P., Specht, J., Johnson, M. L., Maas, M., & Saylor, D. (1997). Caregiving: Concept analysis and outcomes. *Scholarly Inquiry for Nursing Practice: An International Journal, 11*(1), 65-76.

Tarlov, A. R., Ware, J. E., Greenfield, S., Nelson, E. C., Perrin, E., & Zubkoff, M. (1989). The medical outcomes study: An application of methods for monitoring the results of medical care. *Journal of the American Medical Association, 262*, 925-930.

Waltz, C. F., Strickland, O. L., & Lenz, E. R. (1991). *Measurement in nursing research* (2nd ed.). Philadelphia: F. A. Davis.

Werley, H., & Lang, N. (1988). *Identification of the nursing minimum data set.* New York: Springer.

Westra, B. L., & Rodgers, B. B. (1991). The concept of integration: A foundation for evaluating outcomes of of nursing care. *Journal of Professional Nursing*, 7, 277–282.

Whitley, G. G. (1989). Anxiety: Defining the diagnosis. *Journal of Psychosocial Nursing, 27*(10), 7–12.

Whitley, G. G. (1992a). Concept analysis of anxiety. *Nursing Diagnosis, 3*(3), 107–116.

Whitley, G. G. (1992b). Concept analysis of fear. *Nursing Diagnosis, 3*(4), 155–161.

Whitley, G. G. (1994). Expert validation and differentiation of the nursing diagnoses anxiety and fear. *Nursing Diagnosis, 5*(4), 143–150.

Whitley, G. G., & Tousman, S. A. (1996). A multivariate approach for validation of anxiety and fear. *Nursing Diagnosis, 7*(3), 116–124.

21

Applications and Future Directions for Concept Development in Nursing

Beth L. Rodgers and Kathleen A. Knafl

A variety of approaches to concept development have been presented in this text. A discussion of the philosophical foundations of concept development provided an overview of some of the major advances associated with this topic over the years. Issues also were identified to assist researchers in selecting techniques appropriate for the intended inquiry and the concept of interest. A comparison of diverse approaches to concept development followed, further enhancing decision making associated with this process.

The methods presented included several distinct approaches to concept analysis that, although they may appear similar, possess significant philosophical differences. Concept analysis is the most familiar of the concept development techniques, and includes Norris's seminal work on "concept clarification," variations of Wilson's (1963) technique, Rodgers' (1989a, 1993) "evolutionary" foundation for concept development, and the simultaneous concept analysis process utilized by Haase and her colleagues to address a domain of related concepts. The hybrid model of Schwartz-Barcott and Kim starts with a systematic literature review and concept analysis and then adds a phase of field research to expand and further clarify the concept through the collection of empirical data in a natural nursing setting. Various examples of this process were provided that show the usefulness of this model in expanding understanding of concepts as diverse as grief and caring. Another approach presented addressed integrated literature reviews, including meta-analysis as a means to develop concepts, probably a less frequently

401

thought of approach that, nonetheless, offers a significant contribution to concept development.

Each of the approaches presented in this text possesses its own philosophical base, and is oriented toward a specific purpose or outcome. Overall, concept development can be conducted along many lines and in various creative ways. It is fair to say, as well, that it is a neverending process. A concept may never be completely "finished"; instead, development must continue as new knowledge, experiences, and contexts emerge. Without continuing effort to develop concepts, progress in nursing may be impeded by a growing quagmire of conceptual problems.

As noted in the introduction to this text, concept development techniques may be just what are needed to resolve significant problems in nursing. However, there is a need to continue evaluating available methods and to create new and innovative approaches to concept development as new problems are identified. Additional work is needed in several areas, including continued exploration of the nature of concepts, which will shed additional light on appropriate means of development. Similarly, there is a need to evaluate the effectiveness of various techniques with the numerous types of concepts that exist (e.g., static, process, aesthetic, empirical concepts). For concept development to be effective, it should provide some release from ambiguity, enhance understanding, and provide direction for continuing development. Ultimately, the resulting concepts must be useful in accomplishing the aims of the discipline and consistent with the needs of nurses in applying those concepts.

OTHER APPLICATIONS FOR CONCEPT DEVELOPMENT TECHNIQUES

For the most part, we have focused this text on the contributions made to nursing knowledge and research through the use of concept development techniques. These contributions are quite significant in themselves. However, while expanding the knowledge base of the discipline through the resolution of significant conceptual problems is an admirable accomplishment, it does not constitute the only use of concept development techniques. We would not be providing a complete picture of the usefulness of concept development if we did not give some attention to these other applications, especially the use of these techniques to clarify ideas on an individual level and as a teaching strategy.

Individual Clarification of Ideas

In some respects, this application of concept development resembles the specific research uses of these methods discussed throughout this text. Although concept development may be an end point in itself when the purpose of inquiry is to clarify or expand a concept, it may also be an important preliminary step in an investigation. The use of concept development in this manner goes beyond the heuristic nature of some applications to assisting in the initial conceptualization of a study. In other cases, such methods have value simply for clarifying thoughts for future scholarly work.

Selecting and defining the appropriate concepts can be a difficult task in the early stages of a study. Yet, it is one of the most significant activities, ultimately affecting everything else in the investigation. For example, research on older adults' return to home after discharge from a hospital might be shaped much differently if the focus were on adaptation, coping, or integration (Westra & Rodgers, 1991). Similarly, Knafl and Deatrick (1987) found that conceptualizing family response to illness in regard to management, rather than the impact of the illness, directed their focus to very different aspects of the experience. These investigators successfully used concept analysis techniques to clarify and refine the concept of family management style (Deatrick & Knafl, 1990; Knafl & Deatrick, 1990). Concept development techniques can be very beneficial in identifying the appropriate focus to generate productive inquiry through clarifying or defining concepts or evaluating the fit of certain concepts with the situation of interest. These approaches may contribute to the development of a useful and coherent definition of key concepts in research, thereby helping the investigator avoid arbitrary or ad hoc definitions. Because methodological rigor and the usefulness of study findings may rest on the definitions used in a study, the contributions of concept development in the initial phases of an investigation cannot be underestimated.

Synthesizing vast amounts of literature, as accomplished through many of the concept development techniques, can be an important task in clarifying individual ideas as well. It is not uncommon for researchers, especially upon entering a new area of interest, to experience some confusion sorting through what may be multiple, diverse approaches to the subject matter. At such times it can be difficult to deal with these often conflicting ideas and either assimilate them into a coherent whole or develop a sound basis for choosing among competing ideas. Frequently, concept development techniques can provide a solid basis for presenting arguments regarding new ways to view a situation or innovative conceptualizations. Anyone who has worked with new investigators as they became mired in the confusion of the initial research stages, or who has had such an experience as they embarked on a new area of inquiry themselves, will recognize the value of concept development strategies for such purposes. We have recommended various concept development techniques on many occasions to students who were experiencing difficulty identifying a research focus, with overwhelmingly positive results.

Such activities have tremendous value in providing a strong basis for research and assisting in critical thought. Interestingly, concept development techniques, especially concept analysis, are becoming incorporated into graduate education in nursing with increasing frequency, perhaps for these very reasons. However, such activities may also account for the misconception that concept development constitutes merely an "academic exercise" (Diers, 1991). Consequently, we want to stress that the benefits and applications of such techniques extend well beyond academic or intellectual interests, as is evident in this text.

Concept Development in Teaching

The contributions of concept development techniques to the clarification of ideas is relevant even outside the context of actual research, particularly in their use as a teaching strategy. Indeed, Wilson's (1963) well-known work on concept analysis was developed for precisely this purpose. In 1988, Balog described his adaptation of the activities of concept analysis to assist health education students to explore and construct their own views of "health." Initially he provided the student group with a list of people of varying abilities and physical or medical conditions (e.g., athlete, person with myopia, paraplegic, person with bronchogenic carcinoma). The students were directed to explain if each hypothetical person on the list was *healthy* or *ill*. Ultimately, the class as a whole constructed lists of the "ingredients" for both the concepts of health and illness and worked to identify the essential criteria for each. This exercise not only assisted the students to construct their own views of health and illness but also, because of the group work involved, enhanced the students' awareness and appreciation of the wide scope of perspectives that individuals possess on this subject.

Other applications of concept development techniques in teaching are in the promotion of critical or analytical thinking. Students can be encouraged to confront key concepts in nursing by adapting some of the concept development strategies. On the undergraduate level, important concepts in nursing, such as the definition of nursing itself, professionalism, competence, collaboration, disease, human response, and diagnosis, can be explored using some of these techniques to help students come to grips with these ideas, obtain a depth of understanding of these concepts, and present a coherent presentation of their profession to others. As students progress to levels of increased clinical involvement, and in graduate nursing education, concepts relevant to patient care situations may be explored in a similar manner. The techniques of concept development may be an effective practical exercise to promote some of the analytical and critical skills appropriate to higher learning and essential to expert nursing practice.

A strength of many of the concept development techniques is the literature review involved in the process. These techniques provide, in most cases, some structure or system for conducting an extensive, in-depth literature review on the concepts of interest. Class projects or papers might provide an opportunity for students to use these techniques, thus presenting the student with a challenge to view the concept from multiple perspectives and to develop an awareness of the diversity of ideas. The process of comparing, contrasting, and eventually synthesizing ideas is an excellent exercise to develop analytical skills. Finally, if students present their own conclusions regarding the concept in some form, they have the opportunity to develop skill in preparing logical arguments and defending their positions in a public forum. As an added benefit, students may be learning an important skill for later involvement in research activities, thus potentially taking some of the mystery out of the research process as well.

Rodgers has presented concept analysis to nurses in clinical settings to develop their awareness and appreciation of this and other types of research and, especially, to instill an attitude that they *can* make an important contribution to the knowledge base of nursing. The processes involved in concept development are in no way simple or easy, as they require considerable powers of reasoning and analytical skill to be carried out well. Nevertheless, they have been perceived by practitioners as less threatening and, therefore, more manageable than a traditional quasi-experimental or experimental investigation. Unfortunately for many clinicians with entry-level education, these more traditional approaches to research constitute the extent of their knowledge about nursing inquiry.

Tadd and Chadwick (1989) also emphasized the contribution of various analytical techniques in the academic setting. Their discussion included various forms of philosophical analysis and was not focused on concept development specifically. However, their discussion added further emphasis to the value of such methods in teaching, particularly for clarifying ideas, increasing awareness of diverse perspectives and the complexity of language, and promoting the development of analytical skills.

One additional dimension addressed by Tadd and Chadwick (1989) included the use of such techniques by faculty involved in curriculum development. As these authors point out, concepts may be "incorporated into nursing curricula without adequate analysis or indeed without asking rather obvious questions about justifying their inclusion" (p. 157). In many instances, it is unreasonable to expect nurse educators to have a consensus on the definitions of important concepts; certainly there is a need for students to develop a tolerance for ambiguity and diversity. In other situations, agreement is both important and possible, for example, agreement on the notion of competence (or, in another common phrase, "safe professional practice"), which may be a hallmark in the evaluation of student performance and progress. Still, Tadd and Chadwick's call for concentrated attention regarding concepts as they are included in nursing curricula sends a significant caution to nurse educators, and demonstrates yet another application of concept development techniques.

Only a few journal articles were found in which concept development techniques were discussed in reference to nursing education. However, even these limited examples demonstrated the value of these methods in the academic setting. As Dungog (1988) points out, "exploratory rather than expository strategies" may be very effective in promoting learning (p. 14) and in producing graduates capable of success in a constantly changing environment (Tadd & Chadwick, 1989).

FUTURE DIRECTIONS FOR CONCEPT DEVELOPMENT IN NURSING

In a 1979 research conference presentation, Downs argued that

> [nurse researchers] have already hurtled into too much clinical and applied research without sufficient attention to the theory on which it is based. . . . Short shrift is given to efforts aimed at producing descriptive material that could result in the construction of sound experiments later on. (Downs, 1980, p. 97)

Several facts could point to the rejection of this quote as bearing any relevance to nursing research now. First, it was presented almost two decades ago, a vast amount of time in discussions of scientific activities and, especially, in view of the development of nursing knowledge that has occurred during this interim. Second, Downs was referring specifically to evaluation research (the focus of the conference), and the lack of "some kind of unifying theory that will place the huge volume of findings into some kind of theoretical juxtaposition" (p. 94). Finally, although Downs did refer directly to theory development, she did not mention the role of concept development in this process.

We would argue that Downs' (1980) admonition is not the least bit misplaced in the context of contemporary nursing investigations. As the hue and cry for more intervention-oriented, outcome-focused research continues to gain volume, there is considerable danger that nurse researchers will not have a sound descriptive base for their research, and that conceptual problems will undermine the apparent success brought about in the resolution of empirical or clinical problems (Laudan, 1977).

Consequently, the balance between empirical advance and conceptual clarity may be lost, and progress becomes illusory, mired in the new dilemmas that are created along the way.

Providing a Descriptive Basis

Concept development techniques can provide an important part of this descriptive base through the various outcomes that are achieved with these methods: accomplishments of a linguistic, communicative, categorical or classificatory, diagnostic, and heuristic nature. The linguistic function emphasizes word use to clarify vocabulary and alternate forms of expression. The communicative aspect may focus on consensus building to improve understanding and the sharing of ideas. Classification constitutes an important function of concepts that, when the concepts are clarified, enables phenomena to be sorted or categorized relative to shared attributes. This process may be used particularly in the development of taxonomic structures, for example, the development of nursing diagnoses (Lunney, 1990). Finally, the heuristic potential of concept development techniques provides direction for further research by generating not only plausible definitions but questions and, sometimes, hypotheses for further research (Rodgers, 1989a, 1989b).

These functions point to the strong basis for further research that can result from the development of concepts. Yet, it is important to avoid constructing an apparent hierarchical notion of research, where description has value only if it leads later to empirical testing. Description is a valuable end point in itself, because of its power in illustrating or increasing sensitivity to experience, and enhancing understanding.

Furthermore, concept development techniques are not limited to description alone. At times, they border on the prescriptive (if we can use that term safely in this context), suggesting not how nurses *should act* or what they *should do,* but how nurses *might think* about a given situation or topic. It is difficult to argue against the merits of improved or, at least, expanded thinking! Of course, thinking is meant here to refer to the entire domain of cognitive activities. Improvement may take the form of clearly better (more useful, appropriate, or effective) ways to think about something or a challenge to the status quo. Both of these are important components of progress.

Attention to Conceptual Problems

New directions for concept development thus include the increased recognition of conceptual problems, the use of appropriate techniques for their resolution, and the continuing expansion and evaluation of methods, along with the creation of additional methods as new and unique types of problems are identified. In recent years, there has been a great deal of attention to (and, for the most part, support for) the idea of a balance in the generation of nursing knowledge. Typically, these discussions have focused on qualitative and quantitative methods as the entities to be weighed (Knafl et al., 1988; Morse, 1991). Although these debates have some merit, we suggest that balance be considered not only in regard to the methods used. Instead, balance is needed among the types of knowledge that are generated and the kinds of problems solved. For our purposes here, we are concerned especially with the attention given to both empirical and conceptual problems. Throughout this text, there are numerous examples of conceptual problems that have a significant impact on nursing knowledge and practice and that, as a result, cannot be ignored in the scientific enterprise of nursing.

This idea of balance is not unlike the anecdote of sawing off the legs of a chair that sits unevenly on the floor. Nurse scholars must be careful that in resolving some problems, the new problems that will be created as a part of the process are not left unattended. More realistically, every problem "solved" undoubtedly will result in new questions. The task, then, is for inquiry to be pursued in a variety of realms, focused on diverse problems, and with methods appropriate to answer the questions deemed important in nursing. At the same time, it is important not only to recognize the contributions of these varied approaches, but to integrate and build upon their unique contributions.

Indeed, as editors, we might be viewed as having created a few additional problems with this book. One of our primary aims was to call attention to a class of problems that previously may have been misunderstood, inadequately recognized, thought to be incapable of resolution, perhaps ignored altogether, or, in some circumstances, given "second class" status. Calling attention to problems, however, seems to be prerequisite to making progress in an area. More important, we have provided a cross section of valuable tools for addressing the problems that may be identified as a result of this work. We hope this text will contribute to increased understanding of these tools, a foundation for reasoned decision making in the design of investigations, and, ultimately, rigorous and defensible inquiry to promote continued, productive investigations. Our intent in this concluding chapter, then, was not to bring closure, but to open doors to enhance concept development in nursing.

REFERENCES

Balog, J. E. (1988). The concept of health and techniques of conceptual analysis. *Health Education, 19*(4), 54–56.

Deatrick, J., & Knafl, K. (1990). Family management behaviors: Concept analysis and refinement. *Journal of Pediatric Nursing, 5,* 15–22.

Diers, D. (1991). On academic exercises. . . . *Image: Journal of Nursing Scholarship, 23,* 70.

Downs, F. S. (1980). Relationship of finding of clinical research and development of criteria: A researcher's perspective. *Nursing Research, 29,* 94-97.

Dungog, E. F. (1988). Concept teaching in nursing. *ANPhi Papers, 23*(1), 12-14.

Knafl, K. A., & Deatrick, J. A. (1987). Conceptualizing family response to a child's chronic illness or disability. *Family Relations, 36,* 300-304.

Knafl, K. A., & Deatrick, J. A. (1990). Family management style: Concept analysis and development. *Journal of Pediatric Nursing, 5,* 4-14.

Knafl, K. A., Pettengill, M. M., Bevis, M. E., & Kirchhoff, K. T. (1988). Blending qualitative and quantitative approaches to instrument development and data collection. *Journal of Professional Nursing, 4*(1), 30-37.

Laudan, L. (1977). *Progress and its problems.* Berkeley: University of California Press.

Lunney, M. (1990). Accuracy of nursing diagnoses: Concept development. *Nursing Diagnosis, 1*(1), 12-17.

Morse, J. M. (1991). *Qualitative nursing research: A contemporary dialogue* (rev. ed.). Newbury Park, CA: Sage.

Rodgers, B. L. (1989a). Concepts, analysis, and the development of nursing knowledge: The evolutionary cycle. *Journal of Advanced Nursing, 14,* 330-335.

Rodgers, B. L. (1989b). Exploring health policy as a concept. *Western Journal of Nursing Research, 11,* 694-702.

Rodgers, B. L. (1993). Concept analysis: An evolutionary view. In B. L. Rodgers & K. A. Knafl (Eds.), *Concept development in nursing: Foundations, techniques, and applications* (pp. 73-92). Philadelphia: W. B. Saunders.

Tadd, W., & Chadwick, R. (1989). Philosophical analysis and its value to the nurse teacher. *Nurse Education Today, 9,* 155-160.

Westra, B. L., & Rodgers, B. L. (1991). The concept of integration: A foundation for evaluating outcomes of nursing care. *Journal of Professional Nursing, 7,* 277-282.

Wilson, J. (1963). *Thinking with concepts.* London: Cambridge University Press.

Bibliography

This bibliography represents a comprehensive and broad cross section of literature with relevance to concept development in nursing. The literature listed in this bibliography is drawn from a wide range of disciplines and reflects a variety of viewpoints and applications of concept development. Items listed were selected primarily for their contribution to understanding the notion of *concepts* in general and for presenting diverse approaches to concept development. For ease of use, this bibliography is divided into two sections. The first includes items that address philosophical viewpoints associated with concept development, along with theoretical and methodological approaches. Methodology and methods are not included in a separate section due to the fact that these cannot be separated from philosophical viewpoints. The later section includes citations that reflect primarily the results of inquiry regarding specific concepts. For multilingual readers, non-English publications are included as well (many of these publications include abstracts written in English).

Philosophy, Theory, and Methodology of Concept Development

Abell, L. D. (1993). The effects of field dependence, past achievement, and instructional design on concept acquisition among college students. (Doctoral Dissertation, Memphis State University). *Dissertation Abstracts International, 53*:9, 3089A–90A DAI No.: DA9239604.

Adam, E. (1985). Toward more clarity in terminology: Frameworks, theories and models. *Journal of Nursing Education, 24*, 151–155.

Adams, E. W., & Adams, W. Y. (1987). Purpose and scientific concept formation. *The British Journal for the Philosophy of Science, 38*, 419–440.

Ahn, W. K., & Medin, D. L. (1992). A two-stage model of category construction. *Cognitive Science, 16*(1), 81–121.

Alston, W. P. (1963). Meaning and use. *Philosophical Quarterly, 13*, 107–124.

Andersson, T. (1995). Toward a dialectic theory of concepts. *Journal of Psycholinguistic Research, 24*, 377–404.

Anisfeld, M. (1968). Disjunctive concepts. *Journal of General Psychology, 78*, 223–228.

Anker, S. (1996). Models, metaphors, and matter: Artists and scientists visualize scientific concepts. *Art Journal, 55*, 33–43.

Aristotle. (1908). *The organon, or logical treatises with the introduction of porphyry* (O. F. Owen, Trans.). London: G. Bell.

Aristotle. (1947). Analytica Posterioria [Posterior analytics]. In R. McKeon (Ed.), *Introduction to Aristotle* (pp. 9–109). New York: Random House.

Aristotle. (1947). De Anima [On the Soul]. In R. McKeon (Ed.), *Introduction to Aristotle* (pp. 145–235). New York: Random House.

Aristotle. (1947). Metaphysica [Metaphysics]. In R. McKeon (Ed.), *Introduction to Aristotle* (pp. 243–296). New York: Random House.

Aristotle. (1984). Categories. In J. Barnes (Ed.), *The complete works of Aristotle* (pp. 3–24). Princeton: Princeton University Press.

Armstrong, S. L., Gleitman, L. R., & Gleitman, H. (1983). What some concepts might not be. *Cognition, 13*, 263–308.

Artinian, B. (1982). Conceptual mapping: Development of the strategy. *Western Journal of Nursing Research, 4*, 379–393.

Avant, K. C. (1991). Paths to concept development in nursing diagnosis. *Nursing Diagnosis, 2*(3), 105–110.

Ayer, A. J. (Ed.). (1959). *Logical positivism*. Glencoe, IL: Free Press.

Baker, W. J., Prideaux, G. D., & Derwing, B. L. (1980). Grammatical properties of sentences as a basis for concept formation. In G. D. Prideaux, B. L. Derwing, & W. J. Baker (Eds.), *Experimental linguistics: Integration of theories and applications* (pp. 121–140). Ghent: Story-Scientia.

Balog, J. E. (1988). The concept of health and techniques of conceptual analysis. *Health Education, 19*(4), 54–56.

Barrett, C. (1963). Concepts and concept formation. *Proceedings of the Aristotelian Society, 63*, 127–144.

Barrett, J. L., & Keil, F. C. (1996). Conceptualizing a nonnatural entity: Anthropomorphism in God concepts. *Cognitive Psychology, 31*, 219–247.

Barsalou, L. W., & Medin, D. L. (1986). Concepts: Static definitions or context-dependent representations? *Cahiers de Psychologie Cognitive, 6*, 187–202.

Bartsch, R. (1985). Concept formation, truth, and norm. In G. Hoppenbrouwers, P. Seuren, & A. J. M. M. Weijters (Eds.), *Meaning and the lexicon* (pp. 417–424). Dordrecht: Foris.

Becker, C. H. (1983). A conceptualization of concept. *Nursing Papers, 15*(2), 51–58.

Beller, M. (1990). Born's probabilistic interpretation: A case study of 'concepts in flux.' *Studies in History and Philosophy of Science, 21*, 563–588.

Benedek, T. G. (1997). William Osler and development of the concept of systemic lupus erythematosus. *Seminars in Arthritis and Rheumatism, 27*(1), 48–56.

Benoliel, J. Q. (1977). Conceptual precision and research about human dying. *Communicating Nursing Research, 9*, 237–243.

Beran, L., & Bernard, O. (1996). [Formal concept analysis]. *Casopis Lekaru Leskych, 135*, 507–509.

Berthold, J. S. (1964). Theoretical and empirical clarification of concepts. *Nursing Science, 2*, 406–422.

Billman, D., & Knutson, J. (1996). Unsupervised concept learning and value systematicity: A complex whole aids learning the parts. *Journal of Experimental Psychology: Learning, Memory, and Cognition, 22*, 458–475.

Bland, H. B. (1968). Health instruction and the concept approach. *Journal of School Health, 38*(1), 50-53.

Bloch, D. (1974). Some crucial terms in nursing: What do they really mean? *Nursing Outlook, 22*, 689-694.

Bloom, P. (1996). Intention, history, and artifact concepts. *Cognition, 60*(1), 1-29.

Bolton, N. (1977). *Concept formation.* New York: Pergamon.

Brennan, S. E., & Clark, H. H. (1996). Conceptual pacts and lexical choice in conversation. *Journal of Experimental Psychology: Learning, Memory, and Cognition, 22*, 1482-1493.

Brent, S. B., Speece, M. W., Lin, C., Dong, Q., et al. (1996). The development of the concept of death among Chinese and U.S. children 3-17 years of age: from binary to "fuzzy" concepts? *Omega: Journal of Death and Dying, 33*(1), 67-83.

Bridgman, P. W. (1951). The nature of some of our physical concepts, part I. *British Journal for the Philosophy of Science, 1*, 257-272.

Bridgman, P. W. (1951). The nature of some of our physical concepts, part II. *British Journal for the Philosophy of Science, 2*, 25-44.

Bridgman, P. W. (1951). The nature of some of our physical concepts, part III. *British Journal for the Philosophy of Science, 2*, 142-160.

Brooks, J. A., & Kleine-Kracht, A. E. (1983). Evolution of a definition of nursing. *Advances in Nursing Science, 5*(4), 51-63.

Brown, H. I. (1991). Epistemic concepts: A naturalistic approach. *Inquiry, 34*, 323-351.

Busemeyer, J., & McDaniel, M. A. (1997). The abstraction of intervening concepts from experience with multiple input-multiple output causal environments. *Cognitive Psychology, 32*(1), 1-48.

Cabrera, A., & Billman, D. (1996). Language-driven concept learning: Deciphering Jabberwocky. *Journal of Experimental Psychology: Learning, Memory, and Cognition, 22*, 539-555.

Capers, C. F. (1986). Some basic facts about models, nursing conceptualizations, and nursing theories. *Journal of Continuing Education in Nursing, 16*(5), 149-154.

Carnap, R. (1956). *Meaning and necessity.* Chicago: University of Chicago Press.

Chinn, P. L., & Jacobs, M. K. (1987). *Theory and nursing: A systematic approach.* St. Louis: Mosby.

Chinn, P. L., & Kramer, M. (1991). *Theory and nursing: A systematic approach* (3rd ed.). St. Louis: Mosby.

Cobern, W. W. (1996). Worldview theory and conceptual change in science education. *Science Education, 80*(5), 579-610.

Dickoff, J., James, P., & Semradek, J. (1975). Research. Part 1: a stance for nursing research—tenacity or inquiry. *Nursing Research, 24*(2), 84-88.

Diers, D. (1979). *Research in nursing practice.* Philadelphia: J. B. Lippincott.

Diers, D. (1991). On academic exercises . . . *Image: Journal of Nursing Scholarship, 23*, 70.

Dubin, R. (1969). *Theory building.* New York: Free Press.

Duldt, B. W., & Giffin, K. (1985). *Theoretical perspectives for nursing.* Boston: Little, Brown & Co.

Edel, A. (1979). *Analyzing concepts in social science.* New Brunswick, NJ: Transaction Books.

Edel, A. (1982). *Aristotle and his philosophy.* Chapel Hill, NC: University of North Carolina Press.

Edwards, S. D. (1997). What is philosophy of nursing? *Journal of Advanced Nursing, 25,* 1089-1093.

Ellis, R. (1968). Symposium on theory development in nursing. Characteristics of significant theories. *Nursing Research, 17,* 217-222.

Endacott, R. (1997). Clarifying the concept of need: A comparison of two approaches to concept analysis. *Journal of Advanced Nursing, 25,* 471-476.

Engelmann, S. (1969). *Conceptual learning.* Belmont, CA: Dimensions.

Falk, J. H. (1997). Testing a museum exhibition design assumption: Effect of explicit labeling of exhibit clusters on visitor concept development. *Science Education, 81,* 679-687.

Fareed, A. (1994). A philosophical analysis of the concept of reassurance and its effect on coping. *Journal of Advanced Nursing, 20,* 870-873.

Fawcett, J. (1978). The 'what' of theory development, *Theory development: What, why and how?* (Vol. No. 15-1708, pp. 17-33). New York: National League for Nursing.

Fawcett, J. (1989). *Analysis and evaluation of conceptual models of nursing* (2nd ed.). Norwalk, CT: Appleton & Lange.

Febbraro, A., & Chrisjohn, R. (1994). A Wittgensteinian approach to the meaning of conflict. In A. Taylor & J. B. Miller (Eds.), *Conflict and gender* (pp. 237-258). Cresskill, NJ: Hampton.

Fehr, B. (1988). Prototype analysis of the concepts of love and commitment. *Journal of Personality and Social Psychology, 55,* 557-579.

Fennell, B. A., & Bennett, J. (1991). Sociolinguistic concepts and literary analysis. *American Speech, 66,* 371-406.

Fleck, L. (Ed.). (1935). *Genesis and development of a scientific fact.* Chicago: University of Chicago Press.

Flew, A. (Ed.). (1960). *Essays in conceptual analysis.* London: Macmillan.

Fodor, J., & Lepore, E. (1996). The red herring and the pet fish: Why concepts still can't be prototypes. *Cognition, 58,* 253-270.

Frege, G. (1952). Function and concept. In P. Geach & M. Black (Eds.), *Translations from the philosophical writings of Gottlob Frege* (pp. 21-41). Oxford: Basil Blackwell.

Frege, G. (1952). Grundgesetze der Arithmetik. In P. Geach & M. Black (Eds.), *Translations from the philosophical writings of Gottlob Frege* (reprint edition, 1970 ed., pp. 159-181). Oxford: Basil Blackwell.

Frege, G. (1952). On concept and object. In P. Geach & M. Black (Eds.), *Translations from the philosophical writings of Gottlob Frege* (pp. 42-55). Oxford: Basil Blackwell.

Frege, G. (1953). *Foundations of arithmetic: A logico-mathematical enquiry into the concept of number* (J. L. Austin, Trans.) (2nd ed.). New York: Philosophical Library.

Frisch, N. (1997). Editorial: What's in a Name? *Nursing Diagnosis, 8*(1), 3.

Frydman, O. (1995). Knowledge about number and knowledge about knowledge: The insides and outsides of our windows. *Cahiers de Psychologie Cognitive [Current Psychology of Cognition], 14,* 764-774.

Gasking, D. (1960). Clusters. *Australian Journal of Philosophy, 38,* 1-36.

Geach, P., & Black, M. (Eds.). (1970). *Translations from the philosophical writings of Gottlob Frege.* Oxford: Basil Blackwell.

Gelman, S. A., & Medin, D. L. (1993). What's so essential about essentialism? A different perspective on the interaction of perception, language, and conceptual knowledge. *Cognitive Development, 8,* 157-167.

Gibbs, J. P. (1972). *Sociological theory construction.* Hinsdale, IL: Dryden.

Gillett, G. R. (1987). Concepts, structures, and meanings. *Inquiry, 30,* 101-112.

Gleitman, L. R., Gleitman, H., Miller, C., & Ostrin, R. (1996). Similar, and similar concepts. *Cognition, 58,* 321-376.

Goldstone, R. L., & Medin, D. L. (1994). Time course of comparison. *Journal of Experimental Psychology: Learning, Memory, and Cognition, 20*(1), 29-50.

Goldstone, R. L., Medin, D. L., & Gentner, D. (1991). Relational similarity and the nonindependence of features in similarity judgments. *Cognitive Psychology, 23,* 222-262.

Goodglass, H., Wingfield, A., & Ward, S. E. (1997). Judgments of concept similarity by normal and aphasic subjects: Relation to naming and comprehension. *Brain and Language, 56*(1), 138-158.

Goodman, N. (1972). Seven strictures on similarity. In N. Goodman (Ed.), *Problems and projects* (pp. 437-447). New York: Bobbs-Merrill.

Goosen, G. M. (1989). Concept analysis: An approach to teaching physiologic variables. *Journal of Professional Nursing, 5*(1), 31-38.

Gordon, M. (1990). Toward theory-based diagnostic categories. *Nursing Diagnosis, 1*(1), 5-11.

Grene, M. (1963). *A portrait of Aristotle.* Chicago: University of Chicago Press.

Griffin, A. P. (1983). A philosophical analysis of caring in nursing. *Journal of Advanced Nursing, 8,* 289-295.

Haase, J. E., Britt, T., Coward, D. D., Leidy, N. K., & Penn, P. E. (1992). Simultaneous concept analysis of spiritual perspective, hope, acceptance and self-transcendence. *Image: Journal of Nursing Scholarship, 24,* 141-147.

Hacking, I. (1985). Rules, scepticism, proof, Wittgenstein. In I. Hacking (Ed.), *Exercises in analysis: Essays by students of Casimir Lewy* (pp. 113-124). Cambridge: Cambridge University Press.

Hadzikadic, M., Hakenewerth, A., Bohren, B., Norton, J., Mehta, B., & Andrews, C. (1996). Concept formation vs. logistic regression: Predicting death in trauma patients. *Artificial Intelligence in Medicine, 8,* 493-504.

Haig, K. (1956). Frege on concepts. *Theoria, 22,* 85-100.

Hall, R. (1961). Conceptual reform—One task of philosophy. *Proceedings of the Aristotelian Society, 61,* 169-188.

Hallett, G. (1967). *Wittgenstein's definition of meaning as use.* New York: Fordham University Press.

Halliday, M. (1997). Two disquisitions on 'concepts.' *The North American Review, 282,* 50-51.

Hamlyn, D. W. (1983). *The theory of knowledge.* London: Macmillan.

Hardy, M. E. (1973). *Theoretical foundations for nursing.* New York: MSS

Hardy, M. E. (1974). Theories: Components, development, evaluation. *Nursing Research, 23,* 100-107.

Harris, H. W., & Schaffner, K. F. (1992). Molecular genetics, reductionism, and disease concepts in psychiatry. *Journal of Medicine and Philosophy, 17,* 127-153.

Harrison, O. A., & Hoffmeister, J. K. (1977). A statistical method for development of subconcepts in nursing. *Nursing Research, 26,* 448-451.

Hartnack, J. (1965). *Wittgenstein and modern philosophy* (Maurice Cranston, Trans.). New York: New York University Press.

Hempel, C. G. (1952). *Fundamentals of concept formation in empirical science.* Chicago: University of Chicago Press.

Hempel, C. G. (1959). The empiricist criterion of meaning. In A. J. Ayer (Ed.), *Logical positivism* (pp. 108-129). Glencoe, IL: Free Press.

Herradura, E. S. (1973). Concept development in nursing process. *Philippines Journal of Nursing, 42,* 230-234.

Higgs, J., & Titchen, A. (1995). The nature, generation and verification of knowledge. *Physiotherapy, 81,* 521-530.

Hinds, P. S. (1984). Inducing a definition of hope through the use of grounded theory methodology. *Journal of Advanced Nursing, 9,* 357-362.

Holsinger, K. E. (1987). Pluralism and species concepts, or when must we agree with one another? *Philosophy of Science, 54,* 480-485.

Holzman, M. (1981). Where is under: From memories of instances to abstract featural concepts. *Journal of Psycholinguistic Research, 10,* 421-439.

Hume, D. (1955). *An inquiry concerning human understanding.* New York: Liberal Arts Press. (Original work published 1748)

Hupcey, J. E., Morse, J. M., Lenz, E. R., & Tason, M. C. (1996). Wilsonian methods of concept analysis: A critique. *Scholarly Inquiry for Nursing Practice, 10,* 185-210.

Ibemesi, F. N. (1988). Alias Okeome-Ochilozua: An analysis of the concept of assumed names in Igbo society. *Africana-Marburgensia, 21*(1), 18-35.

Jacox, A. (1974). Theory construction in nursing: An overview. *Nursing Research, 23,* 4-13.

Jaeger, J. J. (1986). Concept formation as a tool for linguistic research. In J. J. Ohala & J. J. Jaeger (Eds.), *Experimental phonology* (pp. 211-237). London: Academic.

Jardine, M. (1996). Sight, sound, and epistemology: The experiential sources of ethical concepts. *Journal of the American Academy of Religion, 64,* 1-25.

Jecker, N. S., & Self, D. J. (1991). Separating care and cure: An analysis of historical and contemporary images of nursing and medicine. *Journal of Medicine and Philosophy, 16,* 285-306.

Johnson, J. S., Shenkman, K. D., Newport, E. L., & Medin, D. L. (1996). Indeterminacy in the grammar of adult language learners. *Journal of Memory and Language, 35,* 335-352.

Johnson, P., & Gott, R. (1996). Constructivism and evidence from children's ideas. *Science Education, 80,* 561-577.

Jones, P. S. (1985). Developing concepts and conceptual frameworks in nursing. *ANPhi Papers, 20*(1-2), 8-14.

Jong, W. R. d. (1995). Kant's analytic judgments and the traditional theory of concepts. *Journal of the History of Philosophy, 33,* 613-641.

Kant, I. (1965). *Critique of Pure Reason* (N. K. Smith, Trans.). New York: St. Martin's Press. (Original work published 1781)

Kaplan, A. (1964). *The conduct of inquiry* (2nd ed.). St. Louis: Mosby.

Keck, J. F. (1986). Terminology of theory development. In A. Marriner (Ed.), *Nursing theorists and their work* (pp. 15-23). St. Louis: Mosby.

Kemp, V. H. (1985). Concept analysis as a strategy for promoting critical thinking. *Journal of Nursing Education, 24,* 382-384.

Kenny, A. (1968). *Descartes: A study of his philosophy.* New York: Random House.

Kerlinger, F. N. (1973). *Foundations of behavioral research* (2nd ed.). New York: Holt, Rinehart & Winston.

Kerr, M. E., Hoskins, L. M., Fitzpatrick, J. J., Warren, J. J., Avant, K. C., Carpenito, L. J., Hurley, M. E., Jakob, D., Lunney, M., Mills, W. C., & Rottkamp, B. C. (1992). Development of definitions for Taxonomy II. *Nursing Diagnosis, 3*(2), 65-71.

Kikuchi, J. F. (1997). Clarifying the nature of conceptualizations about nursing. *Canadian Journal of Nursing Research, 29*(1), 97-110.

Kim, H. S. (1983). *The nature of theoretical thinking in nursing.* Norwalk, CT: Appleton-Century-Crofts.

King, I. M. (1975). A process of developing concepts for nursing through research. In P. Verhonick (Ed.), *Nursing Research I* (pp. 25-43). Boston: Little, Brown & Co.

King, I. M. (1988). Concepts: Essential elements of theories. *Nursing Science Quarterly, 1*, 22-25.

Klee, R. L. (1984). Micro-determinism and concepts of emergence. *Philosophy of Science, 51*, 44-63.

Kovecses, Z. (1994). Tocqueville's Passionate 'Beast': A linguistic analysis of the concept of American democracy. *Metaphor and Symbolic Activity, 9*, 113-133.

Kramer, M. K. (1993). Concept clarification and critical thinking: Integrated processes. *Journal of Nursing Education, 32*, 406-414.

Kripke, S. A. (1980). *Naming and necessity.* Oxford: Basil Blackwell.

Kristjanson, L. J. (1992). Conceptual issues related to measurement in family research. *Canadian Journal of Nursing Research, 24*(3), 37-51.

Laudan, L. (1977). *Progress and its problems.* Berkeley: University of California Press.

Leminen, A. (1975). [On concepts and how to define them (author's transl)]. *Sairaanhoidon Vuosikirja [The Yearbook of Nursing], 12*, 22-37.

Lenneberg, E. H. (1962). The relationship of language to the formation of concepts. *Synthese, 14*, 104-109.

Le-Ny, J. F. (1991). Coherence in semantic representations: Text comprehension and acquisition of concepts. In G. Denhiere & J.-P. Rossi (Eds.), *Text and text processing* (pp. 205-221). Amsterdam: North-Holland.

Locke, J. (1975). *An essay concerning human understanding.* Oxford: Oxford University Press. (Original work published 1690)

Longford, C. H. (1949). The nature of formal analysis. *Mind, 58*, 210-214.

Lowe, J. A. (1997). Scientific concept development in Solomon island students: A comparative analysis. *International Journal of Science Education, 19*, 743-759.

Lunney, M. (1990). Accuracy of nursing diagnoses: Concept development. *Nursing Diagnosis, 1*(1), 12-17.

Lycan, W. G. (1986). Two concepts of reduction: Modal realism at risk. *The Journal of Philosophy, 83*, 693-694.

MacGregor, J. N. (1987). Incremental category learning without external information: An algorithm for category-opening internal learning (COIL). *The British Journal of Psychology, 87*, 81-103.

Mackie, P. (1994). Sortal concepts and essential properties. *The Philosophical Quarterly, 44*, 311-333.

Madden, B. P. (1990). The hybrid model for concept development: Its value for the study of therapeutic alliance. *Advances in Nursing Science, 12*(3), 75-87.

Magnus, D. Theory, practice, and epistemology in the development of species concepts. *Studies in History and Philosophy of Science, 27*, 521-545.

Margolis, E. A. (1996). Concepts and the innate mind. (Doctoral dissertation, Rutgers University, 1995). *Dissertation Abstracts International, 57:2*, 715A. DAI No.: DA9618882.

Marks, L. E. (1996). On perceptual metaphors. *Metaphor and Symbolic Activity, 11*(1), 39-66.

Martin, M. G. F. (1992). Perception, concepts, and memory. *The Philosophical Review, 101*, 745-763.

Matravers, D. (1996). Aesthetic concepts and aesthetic experiences. *The British Journal of Aesthetics, 36*, 265-277.

McCloskey, M. E., & Glucksberg, S. (1978). Natural categories: Well defined or fuzzy sets? *Memory & Cognition, 6*, 462-472.

McDonald, J. L., & MacWhinney, B. (1991). Levels of learning: A comparison of concept formation and language acquisition. *Journal of Memory and Language, 30*, 407-430.

Medin, D. L. S., Edward, E. (1984). Concepts and concept formation. *Annual Review of Psychology, 35*, 113-138.

Medin, D. L. (1989). Concepts and conceptual structure. *American Psychologist, 44*, 1469-1481.

Medin, D. L., Ahn, W. K., Bettger, J., Florian, J., et al. (1990). Safe takeoffs—soft landings. *Cognitive Science, 14*, 169-178.

Medin, D. L., & Bettger, J. G. (1991). Sensitivity to changes in base-rate information. *American Journal of Psychology, 104*, 311-332.

Medin, D. L., & Bettger, J. G. (1994). Presentation order and recognition of categorically related examples. *Psychonomic Bulletin and Review, 1*, 250-254.

Medin, D. L., Goldstone, R. L., & Gentner, D. (1993). Respects for similarity. *Psychological Review, 100*, 254-278.

Medin, D. L., Goldstone, R. L., & Markman, A. B. (1995). Comparison and choice: Relations between similarity processes and decision processes. *Psychonomic Bulletin and Review, 2*, 1-19.

Medin, D. L., Lynch, E. B., Coley, J. D., & Atran, S. (1997). Categorization and reasoning among tree experts: Do all roads lead to Rome? *Cognitive Psychology, 32*, 49-96.

Medin, D. L., & Schaffer, M. M. (1978). Context theory of classification learning. *Psychological Review, 85*, 207-238.

Meleis, A. I. (1985). *Theoretical nursing*. Philadelphia: J. B. Lippincott.

Meleis, A. I. (1997). *Theoretical Nursing* (3rd ed.). Philadelphia: J. B. Lippincott.

Mendelsohn, R. L. (1981). Frege on predication. In P. A. French, J. T. E. Uehling, & H. K. Wettstein (Eds.), *Midwest Studies in Philosophy* (Vol. 6, pp. 69-80). Minneapolis: University of Minnesota Press.

Meyer, I., & Mackintosh, K. (1996). Refining the terminographer's concept-analysis methods: How can phraseology help? *Terminology: International Journal of Theoretical and Applied Issues in Specialized Communication, 3*(1), 1-26.

Michael, E., & Michael, F. S. (1989). Two early modern concepts of mind: Reflecting substance vs. thinking substance. *Journal of the History of Philosophy, 27*, 29-48.

Millar, A. (1991). Concepts, experience and inference. *Mind, 100*, 495-505.

Millar, A. (1994). Possessing concepts. *Mind, 103*, 72-82.

Mizuno, H. (1973). [Medicine and civilization. 8. Changes in concept formation in the modern society]. *Kangogaku Zasshi [Japanese Journal of Nursing], 37*, 1060-1064.

Montare, A. (1994). Knowledge acquired from learning: New evidence of hierarchical conceptualization. *Perceptual and Motor Skills, 79*, 975-993.

Mordacci, R. (1995). Health as an analogical concept. *Journal of Medicine and Philosophy, 20*, 475-497.

Morse, J. M. (1995). Exploring the theoretical basis of nursing using advanced techniques of concept analysis. *Advances in Nursing Science, 17*(3), 31-46.

Morse, J. M., Hupcey, J. E., Mitcham, C., & Lenz, E. R. (1996). Concept analysis in nursing research: A critical appraisal. *Scholarly Inquiry for Nursing Practice, 10*, 253-277.

Morse, J. M., Mitcham, C., Hupcey, J. E., & Tason, M. C. (1996). Criteria for concept evaluation. *Journal of Advanced Nursing, 24*, 385-390.

Mundle, C. W. K. (1963). Mental concepts. *Mind, 72*, 577-580.

Murphy, G., & Ross, B. H. (1994). Predictions from uncertain categorizations. *Cognitive Psychology, 27*, 148-193.

Murphy, G. L., & Allopenna, P. D. (1994). The locus of knowledge effects in concept learning. *Journal of Experimental Psychology: Learning, Memory and Cognition, 20*, 904-919.

Nersessian, N. J. (1984). The creation of scientific concepts. *Studies in History and Philosophy of Science, 15*, 175-212.

Newby, T. J., Ertmer, P. A., & Stepich, D. A. (1995). Instructional analogies and the learning of concepts. *Educational Technology Research and Development, 43*(1), 5-18.

Nieuwhof, H. (1994). Arguments and concepts. *Journal of Linguistics, 30*, 253-267.

Norris, C. M. (1982). *Concept clarification in nursing*. Rockville, MD: Aspen.

Nursing Development Conference Group. (1973). *Concept formalization in nursing: Process and Product*. Boston: Little, Brown & Co.

Nussbaum, C. (1990). Concepts, judgments, and unity in Kant's metaphysical deduction of the relational categories. *Journal of the History of Philosophy, 28*, 89-103.

Osherson, D. N., & Smith, E. E. (1981). On the adequacy of prototype theory as a theory of concepts. *Cognition, 9*, 35-38.

Oshima, H. H. (1983). A metaphorical analysis of the concept of mind in the Chuang-tzu. In V. H. Mair (Ed.), *Experimental essays on Chuang-tzu* (pp. 63-84). Honolulu: University of Hawaii Center for Asian & Pacific Studies.

Outhwaite, W. (1982). *Concept formation in social science*. London: Routledge and Kegan Paul.

Paley, J. (1996). How not to clarify concepts in nursing. *Journal of Advanced Nursing, 24*, 572-578.

Papanoustsos, E. P. (1962). Concepts in transformation. *The Philosophical Quarterly, 12*, 329-336.

Parse, R. R. (1987). *Nursing science: Major paradigms, theories, and critiques*. Philadelphia: W. B. Saunders.

Parse, R. R. (1997). Concept inventing: Unitary creations [editorial]. *Nursing Science Quarterly, 10*, 63-64.

Peacocke, C. (1991). The metaphysics of concepts. *Mind, 100*, 525-545.

Peacocke, C. (1992). A study of concepts. Cambridge, MA: The MIT Press.

Philipse, H. (1994). Peacocke on concepts. *Inquiry (Oslo, Norway), 37*, 225-252.

Phillips, P. (1993). A deconstruction of caring. *Journal of Advanced Nursing, 18*, 1554-1558.

Pollock, M. B. (1971). Speaking of concepts. *Journal of School Health, 41*, 283-286.

Price, H. H. (1953). *Thinking and experience.* London: Hutchinson House.

Prudovsky, G. (1997). Can we ascribe to past thinkers concepts they had no linguistic means to express? *History and Theory, 36*(1), 15-31.

Putnam, H. (1957). Psychological concepts, explication, and ordinary language. *Journal of Philosophy, 54*, 94-100.

Putnam, H. (1975). *Mind, language, and reality: Philosophical papers.* (Vol. 2). Cambridge: Cambridge University Press.

Quine, W. V. (1960). *Word and object.* Cambridge, MA: MIT Press.

Randall, J. H. (1960). *Aristotle.* New York: Columbia University Press.

Reckling, J. B. (1994). Conceptual analysis of rights using a philosophic inquiry approach. *Image: Journal of Nursing Scholarship, 26*, 309-314.

Reed, C. L., & Vinson, N. G. (1996). Conceptual effects on representational momentum. *Journal of Experimental Psychology: Human Perception and Performance, 22*, 839-850.

Reynolds, P. D. (1971). *A primer in theory construction.* New York: Bobbs-Merrill.

Reynolds, S., Martin, K., & Groulx, J. (1995). Patterns of understanding. *Educational Assessment, 3*, 363-371.

Richardson, K. (1987). The coding of relations versus the coding of independent cues in concept formation. *The British Journal of Psychology, 78*, 519-544.

Richman, R. J. (1965). Concepts without criteria. *Theoria, 31*, 65-85.

Rickert, H. (1986). *The limits of concept formation in natural science*: A logical introduction to the historical sciences (G. Oakes, Ed. & Trans.). Cambridge: Cambridge University Press.

Rodgers, B. L. (1989). The use and application of concepts in nursing: The case of health policy. (Doctoral dissertation, University Of Virginia, 1987). *Dissertation Abstracts International, B 49/11*, 4756. (AAC#8903985)

Rodgers, B. L. (1989). Concepts, analysis and the development of nursing knowledge: The evolutionary cycle. *Journal of Advanced Nursing, 14*, 330-335.

Rodgers, B. L. (1991). Using concept analysis to enhance clinical practice and research. *DCCN: Dimensions of Critical Care Nursing, 10*(1), 28-34.

Rodgers, B. L., & Knafl, K. A. (Eds.). (1993). *Concept development in nursing: Foundations, techniques, and applications.* Philadelphia: W. B. Saunders.

Rorty, R. (1961). Pragmatism, categories and language. *Philosophical Review, 70*, 197-223.

Rorty, R. (1979). *Philosophy and the mirror of nature.* Princeton: Princeton University Press.

Rosch, E. (1975). Cognitive representation of semantic categories. *Journal of Experimental Psychology, 104*, 192-233.

Rosch, E., & Mervis, C. B. (1975). Family resemblances: Studies in the internal structure of categories. *Cognitive Psychology, 7*, 573-605.

Russell, B. (1914). *Our knowledge of the external world*. Chicago: Open Court.

Ryle, G. (1949). *The concept of mind*. Chicago: University of Chicago Press.

Ryle, G. (1971). *Collected papers* (Vols. 1-2). London: Hutchinson House.

Sandelowski, M., Docherty, S., & Emden, C. (1997). Qualitative metasynthesis: Issues and techniques. *Research in Nursing and Health, 20*, 365-371.

Sartori, G. (1984). *Social science concepts: A systematic analysis*. Beverly Hills, CA: Sage.

Schlick, M. (1959). The turning point in philosophy. In A. J. Ayer (Ed.), *Logical positivism* (pp. 53-59). Glencoe, IL: Free Press.

Schrader, G. (1957). Kant's theory of concepts. *Kantstudien, 49*, 264-278.

Schroth, M. L. (1984). Disjunctive concept formation: S-R hypothesis versus cognitive theory. *The Journal of General Psychology, 110*, 87-92.

Schroth, M. L. (1997). The effects of different training conditions on transfer in concept formation. *The Journal of General Psychology, 124*, 157-165.

Schwartz-Barcott, D., & Kim, H. S. (1986). A hybrid model for concept development. In P. L. Chiinn (Ed.), *Nursing research methodology: Issues and implementation* (pp. 91-101). Rockville, MD: Aspen.

Sedivy, S. (1996). Must conceptually informed perceptual experience involve non-conceptual content? *Canadian Journal of Philosophy, 26*, 413-431.

Seigfried, C. H. (1990). The pragmatist sieve of concepts: Description versus interpretations. *The Journal of Philosophy, 87*, 585-592.

Shimamune, S., & Malott, R. W. (1994). An analysis of concept learning: Simple conceptual control and definition-based conceptual control. *Analysis of Verbal Behavior, 12*, 67-78.

Smith, E. E., & Medin, D. L. (1981). *Categories and concepts*. Cambridge, MA: Harvard University Press.

Sokal, R. R. (1974). Classification: Purposes, principles, progress, prospects. *Science, 185*, 1115-1123.

Sokolowski, R. L. (1987). Exorcising concepts. *The Review of Metaphysics, 40*, 451-463.

Soltis, J. (1978). *An introduction to the analysis of educational concepts*. Reading, MA: Addison-Wesley.

Sophian, C. (1995). The trouble with competence models. *Cahiers de Psychologie Cognitive [Current Psychology of Cognition], 14*, 753-759.

Spalding, T. L., & Murphy, G. L. (1996). Effects of background knowledge on category construction. *Journal of Experimental Psychology: Learning, Memory, and Cognition, 22*, 525-538.

Steimann, F. (1998). Dependency parsing for medical language and concept representation. *Artifial Intelligence in Medicine, 12*(1), 77-86.

Stevens, B. (1984). *Nursing theory: Analysis, application and evaluation* (2nd ed.). Boston: Little, Brown & Co.

Strawson, P. F. (1959). *Individuals: An essay in descriptive metaphysics*. London: Methuen & Co.

Sullivan, T. D. (1982). Concepts. *New Scholasticism, 56*, 146-168.

Summers, S. (1992). Validation of concepts: The next step in instrument development for postanesthesia studies. *Journal of Post Anesthesia Nursing, 7*, 346-351.

Tadd, W., & Chadwick, R. (1989). Philosophical analysis and its value to the nurse teacher. *Nurse Education Today, 9*, 155-160.

Torres, G., & Yura, H. (1975). The meaning and functions of concepts and theories within education and nursing. *NLN Publ*(15-1558), 1-8.

Toulmin, S. (1972). *Human Understanding*. Princeton, NJ: Princeton University Press.

Trandel-Korenchuck, D. M. (1986). Concept development in nursing research. *Nursing Administration Quarterly, 11*(1), 1–9.

Turner, C.W. (1995). Multiple representations of concept formation. (Doctoral dissertation, University of Florida, 1993). *Dissertation Abstracts International, B 55/7*, 3045. (DA9432041)

Vichot, R. J. (1988). John Dewey's theory of concept formation: An ideology of symbols. *Philosophy Today, 32*, 5–16.

Vincent, P. (1975). Some crucial terms in nursing—A second opinion. *Nursing Outlook, 23*(1), 46–48.

Walker, L. O., & Avant, K. C. (1983). *Strategies for theory construction in nursing*. Norwalk, CT: Appleton-Century-Crofts.

Walker, L. O., & Avant, K. C. (1988). *Strategies for theory construction in nursing* (2nd ed.). Norwalk, CT: Appleton & Lange.

Watson, J. (1979). *Nursing: The philosophy and science of caring*. Boston: Little, Brown, & Co.

Watson, J. (1985). *Nursing: Human science and human care*. Norwalk, CT: Appleton-Century-Crofts.

Wautier, G., & Westman, A. S. (1995). Relationships between learning styles and solutions based on analogies or background knowledge. *Psychological Reports, 77*, 1115–1120.

Weisberg, P., & Thiesfeldt, R. M. (1996). Teaching conceptual knowledge with multiple-related exemplars: Enhancement of concept formation, transfer, and absence of stimulus overselection. *Psychological Reports, 78*, 235–241.

Weitz, M. (1977). *The opening mind*. Chicago: University of Chicago Press.

Weitz, M. (1981). Ryle's theories of concepts. In T. E. U. P. A. French, Jr., H. K. Wettstein (Ed.), *Midwest Studies in Philosophy* (Vol. 6, pp. 321–334). Minneapolis: University of Minnesota Press.

Weitz, M. (1983). Descartes's theory of concepts. In T. E. U. P. A. French, Jr., & H. K. Wettstein (Ed.), *Midwest Studies in Philosophy* (Vol. 8, pp. 89–103). Minneapolis: University of Minnesota Press.

Whitley, G. G. (1995). Concept analysis as foundational to nursing diagnosis research. *Nursing Diagnosis, 6*, 91–92.

Wildes, K. W. (1993). Concepts, comparisons, and controversies. *The Journal of Medicine and Philosophy, 18*, 431–436.

Wilson, F. (1985). Dispositions defined: Harre and Madden on analyzing disposition concepts. *Philosophy of Science, 52*, 591–607.

Wilson, J. (1963). *Thinking with concepts*. London: Cambridge University Press.

Wilson, J. (1985). The inevitability of certain concepts (including education): A reply to Robin Barrow. *Educational Theory, 35*, 203–204.

Wisniewski, E. J., & Medin, D. L. (1994). On the interaction of theory and data in concept learning. *Cognitive Science, 18*, 221–281.

Wisniewski, E. J., Imai, M., & Casey, L. (1996). On the equivalence of superordinate concepts. *Cognition, 60*, 269–298.

Wittgenstein, L. (1968). *Philosophical investigations* (G. E. M. Anscombe, Trans.) (3rd ed.). New York: Macmillan.

Wittgenstein, L. (Ed.). (1979). *Notebooks: 1914–1916* (2nd ed.). Chicago: University of Chicago Press.

Wittgenstein, L. (1981). *Tractatus Logico-philosophicus* (D. F. Pears & B. F. McGuiness, Trans.). Great Britain: Whitstable Litho.

Woodfield, A. (1993). Do your concepts develop? *Philosophy, suppl 34*, 41-67.

Woodfield, A. (1994). Does concept-acquisition depend on language learning? *Pragmatics and Cognition, 2*, 307-325.

Woolhouse, R. S. (1971). *Locke's philosophy of science and knowledge*. Oxford: Basil Blackwell.

Wuest, J. (1994). A feminist approach to concept analysis. *Western Journal of Nursing Resarch, 16*, 577-586.

Wulfert, E. G., David, E., Dougher, M. J. (1994). Third-order equivalence classes. *The Psychological Record, 44*, 411-439.

Yolton, J. W. (1960). Concept analysis. *Kantstudien, 52*, 467-484.

Young, J. M. (1994). Synthesis and the content of pure concepts in Kant's first Critique. *Journal of the History of Philosophy, 32*, 331-357.

Zepp, R. A. (1986). Concept formation and verbalization. *Perceptual and Motor Skills, 62*, 370.

Zweiling, K. (1962). Language, thinking and reality. *Logique et Analyse, 5*, 287-290.

Inquiry Related to Specific Concepts

Ackoff, R. L. (1982). Our changing concept of planning. *Journal of Nursing Administration, 12*(10), 35-40.

Acton, G. J., Irvin, B. L., Jensen, B. A., Hopkins, B. A., & Miller, E. W. (1997). Explicating middle-range theory through methodological diversity. *Advances in Nursing Science, 19*(3), 78-85.

Agababa, P. (1992). [Proposition of a new concept: "sequence of communication"]. *Annales Medico Psychologiques, 150*, 355-357.

Agar, N. (1997). Biocentrism and the concept of life. *Ethics, 108*, 147-168.

Ailinger, R. L., & Causey, M. E. (1995). Health concept of older Hispanic immigrants. *Western Journal of Nursing Research, 17*, 605-613.

Ali, M. M. (1997). The concept of modernization: An analysis of contemporary Islamic thought. *The American Journal of Islamic Social Sciences, 14*(1), 13-26.

All, A. C., & Havens, R. L. (1997). Cognitive/concept mapping: A teaching strategy for nursing. *Journal of Advanced Nursing, 25*, 1210-1219.

Allan, H. T. (1993). Feminism: A concept analysis. *Journal of Advanced Nursing, 18*, 1547-1553.

Alligood, M. R. (1992). Empathy: The importance of recognizing two types. *Journal of Psychosocial Nursing and Mental Health Services, 30*(3), 14-17.

Allmark, P. (1995). Can there be an ethics of care? *Journal of Medical Ethics, 21*(1), 19-24.

Anderson, N. A. (1988). *Caregiving, gender and moral responsibility: A nursing conceptual analysis of women's care of the elderly infirm*. Unpublished doctoral dissertation, Adelphi University.

Anderson, S. C. (1994). A critical analysis of the concept of codependency. *Social Work, 39*, 677-685.

Andersson, E. P. (1995). Marginality: Concept or reality in nursing education? *Journal of Advanced Nursing, 21*, 131-136.

Appleton, J. V. (1994). The concept of vulnerability in relation to child protection: Health visitors' perceptions. *Journal of Advanced Nursing, 20*, 1132-1140.

Arakelian, M. (1980). An assessment and nursing application of the concept of locus of control. *Advances in Nursing Science, 3*(1), 25-42.

Asante, M. K. (1992). Afrocentric concepts in African historiography: A review essay. *Research in African Literatures, 23*, 191-195.

Ashmore, R., & Ramsamy, S. (1993). The concept of the "gaze" in mental health nursing. *Senior Nurse, 13*, 46-49.

Attree, M. (1993). An analysis of the concept "quality" as it relates to contemporary nursing care. *International Journal of Nursing Studies, 30*, 355-369.

Attree, M. (1996). Towards a conceptual model of "quality care." *International Journal of Nursing Studies, 33*(1), 13-28.

Atwood, R. K., & Atwood, V. A. (1996). Preservice elementary teachers' conceptions of the causes of seasons. *Journal of Research in Science Teaching, 33*, 553-563.

Aucoin-Gallant, G. (1996). [The learning needs of the cancer patient: A conceptual analysis]. *Canadian Oncology Nursing Journal, 6*(1), 14-17.

Avant, K. (1979). Nursing diagnosis: Maternal attachment. *Advances in Nursing Science, 2*(1), 45-55.

Baggs, J. G., & Schmitt, M. H. (1997). Nurses' and resident physicians' perceptions of the process of collaboration in an MICU. *Research in Nursing and Health, 20*, 71-80.

Baier, M., & Welch, M. (1992). An analysis of the concept of homesickness. *Archives of Psychiatric Nursing, 6*(1), 54-60.

Ballou, K. A. (1998). A concept analysis of autonomy. *Journal of Professional Nursing, 14*, 102-110.

Balog, J. E. (1988). The concept of health and techniques of conceptual analysis. *Health Education, 19*(4), 54-56.

Barnard, A. (1996). Technology and nursing: An anatomy of definition. *International Journal of Nursing Studies, 33*(4), 433-441.

Barnes, C. (1997). Creating our own heritage: Concepts of companies. *Dance Magazine, 71*(June), 56-61.

Barnum, B. S. (1995). Spirituality in nursing: Everything old is new again. *Nursing Leadership Forum, 1*(1), 24-30. [corrected, published erratum appears in *1*(2), 68]

Bartlett, B. J. (1994). A concept analysis of hopelessness. In R. M. Carroll-Johnson & M. Paquette (Eds.), *Classification of Nursing Diagnosis: Proceedings of the Tenth Conference* (p. 398). Philadelphia: J. B. Lippincott.

Battenfield, B. L. (1984). Suffering: A conceptual description and content analysis of an operational schema. *Image: Journal of Nursing Scholarship, 16*, 36-41.

Baziak, A. T. (1966). Concept-attainment in a practice setting. *Perspectives in Psychiatric Care, 4*(3), 32-44.

Beck, C. T. (1982). The conceptualization of power. *Advances in Nursing Science, 4*(2), 1-17.

Beck, C. T. (1996). A concept analysis of panic. *Archives of Psychiatric Nursing, 10*, 265-275.

Beck, P. (1975). [The health-disease concept]. *Zeitschrift Fur Krankenpflege. Revue Suisse Des Infirmieres, 68*(2), 45, 57.

Beck, P. (1975). [Health-illness concept: Health, illness and care personnel]. *Zeitschrift Fur Krankenpflege. Revue Suisse Des Infirmieres, 68*(4), 125-126.

Becker, C. H. (1983). A conceptualization of concept. *Nursing Papers, 15*(2), 51-58.

Beeber, L. S., & Schmitt, M. H. (1986). Cohesiveness in groups: A concept in search of a definition. *Advances in Nursing Science, 8*(2), 1-11.

Bennett, J. A. (1995). "Methodological notes on empathy": Further considerations. *Advances in Nursing Science, 18*(1), 36-50.

Benoliel, J. Q. (1972). The concept of care for a child with leukemia. *Nursing Forum, 11*(2), 194-204.

Benor, D. J. (1995). Spiritual healing: A unifying influence in complementary therapies. *Complementary Therapies in Medicine, 3*, 234-238.

Berterö, C., Eriksson, B. E., & Ek, A. C. (1997). A substantive theory of quality of life of adults with chronic leukaemia. *International Journal of Nursing Studies, 34*(1), 9-16.

Betz, C. L., & Poster, E. C. (1984). Children's concepts of death: Implications for pediatric practice. *Nursing Clinics of North America, 19*, 341-349.

Beyea, S. C. (1990). Concept analysis of feeling: A human response pattern. *Nursing Diagnosis, 1*(3), 97-101.

Black, P., McKenna, H., & Deeny, P. (1997). A concept analysis of the sensoristrain experienced by intensive care patients. *Intensive Critical Care Nursing, 13*, 209-215.

Bohlander, J. R. (1995). Differentiation of self: An examination of the concept. *Issues in Mental Health Nursing, 16*, 165-184.

Bond, A. E. (1996). Quality of life for critical care patients: A concept analysis. *American Journal of Critical Care, 5*, 309-313.

Boschma, G. (1994). The meaning of holism in nursing: Historical shifts in holistic nursing ideas. *Public Health Nursing, 11*, 324-330.

Bottomley, A., & Jones, L. (1997). Social support and the cancer patient—a need for clarity. *European Journal of Cancer Care (Engl), 6*(1), 72-77.

Bottorff, J. L., Gogag, M., & Engelberg Lotzkar, M. (1995). Comforting: Exploring the work of cancer nurses. *Journal of Advanced Nursing, 22*, 1077-1084.

Boulanger, J., & Goulet, C. (1994). Nursing parents' relationship with the newborn [French]. *Canadian Nurse, 90*(4), 44-48.

Bowles, N. (1995). A critical appraisal of preceptorship. *Nursing Standard, 9*(45), 25-28.

Boyd, C. (1985). Toward an understanding of mother-daughter identification using concept analysis. *Advances in Nursing Science, 7*(3), 78-86.

Boykin, A., & Schoenhofer, S. (1990). Caring in nursing: Analysis of extant theory. *Nursing Science Quarterly, 3*, 149-155.

Brabant, S., Forsyth, C. J., & McFarlain, G. (1994). Defining the family after the death of a child. *Death Studies, 18*, 197-206.

Bradley, S. F. (1996). Processes in the creation and diffusion of nursing knowledge: An examination of the developing concept of family-centred care. *Journal of Advanced Nursing, 23*, 722-727.

Brennan, M. (1997). A concept analysis of consent. *Journal of Advanced Nursing, 25*, 477-484.

Brent, S. B., Speece, M. W., Lin, C., Dong, Q., et al. (1996). The development of the concept of death among Chinese and U.S. children 3-17 years of age: from binary to "fuzzy" concepts? *Omega: Journal of Death and Dying, 33*(1), 67-83.

Bricker, P. L., & Fleischer, C. G. (1993). Social support as experienced by

Roman Catholic priests: The influence of vocationally imposed network restrictions. *Issues in Mental Health Nursing, 14*, 219-234.

Brooks, J. A., & Kleine-Kracht, A. E. (1983). Evolution of a definition of nursing. *Advances in Nursing Science, 5*(4), 51-63.

Browne, A. (1993). A conceptual clarification of respect. *Journal of Advanced Nursing, 18*, 211-217.

Browne, A. J. (1995). The meaning of respect: A First Nations perspective. *Canadian Journal of Nursing Research, 27*(4), 95-109.

Browne, A. J. (1997). A concept analysis of respect: Applying the Hybrid Model in cross-cultural settings. *Western Journal of Nursing Research, 19*(6), 762.

Brownell, M. J. (1984). The concept of crisis: Its utility for nursing. *Advances in Nursing Science, 6*(3), 10-21.

Brubaker, B. H. (1983). Health promotion: A linguistic analysis. *Advances in Nursing Science, 5*(3), 1-14.

Bruni, N. (1997). The nurse educator as teacher: Exploring the construction of the 'reluctant instructor.' *Nursing Inquiry, 4*(1), 34-40.

Buchanan, S., & Ross, E. K. (1995). A concept analysis of caring. *Perspectives, 19*(3), 3-6.

Buchmann, W. F. (1997). Adherence: A matter of self-efficacy and power. *Journal of Advanced Nursing, 26*, 132-137.

Burch, S. (1994). Consciousness: How does it relate to health? *Journal of Holistic Nursing, 12*(1), 101-116.

Burch, T. A. C. (1990). A definition of scholarship by doctorally prepared nurse faculty. (Doctoral dissertation, University Of Illinois at Chicago, Health Sciences Center, 1989). *Dissertation Abstracts International, B 51/01*, 142.

Burke, M. L., Hainsworth, M. A., Eakes, G. G., & Lindgren, C. L. (1992). Current knowledge and research on chronic sorrow: A foundation for inquiry. *Death Studies, 16*, 231-245.

Burkhardt, M. A. (1989). Spirituality: An analysis of the concept. *Holistic Nursing Practice, 3*(3), 69-77.

Burnside, I., & Haight, B. K. (1992). Reminiscence and life review: Analysing each concept. *Journal of Advanced Nursing, 17*, 855-862.

Burrows, D. E. (1997). Facilitation: A concept analysis. *Journal of Advanced Nursing, 25*, 396-404.

Byrd, M. E. (1995). A concept analysis of home visiting. *Public Health Nursing, 12*(2), 83-89.

Cahill, J. (1996). Patient participation: A concept analysis. *Journal of Advanced Nursing, 24*, 561-571.

Campbell, L. (1987). Hopelessness: A concept analysis. *Journal of Psychosocial Nursing and Mental Health Services, 25*(2), 18-22.

Carlson-Sabelli, L. (1987). Role reversal: A concept analysis and reinterpretation of the research literature. *Journal of Group Psychotherapy, Psychodrama & Sociometry, 41*(4), 139-152.

Carnes, B. A. (1984). Concept analysis: Dependence. *Critical Care Quarterly, 6*(4), 29-39.

Carnevali, D., & Brueckner, S. (1970). Immobilization—reassessment of a concept. *American Journal of Nursing, 70*, 1502-1507.

Caroline, H. A. (1993). Explorations of close friendship: A concept analysis. *Archives of Psychiatric Nursing, 7*, 236-243.

Carr, G. (1996). Themes relating to sexuality that emerged from a discourse analysis of the Nursing Times during 1980-1990. *Journal of Advanced Nursing, 24,* 196-212.

Carr, J. M., & Clarke, P. (1997). Development of the concept of family vigilance. *Western Journal of Nursing Research, 19*(6), 726-739.

Caspari, S. (1997). [Holism—more than a concept with which to cloak oneself]. *Tidskriftet Sykeplelen, 85*(20), 56-8.

Cassidy, V. R. (1996). Moral competency, *Annual Review of Nursing Research, 14,* 181-204.

Cella, D. F. (1992). Quality of life: The concept. *Journal of Palliative Care, 8*(3), 8-13.

Chadderton, H. (1995). An analysis of the concept of participation within the context of health care planning. *Journal of Nursing Management, 3,* 221-228.

Cheek, J., Gibson, T., & Heartfield, M. (1993). Holism, care and nursing: Points of reflection during the evolution of a philosophy of nursing statement. *Contemporary Nurse: A Journal for the Australian Nursing Profession, 2*(2), 68-72.

Chodil, J., & Williams, B. (1970). The concept of sensory deprivation. *Nursing Clinics of North America, 5,* 453-465.

Clawson, J. A. (1996). A child with chronic illness and the process of family adaptation. *Journal of Pediatric Nursing: Nursing Care of Children and Families, 11*(1), 52-61.

Clifford, C. (1996). Role: A concept explored in nursing education. *Journal of Continuing Education in Nursing, 27*(1), 17-27.

Cody, W. K. (1991). Multidimensionality: Its meaning and significance. *Nursing Science Quarterly, 4,* 140-141.

Coler, M. S. (1994). Achieving linguistic clarity: A model to aid translations. *Nursing Diagnosis, 5*(3), 102-105.

Coler, M. S. (1996). PERC: A nursing syndrome for AIDS. *Nursing Diagnosis, 7*(1), 19-23.

Cooley, M. E. (1998). Quality of life in persons with non-small cell lung cancer: A concept analysis. *Cancer Nursing, 21,* 151-161.

Coward, D. D. (1996). Self-transcendence and correlates in a healthy population. *Nursing Research, 45*(2), 116-121.

Cowles, K. V. (1984). Life, death, and personhood. *Nursing Outlook, 32,* 169-172.

Cowles, K. V. (1996). Cultural perspectives of grief: An expanded concept analysis. *Journal of Advanced Nursing, 23,* 287-294.

Cowles, K. V., & Rodgers, B. L. (1991). The concept of grief: A foundation for nursing practice and research. *Research in Nursing and Health, 14,* 119-127.

Coyne, I. T. (1996). Parent participation: A concept analysis. *Journal of Advanced Nursing, 23,* 733-740.

Crawford, G. (1982). The concept of patterns in nursing: Conceptual development and measurement. *Advances in Nursing Science, 5*(4), 1-6.

Crespo-Fierro, M. (1997). Compliance/adherence and care management in HIV disease. *Journal of the Association of Nurses AIDS Care, 8*(4), 43-54.

Cross, K. D. (1996). An analysis of the concept facilitation. *Nurse Education Today, 16,* 350-355.

Cupples, S. A. (1992). Pain as "hurtful experience": A philosophical analysis and implications for holistic nursing care. *Nursing Forum, 27*(1), 5-11.

Curley, M. A. (1997). Mutuality—an expression of nursing presence. *Journal of Pediatric Nursing, 12,* 208-213.

Cutcliffe, J. R. (1997). The nature of expert psychiatric nurse practice: A grounded theory study. *Journal of Clinical Nursing, 6,* 325-332.

Davies, S., Laker, S., & Ellis, L. (1997). Promoting autonomy and independence for older people within nursing practice: A literature review. *Journal of Advanced Nursing, 26,* 408-417.

Davis, G. C. (1992). The meaning of pain management: A concept analysis. *Advances in Nursing Science, 15*(1), 77-86.

de Carvalho, E. C., & Coler, M. S. (1995). Diagnoses of the human response pattern, communicating: A proposal for revision. *Nursing Diagnosis, 6,* 155-160.

de Jong-Gierveld, J. (1989). Personal relationships, social support, and loneliness. *Journal of Social and Personal Relationships, 6,* 197-221.

DeFeo, D. J. (1990). Change: A central concern of nursing. *Nursing Science Quarterly, 3,* 88-94.

Delisle, I. (1976). [The concept health; art of living of pediatric nurses]. *Infirmiere Canadienne, 18*(6), 19-21.

Diez Manrique, J. F., Garcia Barredo Perez, R., Garcia Usieto, E., Pena Martin, C., & Vazquez Barquero, J. L. (1993). [Bibliographic analysis of the concept "alcohol-related problems"]. *Actas Luso-Espanolas De Neurologia Psiquiatria Y Ciencias Afines, 21*(2), 44-50.

Dolfman, M. L. (1973). The concept of health: An historic and analytic examination. *Journal of School Health, 43,* 491-497.

Doona, M. E., Haggerty, L. A., & Chase, S. K. (1997). Nursing presence: An existential exploration of the concept. *Scholarly Inquiry for Nursing Practice, 11,* 3-16.

dos Santos, S. R., Barbosa, M. Z. U., & Coler, M. S. (1994). An analysis of the axial concept as proposed by the NANDA Taxonomy Committee related to community diagnoses of a rural community in northeastern Brazil. In R. M. Carroll-Johnson & M. Paquette (Eds.), *Classification of nursing diagnoses: Proceedings of the tenth conference* (pp. 375-376). Philadelphia: J. B. Lippincott.

Dougherty, C. (1997). Reconceptualization of the nursing diagnosis decreased cardiac output. *Nursing Diagnosis, 8*(1), 29-36.

Draper, P. (1992). Quality of life as quality of being: An alternative to the subject-object dichotomy. *Journal of Advanced Nursing, 17,* 965-970.

Drew, B. L. (1990). Differentiation of hopelessness, helplessness, and powerlessness using Erik Erikson's "Roots of virtue." *Archives of Psychiatric Nursing, 4,* 332-337.

Duffy, M. E. (1987). The concept of adaptation: Examining alternatives for the study of nursing phenomena. *Scholarly Inquiry for Nursing Practice, 1,* 179-192.

Duquette, A. M. (1997). Adaptation: A concept analysis. *Journal of School Nursing, 13*(3), 30-33.

Dyer, J. G., & McGuinness, T. M. (1996). Resilience: Analysis of the concept. *Archives of Psychiatric Nursing, 10,* 276-282.

Dyson, J., Cobb, M., & Forman, D. (1997). The meaning of spirituality: A literature review. *Journal of Advanced Nursing, 26,* 1183-1188.

Egan, M. P. (1997). Contracting for safety: A concept analysis. *Crisis, 18*(1), 17-23.

Elliott-Schmidt, R., & Strong, J. (1997). The concept of well-being in a rural setting: Understanding health and illness. *Australian Journal of Rural Health, 5*(2), 59-63.

Emblen, J. D. (1992). Religion and spirituality defined according to current use in nursing literature. *Journal of Professional Nursing, 8*(1), 41-47.

Endacott, R. (1997). Clarifying the concept of need: A comparison of two approaches to concept analysis. *Journal of Advanced Nursing, 25,* 471-476.

Ens, I. C. (1997). An analysis of the concept of countertransference. *Archives of Psychiatric Nursing, 12,* 273-281.

Eriksen, L. R. (1995). Patient satisfaction with nursing care: Concept clarification. *Journal of Nursing Measurement, 3*(1), 59-76.

Eriksson, K. (1993). Different forms of caring communion. *Nursing Science Quarterly, 5,* 93.

Estabrooks, C. A., & Morse, J. M. (1992). Toward a theory of touch: The touching process and acquiring a touching style. *Journal of Advanced Nursing, 17,* 448-456.

Evans, S. K. (1979). Descriptive criteria for the concept of depleted health potential. *Advances in Nursing Science, 1*(3), 67-74.

Fagermoen, M. S. (1997). Professional identity: Values embedded in meaningful nursing practice. *Journal of Advanced Nursing, 25,* 434-441.

Faller, N. A. (1993). (Non)compliance. *Ostomy/Wound Management, 39*(3), 35-38.

Fareed, A. (1994). A philosophical analysis of the concept of reassurance and its effect on coping. *Journal of Advanced Nursing, 20,* 870-873.

Faresjo, T., Svardsudd, K., & Tibblin, G. (1997). The concept of status incongruence revisited: A 22-year follow-up of mortality for middle-aged men. *Scandinavian Journal of Social Medicine, 25*(1), 28-32.

Fealy, G. M. (1995). Professional caring: The moral dimension. *Journal of Advanced Nursing, 22,* 1135-1140.

Fealy, G. M. (1997). The theory-practice relationship in nursing: An exploration of contemporary discourse. *Journal of Advanced Nursing, 25,* 1061-1069.

Febbraro, A., & Chrisjohn, R. (1994). A Wittgensteinian approach to the meaning of conflict. In A. Taylor & J. B. Miller (Eds.), *Conflict and gender* (pp. 237-258). Cresskill, NJ: Hampton.

Fedoryka, K. (1997). Health as a normative concept: Towards a new conceptual framework. *Journal of Medicine and Philosophy, 22,* 143-160.

Fehr, B. (1988). Prototype analysis of the concepts of love and commitment. *Journal of Personality and Social Psychology, 55,* 557-579.

Fehring, R. J., Miller, J. F., & Shaw, C. (1997). Spiritual well-being, religiosity, hope, depression, and other mood states in elderly people coping with cancer. *Oncology Nursing Forum, 24,* 663-671.

Felce, D. (1997). Defining and applying the concept of quality of life. *Journal of Intellectual Disability Research, 41*(Pt 2), 126-135.

Ferrans, C. E. (1992). Conceptualizations of quality of life in cardiovascular research. *Progress in Cardiovascular Nursing, 7*(2), 2-6.

Fetsch, S. H. (1991). *Advocacy in pediatric nursing: A qualitative study.* University of Kansas.

Field, E. R. (1960). Authority: A select power. *Advances in Nursing Science, 3*(1), 69-83.

Fife, B. L. (1994). The conceptualization of meaning in illness. *Social Science and Medicine, 38,* 309-316.

Finley, N. J., & Norman, R. L. (1997). The concept of social parallax. *Women and Language, 20*, 5-8.

Fitzgerald, M. H., & Mullavey, O. B. C. (1996). Analysis of student definitions of culture. *Physical and Occupational Therapy in Geriatrics, 14*(1), 67-89.

Fleming, V. E. M. (1998). Autonomous or automatons? An exploration through history of the concept of a autonomy in midwifery in Scotland and New Zealand. *Nursing Ethics, 5*, 43-51.

Forrest, S. (1993). Toward understanding the self. *Nursing Forum, 28*(2), 5-10.

Forsyth, G. L. (1980). Analysis of the concept of empathy: Illustration of one approach. *Advances in Nursing Science, 2*(2), 33-42.

Fowler, M. E. (1998). Recognizing the phenomenon of readiness: Concept analysis and case study. *The Journal of the Association of Nurses in AIDS, 9*(3), 72-76.

Fowler, S. B. (1995). Hope: Implications for neuroscience nursing. *Journal of Neuroscience Nursing, 27*, 298-304.

Fowler, S. B. (1997). Health promotion in chronically ill older adults. *Journal of Neuroscience Nursing, 29*(1), 39-43.

Frank, J. (1984). Interview with Jerome Frank, Ph.D., M.D. Exploring concepts of influence, persuasion, and healing. *Journal of Psychosocial Nursing and Mental Health Services, 22*(9), 32-34; 36-37.

Frederickson, K. (1993). Using a nursing model to manage symptoms: Anxiety and the Roy adaptation model. *Holistic Nursing Practice, 7*(2), 36-43.

Friedemann, M. L. (1989). The concept of family nursing. *Journal of Advanced Nursing, 14*, 211-216.

Fuller, J. G. (1991). *A conceptualization of presence as a nursing phenomenon.* Unpublished doctoral dissertation, University of Utah.

Fulton, G., Madden, C., & Minichiello, V. (1996). The social construction of anticipatory grief. *Social Science and Medicine, 43*, 1349-1358.

Galante, C. M. (1991). *Strategic management in nursing: A concept analysis.* Unpublished doctoral dissertation, George Mason University.

Gallagher, S. (1997). Surviving redesign: Basic concepts of patient-focused care and their application to WOC nursing. *Journal of Wound, Ostomy, and Continence Nursing, 24*, 132-136.

Gallop, R., McCay, E., & Esplen, M. J. (1992). The conceptualization of impulsivity for psychiatric nursing practice. *Archives of Psychiatric Nursing, 6*, 366-373.

Geissler, E. M. (1984). Crisis: What it is and is not. *Advances in Nursing Science, 6*(4), 1-9.

Gibson, C. H. (1991). A concept analysis of empowerment. *Journal of Advanced Nursing, 16*, 354-361.

Gibson, C. (1998). The concept of community: Implications for community care. *Nursing Standard, 12*(34), 40-43.

Giedt, J. F. (1997). Guided imagery: A psychoneuroimmunological intervention in holistic nursing practice. *Journal of Holistic Nursing, 15*, 112-127.

Gift, H. C., Atchison, K. A., & Dayton, C. M. (1997). Conceptualizing oral health and oral health-related quality of life. *Social Science and Medicine, 44*, 601-608.

Gilje, F. (1992). Being there: An analysis of the concept of presence. In D. A. Gaut (Ed.), *The presence of caring in nursing* (pp. 53-67). New York: National League for Nursing PUBL 1992 #15-2465.

Goddard, N. C. (1995). "Spirituality as integrative energy": A philosophical analysis as requisite precursor to holistic nursing practice. *Journal of Advanced Nursing, 22*, 808-815.

Golberg, B. (1998). Connection: An exploration of spirituality in nursing care. *Journal of Advanced Nursing, 27*, 836-842.

Goodwin, L. D. (1997). Changing conceptions of measurement validity. *Journal of Nursing Education, 36*, 102-107.

Graham, C. A., & Smith, M. M. (1984). Operationalizing the concept of sexuality comfort: Applications for sexuality educators. *Journal of School Health, 54*, 439-442.

Graham, I. W. (1992). Reconstructing nursing: A coronary care perspective of the primary nurse philosophy. *Intensive and Critical Care Nursing, 8*, 118-124.

Gravelle, A. M. (1997). Caring for a child with a progressive illness during the complex chronic phase: Parents' experience of facing adversity. *Journal of Advanced Nursing, 25*, 738-745.

Green, J. A. (1979). Science, nursing, and nursing science: A conceptual analysis. *Advances in Nursing Science, 2*(1), 57-64.

Green-Hernandez, C. (1997). Application of caring theory in primary care: A challenge for advanced practice. *Nursing Administration Quarterly, 21*(4), 77-82.

Gresham, M. L. (1976). The infantilization of the elderly: A developing concept. *Nursing Forum, 15*, 195-210.

Griffin, A. P. (1983). A philosophical analysis of caring in nursing. *Journal of Advanced Nursing, 8*, 289-295.

Gropper, E. I. (1992). Promoting health by promoting comfort. *Nursing Forum, 27*(2), 5-8.

Guice, E. D. (1992). *The effect of instruction in concept analysis on critical thinking skills and moral reasoning decisions of senior baccalaureate nursing students.* Unpublished doctoral dissertation, University of Alabama.

Gumbrecht, H. U. (1993). Everyday-world and life-world as philosophical concepts: A genealogical approach. *New Literary History, 24*, 745-761.

Haddock, J. (1996). Towards further clarification of the concept 'dignity.' *Journal of Advanced Nursing, 24*, 924-931.

Hagerty, B. M., Lynch Sauer, J., Patusky, K. L., Bouwsema, M., & Collier, P. (1992). Sense of belonging: A vital mental health concept. *Archives of Psychiatric Nursing, 6*, 172-177.

Haggman Laitila, A., & Pietila, A. M. (1993). [Life control, the core of being healthy. Theoretical-empirical definition of the concept "life control"]. *Hoitotiede, 5*(1), 2-10.

Hahn, A. F. (1997). Guillain-Barré syndrome: An evolving concept. *Current Opinions in Neurology, 10*, 363-365.

Hahn, R. A. (1997). The nocebo phenomenon: Concept, evidence, and implications for public health. *Preventive Medicine, 26*, 607-611.

Haight, B. K., & Warren, J. (1991). Apathy: Development of a nursing diagnosis. *Applied Nursing Research, 4*, 186-187.

Hakulinen, T., & Paunonen, M. (1994). [Analysis of the concept of family nursing. Family systems nursing and family-centered nursing as closely related concepts]. *Hoitotiede, 6*(2), 58-65.

Hall, J. M., Stevens, P. E., & Meleis, A. I. (1994). Marginalization: A guiding concept for valuing diversity in nursing knowledge development. *Advances in Nursing Science, 16*(4), 23-41.

Ham Ying, S. (1993). Analysis of the concept of holism within the context of nursing. *British Journal of Nursing, 2*, 771-775.

Hanchett, E. S. (1992). Concepts from Eastern philosophy and Rogers' science of unitary human beings. *Nursing Science Quarterly, 5*, 164-170.

Hawks, J. H. (1991). Power: A concept analysis. *Journal of Advanced Nursing, 16*, 754-762.

Hawks, J. H. (1992). Empowerment in nursing education: Concept analysis and application to philosophy, learning and instruction. *Journal of Advanced Nursing, 17*, 609-618.

Henderson, V. (1984). [My concept of nursing. A concept which varies according to culture]. *Soins (Paris)*(440), 35-40.

Hendricks-Ferguson, V. L. (1997). An analysis of the concept of hope in the adolescent with cancer. *Journal of Pediatric Oncology Nursing, 14*(2), 73-80.

Henneman, E. A., Lee, J. L., & Cohen, J. I. (1995). Collaboration: A concept analysis. *Journal of Advanced Nursing, 21*, 103-109.

Henry, C. (1987). Persons and humans. *Journal of Advanced Nursing, 12*, 754-762.

Henry, C., & Tuxill, A. C. (1987). Concept of the person: Introduction to the health professionals. *Journal of Advanced Nursing, 12*, 245-249.

Henson, R. H. (1997). Analysis of the concept of mutuality. *Image: Journal of Nursing Scholarship, 29*, 77-81.

Hertz, J. E. (1996). Conceptualization of perceived enactment of autonomy in the elderly. *Issues in Mental Health Nursing, 17*, 261-273.

Hewison, A. (1996). Organizational culture: A useful concept for nurse managers? *Journal of Nursing Management, 4*(1), 3-9.

Hinds, G., & Moyer, A. (1997). Support as experienced by patients with cancer during radiotherapy treatments. *Journal of Advanced Nursing, 26*, 371-379.

Hinds, P. S. (1984). Inducing a definition of hope through the use of grounded theory methodology. *Journal of Advanced Nursing, 9*, 357-362.

Hines, D. R. (1992). Presence: Discovering the artistry in relating. *Journal of Holistic Nursing, 10*(4), 294-305.

Hirter, J., & Van Nest, R. L. (1995). Vigilance: A concept and a reality. *CRNA: The Clinical Forum for Nurse Anesthetists, 6*(2), 96-98.

Hockenberry-Eaton, M., Manteuffel, B., & Bottomley, S. (1997). Development of two instruments examining stress and adjustment in children with cancer. *Journal of Pediatric Oncology Nursing, 14*, 178-185.

Hoffer, J. (1994). Concept analysis of communication in families. In R. M. Carroll-Johnson & M. Paquette (Eds.), *Classification of nursing diagnoses: Proceedings of the tenth conference* (p. 399). Philadelphia: J. B. Lippincott.

Hoffmann, G. S. (1969). The concept of love. *Nursing Clinics of North America, 4*, 663-672.

Holmes, C. A., & Warelow, P. J. (1997). Culture, needs and nursing: A critical theory approach. *Journal of Advanced Nursing, 25*, 463-470.

Hoover, D. (1995). Impaired personal boundaries: A proposed nursing diagnosis. *Perspectives in Psychiatric Care, 31*(3), 9-13.

Hoover, D., & Norris, J. (1996). Validation study for impaired personal boundaries, proposed nursing diagnosis. *Nursing Diagnosis, 7*, 147-151.

Horowitz, M., Sonneborn, D., & Sugahara, C. (1996). Self-regard: A new measure. *The American Journal of Psychiatry, 153*, 382-385.

Hupcey, J. E. (1998). Social support: Assessing conceptual coherence. *Qualitative Health Research, 8*, 304-318.

Hutchings, D. (1997). The hardiness of hospice nurses. *American Journal of Hospice and Palliative Care, 14*, 110-113.

Hutchison, P., & Nogradi, G. (1996). The concept and nature of community development in recreation and leisure. *Journal of Applied Recreation Research, 21*(2), 93-130.

Ikuenobe, P. (1997). The parochial universalist conception of 'philosophy' and 'African philosophy.' *Philosophy East and West, 47*, 189-210.

Irvine, R., & Graham, J. (1994). Deconstructing the concept of profession: A prerequisite to carving a niche in a changing world. *Australian Occupational Therapy Journal, 41*(1), 9-18.

Jackson, B. S. (1993). Hope and wound healing. *Journal of ET Nursing, 20*(2), 73-77.

Jacob, S. R. (1993). An analysis of the concept of grief. *Journal of Advanced Nursing, 18*, 1787-1794.

Jacobs, P. M., Ott, B., Sullivan, B., Ulrich, Y., & Short, L. (1997). An approach to defining and operationalizing critical thinking. *Journal of Nursing Education, 36*(1), 19-22.

Jansen, G., Dassen, T., & Moorer, P. (1997). The perception of aggression. *Scandinavian Journal of Caring Sciences, 11*(1), 51-55.

Janssen, H. J. E. M., Cuisinier, M. C. J., & Hoogduin, K. A. L. (1996). A critical review of the concept of pathological grief following pregnancy loss. *Omega: Journal of Death and Dying, 33*(1), 21-42.

Jasper, M. A. (1994). Expert: A discussion of the implications of the concept as used in nursing. *Journal of Advanced Nursing, 20*, 769-776.

Jassak, P. F., & Knafl, K. A. (1990). Quality of family life: Exploration of a concept. *Seminars in Oncology Nursing, 6*, 298-302.

Jenner, C. A. (1997). The art of nursing: A concept analysis. *Nursing Forum, 32*(4), 5-11.

Johns, J. L. (1996). A concept analysis of trust. *Journal of Advanced Nursing, 24*(1), 76-83.

Johnson, J. M. (1992). The tendency for temperament to be "temperamental": Conceptual and methodological considerations. *Journal of Pediatric Nursing: Nursing Care of Children and Families, 7*, 347-353.

Johnson, M. (1997). Observations on the neglected concept of intervention in nursing research. *Journal of Advanced Nursing, 25*, 23-29.

Johnson, R. N. (1996). Kant's conception of merit. *Pacific Philosophical Quarterly, 77*, 310-334.

Jones, J. A. (1983). Where angels fear to tread—nursing and the concept of creativity. *Journal of Advanced Nursing, 8*, 405-411.

Jones, R. A. (1997). Multidisciplinary collaboration: Conceptual development as a foundation for patient-focused care. *Holistic Nursing Practice, 11*(3), 8-16.

Kahn, D. L., & Steeves, R. H. (1986). The experience of suffering: Conceptual clarification and theoretical definition. *Journal of Advanced Nursing, 11*, 623-631.

Kahn, D. L., & Steeves, R. H. (1988). Caring and practice: Construction of the nurse's world. *Scholarly Inquiry for Nursing Practice, 2*, 201-216.

Kane, C. F. (1988). Family social support: Toward a conceptual model. *Advances in Nursing Science, 10*(2), 18-25.

Kaplan, L., Ade Ridder, L., Hennon, C. B., Brubaker, E., & Brubaker, T. (1995). Preliminary typology of couplehood for community-dwelling wives: "I" versus "we." *International Journal of Aging and Human Development, 40,* 317-337.

Keller, M. J. (1981). Toward a definition of health. *Advances in Nursing Science, 4,* 43-64.

Kelley, J. H., & Frisch, N. C. (1994). A transcultural concept analysis of social isolation. In R. M. Carroll-Johnson & M. Paquette (Eds.), *Classification of nursing diagnosis: proceedings of the tenth conference* (pp. 232-233). Philadelphia: J. B. Lippincott.

Kelly-Powell, M. L. (1997). Personalizing choices: Patients' experiences with making treatment decisions. *Research in Nursing and Health, 20,* 219-227.

Kerr, N. J. (1985). Behavioral manifestations of misguided entitlement. *Perspectives in Psychiatric Care, 23*(1), 5-15.

Kersbergen, A. L. (1997). Defining managed care in an evolving health care environment. (Doctoral dissertation, University of Wisconsin-Milwaukee, 1996). *Dissertation Abstracts International, B 57/12,* 7450. (AAC#9717140)

Keyser, P. K. (1989). *From angels to advocates: The concept of virtue in nursing ethics from 1870 to 1980.* Unpublished doctoral dissertation, University of Texas at Dallas.

Kienle, G. S., & Kiene, H. (1996). Placebo effect and placebo concept: A critical methodological and conceptual analysis of reports on the magnitude of the placebo effect. *Alternative Therapies in Health and Medicine, 2*(6), 39-54.

Kikuchi, J. F. (1997). Clarifying the nature of conceptualizations about nursing. *Canadian Journal of Nursing Research, 29*(1), 97-110.

Kindleman, B. (1993). The concept of hope: Implications for nursing. *CAET Journal, 12*(1), 7-10.

King, I. M. (1992). King's theory of goal attainment. *Nursing Science Quarterly, 5,* 19-26.

King, K. A. (1997). Self-concept and self-esteem: A clarification of terms. *Journal of School Health, 67*(2), 68-70.

King, L., & Appleton, J. V. (1997). Intuition: A critical review of the research and rhetoric. *Journal of Advanced Nursing, 26,* 194-202.

Kissinger, J. A. (1998). Overconfidence: A concept analysis. *Nursing Forum, 33*(2), 18-26.

Kita, A. (1997). [Characteristics of the social support for pregnant women in Japan—according to concept of four kinds of social support]. *Nihon Kango Kagakkai Shi [Journal of Academy of Nursing Science], 17*(1), 8-21.

Kleinpell, R. M. (1991). Concept analysis of quality of life. *Dimensions of Critical Care Nursing, 10,* 223-229.

Knafl, K. A., & Deatrick, J. A. (1986). How families manage chronic conditions: An analysis of the concept of normalization. *Research in Nursing and Health, 9*(3), 215-222.

Knafl, K. A., & Deatrick, J. A. (1990). Family management style: Concept analysis and development. *Journal of Pediatric Nursing, 5*(1), 4-14.

Knapik-Smith, M., & Bennett, G. (1997). Moderate drinking in women: A concept analysis. *Issues in Mental Health Nursing, 18,* 285-301.

Ko, N. Y., Shiau, C., & Sheu, S. L. (1997). [Uncertainty: A concept analysis]. *Hu Li Tsa Chih [Journal of Nursing], 44*(1), 92-97.

Kolanowski, A. M. (1991). Restlessness in the elderly: A concept analysis. In P. L. Chinn (Ed.), *Anthology on caring* (pp. 345-353). New York: National League for Nursing Vol. 2392.

Kolanowski, A. M. (1995). Disturbing behaviors in demented elders: A concept synthesis. *Archives of Psychiatric Nursing, 9*(4), 188-194.

Kolcaba, K. Y. (1991). A taxonomic structure for the concept comfort. *Image: Journal of Nursing Scholarship, 23*, 237-240.

Kolcaba, K. Y. (1992). Gerontological nursing: The concept of comfort in an environmental framework. *Journal of Gerontological Nursing, 18*(6), 33-38.

Kolcaba, K. Y. (1992). Holistic comfort: Operationalizing the construct as a nurse-sensitive outcome. *Advances in Nursing Science, 15*(1), 1-10.

Kolcaba, K. Y., & Kolcaba, R. J. (1991). An analysis of the concept of comfort. *Journal of Advanced Nursing, 16*, 1301-1310.

Kontz, M. (1991). A proposed model for assessing compliance with the unitary man/human framework based on an analysis of the concept of compliance. In R. M. Carroll-Johnson (Ed.), *Classification of nursing diagnoses: Proceedings of the ninth conference held in Orlando, FL, 1990.* Philadelphia: J. B. Lippincott.

Kovacs, J. (1989). Concepts of health and disease. *The Journal of Medicine and Philosophy, 14*, 261-267.

Kulbok, P. A., & Baldwin, J. H. (1992). From preventive health behavior to health promotion: advancing a positive construct of health. *Advances in Nursing Science, 14*(4), 50-64.

Kulbok, P. A., Baldwin, J. H., Cox, C. L., & Duffy, R. (1997). Advancing discourse on health promotion: Beyond mainstream thinking. *Advances in Nursing Science, 20*(1), 12-20.

Laatu, S., Portin, R., Revonsuo, A., Tuisku, S., & Rinne, J. (1997). Knowledge of concept meanings in Alzheimer's disease. *Cortex, 33*(1), 27-45.

Laffrey, S. C., Loveland Cherry, C. J., & Winkler, S. J. (1986). Health behavior: Evolution of two paradigms. *Public Health Nursing, 3*(2), 92-100.

Lamb, M. A. (1998). Concept analysis of relating: A human response pattern. *Nursing Diagnosis, 9*(1), 15-22.

Langford, C. P. H., Bowsher, J., Maloney, J. P., & Lillis, P. P. (1997). Social support: A conceptual analysis. *Journal of Advanced Nursing, 25*, 95-100.

Lea, A., & Watson, R. (1996). Caring research and concepts: A selected review of the literature. *Journal of Clinical Nursing, 5*(2), 71-77.

Lea, A., Watson, R., & Deary, I. J. (1998). Caring in nursing: a multivariate analysis. *Journal of Advanced Nursing, 28*(3), 662.

Lee, H. J. (1983). Analysis of a concept: Hardiness. *Oncology Nursing Forum, 10*(4), 32-35.

Lee, T. B. (1997). Surveillance in acute care and nonacute care settings: current issues and concepts. *American Journal of Infection Control, 25*, 121-124.

Leininger, M. (1967). The culture concept and its relevance to nursing. *Journal of Nursing Education, 6*(2), 27-37.

Le Moigne, J. L. (1997). [Concept formation, in and by the organization, the assumed action in its complexity]. *Recherche En Soins Infirmiers, 51*, 25-41.

LeMone, P. (1991). Analysis of a human phenomenon: Self-concept. *Nursing Diagnosis, 2*(3), 126-130.

Lerdal, A. (1998). A concept analysis of energy. Its meaning in the lives of three individuals with chronic illness. *Scandinavian Journal of Caring Sciences, 12*(1), 3-10.

Lindgren, C. L., Burke, M. L., Hainsworth, M. A., & Eakes, G. G. (1992). Chronic sorrow: A lifespan concept. *Scholarly Inquiry for Nursing Practice, 6*, 27–42.

Lindley Davis, B. (1991). Process of dying: Defining characteristics. *Cancer Nursing, 14*(6), 328–333.

Lindsey, E., & Hills, M. (1992). An analysis of the concept of hardiness. *Canadian Journal of Nursing Research, 24*(1), 39–50.

Lippman, L. (1977). "Normalization" and related concepts: Words and ambiguities. *Child Welfare, 56*, 301–310.

Longway, I. M. (1972). Curriculum concepts—an historical analysis. *Nursing Outlook, 20*(2), 116–120.

Low, J. (1996). The concept of hardiness: A brief but critical commentary. *Journal of Advanced Nursing, 24*, 588–590.

Loyer, R. (1995). Spirituality in nursing: Towards a definition. *Australian Journal of Holistic Nursing, 2*(1), 31–37.

Lugton, J. (1997). The nature of social support as experienced by women treated for breast cancer. *Journal of Advanced Nursing, 25*, 1184–1191.

Lutzen, K., da Silva, A. B., & Nordin, C. (1995). An analysis of some dimensions of the concept of moral sensing exemplified in psychiatric care...including commentary by Katims I. *Scholarly Inquiry for Nursing Practice, 9*, 57–70.

Lyons, P. (1997). Larry Brown's Joe and the uses and abuses of the "region" concept. *Studies in American Fiction, 25*, 101–124.

Maas, M. L., Johnson, M., & Moorhead, S. (1996). Classifying nursing-sensitive patient outcomes. *Image: Journal of Nursing Scholarship, 28*, 295–301.

Maben, J., & Clark, J. M. (1995). Health promotion: A concept analysis. *Journal of Advanced Nursing, 22*, 1158–1165.

Mahon, P. Y. (1996). An analysis of the concept "patient satisfaction" as it relates to contemporary nursing care. *Journal of Advanced Nursing, 24*, 1241–1248.

Mahon, S. M. (1994). Concept analysis of pain: Implications related to nursing diagnosis. *Nursing Diagnosis, 5*(1), 14–25.

Maibach, E., & Murphy, D. A. (1995). Self-efficacy in health promotion research and practice: Conceptualization and measurement. *Health Education Research, 10*(1), 37–50.

Mairis, E. D. (1994). Concept clarification in professional practice—dignity. *Journal of Advanced Nursing, 19*, 947–953.

Malloy, G. B., & Berkery, A. C. (1993). Codependency: A feminist perspective. *Journal of Psychosocial Nursing and Mental Health Services, 31*(4), 15–19.

Mammen, S. (1973). The concept of self-care. *Nursing Journal of India, 64*(11), 375 passim.

Manciaux, M. (1973). A new concept—family care. *International Nursing Review, 20*(3), 85–88 passim.

Mansen, T. J. (1993). The spiritual dimension of individuals: Conceptual development. *Nursing Diagnosis, 4*, 140–147.

Mansfield, E. (1973). Empathy: Concept and identified psychiatric nursing behavior. *Nursing Research, 22*, 525–530.

Marck, P. (1990). Therapeutic reciprocity: A caring phenomenon. *Advances in Nursing Science, 13*(1), 49–59.

Mardell, A. (1996). Advocacy: Exploring the concept. *British Journal of Theatre Nursing, 6*(7), 34–36.

Martsolf, D. S., & Mickley, J. R. (1998). The concept of spirituality in nursing theories: Differing world-views and extent of focus. *Journal of Advanced Nursing, 27*, 294-303.

Matravers, D. (1996). Aesthetic concepts and aesthetic experiences. *The British Journal of Aesthetics, 36*, 265-277.

Matteson, P., & Hawkins, J. W. (1990). Concept analysis of decision making. *Nursing Forum, 25*(2), 4-10.

McCance, T. V., McKenna, H. P., & Boore, J. R. P. (1997). Caring: Dealing with a difficult concept. *International Journal of Nursing Studies, 34*, 241-248.

McCormack, B. (1992). Intuition: Concept analysis and application to curriculum development. Concept analysis, part 1. *Journal of Clinical Nursing, 1*, 339-344.

McCormack, B. (1993). Intuition: Concept analysis and application to curriculum development. Application to curriculum development, part 2. *Journal of Clinical Nursing, 2*, 11-17.

McDaniel, R. W., & Bach, C. A. (1994). Quality of life: A concept analysis. *Rehabilitation Nursing Research, 3*(1), 18-22.

McHaffie, H. E. (1992). Coping: An essential element of nursing. *Journal of Advanced Nursing, 17*(8), 933-940.

McSherry, W., & Draper, P. (1998). The debates emerging from the literature surrounding the concept of spirituality as applied to nursing. *Journal of Advanced Nursing, 27*, 683-691.

Meeberg, G. A. (1993). Quality of life: A concept analysis. *Journal of Advanced Nursing, 18*(1), 32-38.

Mehta, M. D. (1997). Risk assessment and sustainable development: Towards a concept of. *Risk: Health, Safety & Environment, 8*(2), 137.

Meize-Grochowski, R. (1984). An analysis of the concept of trust. *Journal of Advanced Nursing, 9*, 563-572.

Mekwa, J. N., Uys, L. R., & Vermaak, M. V. (1992). A concept analysis of nurses' commitment to patient care. *Curationis, 15*(3), 7-11.

Messias, D. K. (1996). Concept development: Exploring undocumentedness. *Scholarly Inquiry for Nursing Practice, 10*, 235-252.

Miles, M. S., & Holditch Davis, D. (1995). Compensatory parenting: How mothers describe parenting their 3-year-old, prematurely born children. *Journal of Pediatric Nursing, 10*, 243-253.

Milligan, R., Lenz, E. R., Parks, P. L., Pugh, L. C., & Kitzman, H. (1996). Postpartum fatigue: Clarifying a concept. *Scholarly Inquiry for Nursing Practice, 10*, 279-291.

Misao, H., Hayama, Y., Hishinuma, M., Iwai, I., & Kaharu, C. (1996). [Analysis of the concept of care/caring-structure of attributes identified from qualitative and quantitative research]. *Seiroka Kango Daigaku Kiyo, 22*, 14-28.

Mitchell, G. J. (1993). Living paradox in Parse's theory. *Nursing Science Quarterly, 6*, 44-51.

Mitchell, G. J. (1996). Pretending: A way to get through the day. *Nursing Science Quarterly, 9*, 92-93.

Mizuno, M. (1997). [The meaning and structure of cancer survivors' perception of their health]. *Nihon Kango Kagakkai Shi [Journal of Academy of Nursing Science], 17*(1), 48-57.

Moch, S. D. (1989). Health within illness: Conceptual evolution and practice possibilities. *Advances in Nursing Science, 11*(4), 23-31.

Moch, S. D. (1998). Health-within-illness: Concept development through research and practice. *Journal of Advanced Nursing, 28*(2), 305.

Mohnkern, S. M. (1992). Presence in nursing: Its antecedents, defining attributes and consequences (Doctoral dissertation, University of Texas at Austin). *Dissertation Abstracts International, B 53/04*, 1787. (AAC# 9225674).

Moloney, M. F. (1997). The meanings of home in the stories of older women. *Western Journal of Nursing Research, 19*, 166–176.

Moore, P. V., & Williamson, G. C. (1984). Health promotion: Evolution of a concept. *Nursing Clinics of North America, 19*, 195–206.

Mordacci, R. (1995). Health as an analogical concept. *Journal of Medicine and Philosophy, 20*, 475–497.

Mornhinweg, G. C., & Voignier, R. R. (1996). Rest. *Holistic Nursing Practice, 10*(4), 54–60.

Morse, J. M., Anderson, G., Bottorff, J. L., Yonge, O. B, Solberg, S. M., & McIlveen, K. H. (1992). Exploring empathy: A conceptual fit for nursing practice? *Image: Journal of Nursing Scholarship, 24*, 273–280.

Morse, J. M., Bottorff, J., Neander, W., & Solberg, S. (1991). Comparative analysis of conceptualizations and theories of caring. *Image: Journal of Nursing Scholarship, 23*, 119–126.

Morse, J. M., & Carter, B. (1996). The essence of enduring and expressions of suffering: The reformulation of self (including commentary by M. M. Rawnsley, with author response). *Scholarly Inquiry for Nursing Practice, 10*, 43–74.

Morse, J. M., & Doberneck, B. (1995). Delineating the concept of hope. *Image: Journal of Nursing Scholarship, 27*, 277–285.

Morse, J. M., & Mitcham, C. (1997). Compathy: The contagion of physical distress. *Journal of Advanced Nursing, 26*, 649–657.

Morse, J. M., Solberg, S., Neander, W., Bottorff, J., & Johnson, J. L. (1990). Concepts of caring and caring as a concept. *Advances in Nursing Science, 13*(1), 1–14.

Mowat, J., & Laschinger, H. K. S. (1994). Self-efficacy in caregivers of cognitively impaired elderly people: A concept analysis. *Journal of Advanced Nursing, 19*, 1105–1113.

Muller, M. E., & Dzurec, L. C. (1993). The power of the name. *Advances in Nursing Science, 15*(3), 15–22.

Mullins, D. L. (1994). Powerlessness: Concept analysis and validation of the defining characteristics. In R. M. Carroll-Johnson & M. Paquette (Eds.), *Classification of Nursing Diagnoses: Proceedings of the Tenth Conference* (pp. 208–210). Philadelphia: J. B. Lippincott.

Musschenga, A. W. (1997). The relation between concepts of quality-of-life, health and happiness. *The Journal of Medicine and Philosophy, 22*, 11–28.

Nagelsmith, L. (1995). Competence: An evolving concept. *Journal of Continuing Education in Nursing, 26*, 245–248.

Narlikar, J. V. (1992). The concepts of "beginning" and "creation" in cosmology. *Philosophy of Science, 59*, 361–371.

Nelson, D. B., & Clements, C. (1988). Preterm infant stimulation: The analysis of a concept. *Journal of Pediatric Health Care, 2*(2), 79–88.

Nemcek, M. A. (1987). Self nurturing: A concept analysis. *AAOHN Journal, 35*, 349–352.

Ness, P. (1997). Understandings of health. How individual perceptions of health affect health promotion needs in organizations. *AAOHN Journal, 45*, 330-336.

Nethercott, S. (1993). A concept for all the family. Family centred care: A concept analysis. *Professional Nurse, 8*, 794-797.

Newbern, V. B., & Krowchuk, H. V. (1994). Failure to thrive in elderly people: A conceptual analysis. *Journal of Advanced Nursing, 19*, 840-849.

Newman, M. A. (1991). Health conceptualizations. *Annual Review of Nursing Research, 43*, 221-243.

Niemann, G., & Michaelis, R. (1996). [Cerebral palsy (I)—an analysis of the concept]. *Klinische Padiatrie, 208*, 276-279.

Noland, L. R. (1991). *Fidelity in health care—emphasis on nursing: A concept analysis.* (Doctoral dissertation, University of Virginia, 1991). *Dissertation Abstracts International, B 53/02*, 7450. (AAC#9219268)

Norman, E. M. (1989). Analysis of the concept of posttraumatic stress disorder. *Journal of Advanced Medical Surgical Nursing, 1*(4), 55-64.

Nystrom, A. E. M. (1995). The concept of cogitation. *Journal of Advanced Nursing, 21*, 364-370.

O'Berle, K., & Davies, B. (1992). Support and caring: Exploring the concepts. *Oncology Nursing Forum, 19*, 763-767.

Ogawa, N. (1997). [Florence Nightingale's concept of home nursing: An analysis of her writings]. *Kango Kenkyu [Japanese Journal of Nursing Research], 30*(1), 63-75.

Olson, R. S. (1985). Normalization: A concept in analysis . . ."re-valuation" of a devalued person. *Rehabilitation Nursing, 10*(6), 22-23.

Ouellet, L. L., & Rush, K. L. (1992). A synthesis of selected literature on mobility: A basis for studying impaired mobility. *Nursing Diagnosis, 3*(2), 72-80.

Ouellet, L. L., & Rush, K. L. (1996). A study of nurses' perceptions of client mobility. *Western Journal of Nursing Research, 18*, 565-579.

Paavilainen, E., Astedt Kurki, P., & Paunonen, M. (1996). Child abuse in families—concept analysis [Finnish]. *Hoitotiede, 8*(3), 111-118.

Panzarine, S. (1985). Coping: Conceptual and methodological issues. *Advances in Nursing Science, 7*, 49-58.

Payne, L. (1983). Health: A basic concept in nursing theory. *Journal of Advanced Nursing, 8*(5), 393-395.

Penrod, J., & Morse, J. M. (1997). Strategies for assessing and fostering hope: The hope assessment guide. *Oncology Nursing Forum, 24*, 1055-1063.

Pepin, J. I. (1992). Family caring and caring in nursing. *Image: Journal of Nursing Scholarship, 24*, 127-131.

Pesut, D. J. (1992). Self-regulation, self-management and self-care. *South Carolina Nurse, 7*(2), 22-23.

Pezza, P. E. (1991). Value concept and value change theory in health education: A conceptual, empirical, methodological review. *Health Values: Achieving High Level Wellness, 15*(4), 3-12.

Phillips, B. B., & Bramlett, M. H. (1994). Integrated awareness: A key to the pattern of mutual process. *Visions: The Journal of Rogerian Nursing Science, 2*(1), 19-34.

Phillips, D. E. (1994). The community concept in long term health care. *Canadian Nursing Home, 5*(3), 10-15.

Phillips, P. (1993). A deconstruction of caring. *Journal of Advanced Nursing, 18*, 1554-1558.

Pickering, A. (1995). Concepts and the mangle of practice: Constructing quaternions. *The South Atlantic Quarterly, 94*, 417–480.

Pidgeon, V. (1985). Children's concepts of illness: Implications for health teaching. *Maternal Child Nursing Journal, 14*(1), 23–35.

Pierce, L. L. (1994). Fear held by caregivers of people with stroke: A concept analysis. *Rehabilitation Nursing Research, 3*(2), 69–74.

Pike, A. W. (1990). On the nature and place of empathy in clinical nursing practice. *Journal of Professional Nursing, 6*, 235–240.

Pilhammar-Andersson, E. (1995). Marginality: Concept or reality in nursing education? *Journal of Advanced Nursing, 21*, 131–136.

Pinch, W. J. (1995). Synthesis: Implementing a complex process. *Nurse Educator, 20*(1), 34–40.

Plantinga, A. (1986). Two concepts of modality: Modal realism and modal reductionism. *The Journal of Philosophy, 83*, 693.

Playle, J. F. (1996). Quality in nurse education: An exploration of the concept of students as customers. *Nurse Education Today, 16*, 215–220.

Pless, B. S., & Clayton, G. M. (1993). Clarifying the concept of critical thinking in nursing. *Journal of Nursing Education, 24*, 425–428.

Polaschek, N. R. (1998). Cultural safety: A new concept in nursing people of different ethnicities. *Journal of Advanced Nursing, 27*, 452.

Polk, L. V. (1997). Toward a middle-range theory of resilience. *Advances in Nursing Science, 19*(3), 1–13.

Pollock, D. (1996). Personhood and illness among the Kulina. *Medical Anthropology Quarterly, 10*, 319–341.

Potari, D., & Spiliotopoulou, V. (1996). Children's approaches to the concept of volume. *Science Education, 80*(3), 341–360.

Potempa, K., Lopez, M., Reid, C., & Lawson, L. (1986). Chronic fatigue. *Image: Journal of Nursing Scholarship, 18*, 165–169.

Powell, A. (1997). Grief and the concept of loss in midwifery practice. Part 1. Normal and abnormal grief. *Professional Care of Mother and Child, 7*(2), 37–39.

Powell, A. (1997). Understanding grief. Grief and the concept of loss in midwifery practice. Part 2. Grief in obstetrics and midwifery. *Professional Care of Mother and Child, 7*(3), 76–78.

Price, V., & Archbold, J. (1997). What's it all about, empathy? *Nurse Education Today, 17*, 106–110.

Proot, I. M., Crebolder, H. F., Abu-Saad, H. H., & Ter Meulen, R. H. (1998). Autonomy in the rehabilitation of stroke patients in nursing homes. A concept analysis. *Scandinavian Journal of Caring Sciences, 12*, 139–145.

Qvarnstrom, U., & Haugen, M. (1987). Analysis of the concept of quality of life. *Scandinavian Journal of Caring Sciences, 1*(2), 47–50.

Ramos, M. C. N. (1992). *Empathy within the nurse-patient relationship.* (Doctoral dissertation, University of Virginia, 1990). *Dissertation Abstracts International, B 52/10*, 5193. (AAC#9131565)

Rawnsley, M. M. (1985). Nursing: The compassionate science. *Cancer Nursing, 8*(Suppl 1), 71–74.

Ream, E., & Richardson, A. (1996). Fatigue: A concept analysis. *International Journal of Nursing Studies, 33*, 519–529.

Reckling, J. B. (1994). Conceptual analysis of rights using a philosophic inquiry approach. *Image: Journal of Nursing Scholarship, 26*, 309–314.

Redeker, N. S., & Mason, D. J. (1994). Perspectives on activity. *Scholarly Inquiry for Nursing Practice, 8,* 277-93.

Reed, P. G., & Leonard, V. E. (1989). An analysis of the concept of self-neglect. *Advances in Nursing Science, 12*(1), 39-53.

Rew, L. (1986). Intuition: Concept analysis of a group phenomenon. *Advances in Nursing Science, 8*(2), 21-28.

Rew, L., & Barrow, E. M. (1987). Intuition: A neglected hallmark of nursing knowledge. *Advances in Nursing Science, 10*(1), 49-62.

Rhodes, V. A. (1997). Criteria for assessment of nausea, vomiting, and retching. *Oncology Nursing Forum, 24*(7 Suppl), 13-19.

Rice, G. E., & Young, L. H. (1994). A folk model of arthritis. *Health Values: Achieving High Level Wellness, 18*(2), 15-27.

Rich, J. A., & Stone, D. A. (1996). The experience of violent injury for young African-American men: The meaning of being a "sucker" [see comments]. *Journal of General Internal Medicine, 11*(2), 77-82.

Richmond, J. P., & McKenna, H. (1998). Homophobia: An evolutionary analysis of the concept as applied to nursing. *Journal of Advanced Nursing, 28,* 362-369.

Riding, T. M. (1997). Normalization: Analysis and application within a special hospital. *Journal of Psychiatric and Mental Health Nursing, 4*(1), 23-28.

Rieder, J. (1997). The institutional overdetermination of the concept of romanticism. *Yale Journal of Criticism, 10,* 145-163.

Riffle, K. L. (1973). Rehabilitation: The evolution of a social concept. *Nursing Clinics of North America, 8,* 665-671.

Rittman, M. R. (1991). Constructing reality: The meanings of "family" in two psychiatric treatment programs. (Doctoral dissertation, University of Florida, 1991). *Dissertation Abstracts International, A 51/10,* 3530. (AAC#9106471)

Roberts, K. T., & Aspy, C. B. (1993). Development of the Serenity Scale. *Journal of Nursing Measurement, 1,* 145-164.

Roberts, K. T., & Fitzgerald, L. (1991). Serenity: Caring with perspective. *Scholarly Inquiry for Nursing Practice, 5,* 127-146.

Roberts, K. T., & Whall, A. (1996). Serenity as a goal for nursing practice. *Image: Journal of Nursing Scholarship, 28,* 359-364.

Robinson, C. A. (1993). Managing life with a chronic condition: The story of normalization. *Qualitative Health Research, 3*(1), 6-28.

Robinson, D. S., & McKenna, H. P. (1998). Loss: An analysis of a concept of particular interest to nursing. *Journal of Advanced Nursing, 27,* 779-784.

Robinson, L., & Mahon, M. M. (1997). Sibling bereavement: A concept analysis. *Death Studies, 21,* 477-499.

Rodgers, B. L. (1989). The use and application of concepts in nursing: The case of health policy. (Doctoral dissertation, University Of Virginia, 1987). *Dissertation Abstracts International, B 49/11,* 4756. (AAC#8903985)

Rodgers, B. L. (1989). Concepts, analysis and the development of nursing knowledge: The evolutionary cycle. *Journal of Advanced Nursing, 14,* 330-335.

Rodgers, B. L. (1989). Exploring health policy as a concept. *Western Journal of Nursing Research, 11,* 694-702.

Rodgers, B. L., & Cowles, K. V. (1991). The concept of grief: A foundation for nursing research and practice. *Research in Nursing and Health, 14,* 119-127.

Rodgers, B. L., & Cowles, K. V. (1991). The concept of grief: An analysis of classical and contemporary thought. *Death Studies, 15*, 443-458.

Rodgers, B. L., & Cowles, K. V. (1997). A conceptual foundation for human suffering in nursing care and research. *Journal of Advanced Nursing, 25*, 1048-1053.

Rodwell, C. M. (1996). An analysis of the concept of empowerment. *Journal of Advanced Nursing, 23*, 305-313.

Roelofs, L. H. (1992). The meaning of leisure for older persons (Doctoral dissertation, University of Illinois at Chicago, Health Sciences Center). *Dissertation Abstracts International, B 52/12*, 6320. (AAC#9213145)

Rogers, A. C. (1997). Vulnerability, health and health care. *Journal of Advanced Nursing, 26*, 65-72.

Rose, P. (1995). Best interests: A concept analysis and its implications for ethical decision-making in nursing. *Nursing Ethics, 2*, 149-160.

Rosenbaum, J. N. (1989). Self-caring: Concept development for nursing. *Recent Advances in Nursing, 24*, 18-31.

Rosenthal Dichter, C. H. (1996). The pediatric physiologic stress response: A concept analysis. *Scholarly Inquiry for Nursing Practice, 10*, 211-234.

Rush, K. L., & Ouellet, L. L. (1993). Mobility: A concept analysis. *Journal of Advanced Nursing, 18*, 486-492.

Russell, C. K., Bunting, S. M., & Gregory, D. M. (1997). Protective care-receiving: The active role of care-recipients. *Journal of Advanced Nursing, 25*, 532-540.

Sadler, J. J. (1995). Analysis and observation of the concept of caring in nursing. (Doctoral dissertation, University of Wisconsin-Milwaukee). *Dissertation Abstracts International, B 56/05*, 2564. (AAC#9528682)

Sarkis, J. M., & Skoner, M. M. (1987). An analysis of the concept of holism in nursing literature. *Holistic Nursing Practice, 2*(1), 61-69.

Schmidt, J. (1972). Availability: A concept of nursing practice. *American Journal of Nursing, 72*, 1086-1089.

Schumacher, K. L., & Meleis, A. I. (1994). Transitions: A central concept in nursing. *Image: Journal of Nursing Scholarship, 26*, 119-127.

Scott, P. A. (1995). Care, attention and imaginative identification in nursing practice. *Journal of Advanced Nursing, 21*, 1196-1200.

Sheldon, L. M. (1996). An analysis of the concept of humour and its application to one aspect of children's nursing. *Journal of Advanced Nursing, 24*, 1175-1183.

Shumaker, S. A., & Brownell, A. (1984). Toward a theory of social support: Closing conceptual gaps. *Journal of Social Issues, 40*, 11-36.

Simmons, S. J. (1989). Health: A concept analysis. *International Journal of Nursing Studies, 26*, 155-161.

Singh, T. A. S., & Srivastava, A. K. (1995). An exploration of children's conception of intelligence. *Journal of Indian Psychology, 13*(2), 47-55.

Sletteboe, A. (1997). Dilemma: A concept analysis. *Journal of Advanced Nursing, 26*, 449-454.

Slevin, E. (1995). A concept analysis of, and proposed new term for, challenging behaviour. *Journal of Advanced Nursing, 21*, 928-934.

Smith, A. (1995). An analysis of altruism: A concept of caring. *Journal of Advanced Nursing, 22*, 785-790.

Smith, J. P. (1983). Concept of nursing literacy: An energizing force in health care. *Journal of Advanced Nursing, 8*, 69-75.

Smith, L. S. (1998). Concept analysis: Cultural competence. *Journal of Cultural Diversity, 5*(1), 4-10.

Söderberg, A., Gilje, F., & Norberg, A. (1997). Dignity in situations of ethical difficulty in intensive care. *Intensive Critical Care Nursing, 13*, 135-144.

Sourial, S. (1997). An analysis of caring. *Journal of Advanced Nursing, 26*, 1189-1192.

St. John, W. (1993). Primary health care: A clarification of the concept and the nursing role. *Contemporary Nurse: A Journal for the Australian Nursing Profession, 2*(2), 73-78.

Stephen, T. (1994). Exploring respect. *CAET Journal, 13*(1), 7-13.

Stephenson, C. (1991). The concept of hope revisited for nursing. *Journal of Advanced Nursing, 16*, 1456-1461.

Stewart, A. L. (1992). Conceptual and methodologic issues in defining quality of life: State of the art. *Progress in Cardiovascular Nursing, 7*(1), 3-11.

Stewart, B. M., & Krueger, L. E. (1996). An evolutionary concept analysis of mentoring in nursing. *Journal of Professional Nursing, 12*, 311-321.

Stubblefield, C. (1995). Optimism: A determinant of health behavior. *Nursing Forum, 30*, 19-24.

Sulg, I. (1974). [The concept of death]. *Tidskrift For Sveriges Sjukskoterskor, 41*(8), 4-11.

Sullivan, G. C. (1993). Towards clarification of convergent concepts: Sense of coherence, will to meaning, locus of control, learned helplessness and hardiness. *Journal of Advanced Nursing, 18*, 1772-1778.

Summers, S. (1992). Concept analysis methodology: Applications to altered level of consciousness. *Journal of Post Anesthesia Nursing, 7*, 273-277.

Sutherland, J. A. (1995). Historical concept analysis of empathy. *Issues in Mental Health Nursing, 16*, 555-566.

Swanson, E. A., Jensen, D. P., Specht, J., Johnson, M. L., Maas, M., & Saylor, D. (1997). Caregiving: Concept analysis and outcomes. *Scholarly Inquiry for Nursing Practice, 11*, 65-76; discussion 77-79.

Sweeney, N. M. (1994). A concept analysis of personal knowledge: Application to nursing education. *Journal of Advanced Nursing, 20*, 917-924.

Symes, L. (1995). Post traumatic stress disorder: An evolving concept. *Archives of Psychiatric Nursing, 9*, 195-202.

Symonds, B. (1991). Sociological issues in the conceptualization of mental illness. *Journal of Advanced Nursing, 16*, 1470-1477.

Tapia Granados, J. A. (1994). [Incidence: concept, terminology and dimensional analysis]. *Medicina Clinica (Barcelona), 103*, 140-142.

Teasdale, K. (1989). The concept of reassurance in nursing. *Journal of Advanced Nursing, 14*, 444-450.

Teel, C. S. (1991). Chronic sorrow: Analysis of the concept. *Journal of Advanced Nursing, 16*, 1311-1319.

Thaler, P. (1997). Concepts of ethnicity in early twentieth-century Norwegian America. *Scandinavian Studies, 69*, 85-103.

Tiesinga, L. J., Dassen, T. W. N., & Halfens, R. J. G. (1996). Fatigue: A summary of the definitions, dimensions, and indicators. *Nursing Diagnosis, 7*(2), 51-62.

Tilden, V. P. (1985). Issues of conceptualizations and measurement of social support in the construction of nursing theory. *Research in Nursing and Health, 8*, 199-206.

Timmerman, G. M. (1991). A concept analysis of intimacy. *Issues in Mental Health Nursing, 12*, 19-30.

Uhle, S. M. (1994). Codependence: Contextual variables in the language of social pathology. *Issues in Mental Health Nursing, 15*, 307-317.

Vallerand, R. J., Deshaies, P., Cuerrier, J. P., Briere, N. M., et al. (1996). Toward a multidimensional definition of sportsmanship. *Journal of Applied Sport Psychology, 8*(1), 89-101.

Wagner, P. J., & Mongan, P. F. (1998). Validating the concept of abuse: Women's perceptions of defining behaviors and the effects of emotional abuse on health indicators. *Archives of Family Medicine, 7*(1), 25-29.

Walton, J. (1996). Spiritual relationships: A concept analysis. *Journal of Holistic Nursing, 14*, 237-250.

Warren, B. J. (1993). Explaining social isolation through concept analysis. *Archives of Psychiatric Nursing, 7*, 270-276.

Watson, S. J. (1991). An analysis of the concept of experience. *Journal of Advanced Nursing, 16*, 1117-1121.

Watt, E. (1997). An exploration of the way in which the concept of patient advocacy is perceived by registered nurses working in an acute care hospital. *International Journal of Nursing Practice, 3*, 119-127.

Weeks, S. K., & O'Connor, P. C. (1994). Concept analysis of family + health = a new definition of family health. *Rehabilitation Nursing, 19*, 207-210.

Wendler, M. C. (1996). Understanding healing: A conceptual analysis. *Journal of Advanced Nursing, 24*, 836-842.

Westra, B. L., & Rodgers, B. L. (1991). The concept of integration: A foundation for evaluating outcomes of nursing care. *Journal of Professional Nursing, 7*, 277-282.

White, S. J. (1997). Empathy: A literature review and concept analysis. *Journal of Clinical Nursing, 6*, 253-257.

Whitley, G. G. (1992). Concept analysis of anxiety. *Nursing Diagnosis, 3*, 107-116.

Whitley, G. G. (1992). Concept analysis of fear. *Nursing Diagnosis, 3*, 155-161.

Whitley, G. G. (1994). Expert validation and differentiation of the nursing diagnoses Anxiety and Fear. *Nursing Diagnosis, 5*, 143-50.

Whitley, G. G. (1995). Where we are now: Concept analysis in nursing diagnosis research. *Nursing Diagnosis, 6*(2), 91-92.

Wiens, A. G. (1993). Patient autonomy in care: A theoretical framework for nursing. *Journal of Professional Nursing, 9*, 95-103.

Wilkinson, J. (1997). Developing a concept analysis of autonomy in nursing practice. *British Journal of Nursing, 6*, 703-707.

Wilson, J., & Retsas, A. (1997). Australian nurses' personal constructs about effective nurses—a repertory grid approach. *Journal of Professional Nursing, 13*, 193-199.

Wing, D. M. (1996). A concept analysis of alcoholic denial and cultural accounts. *Advances in Nursing Science, 19*(2), 54-63.

Wiseman, T. (1996). A concept analysis of empathy. *Journal of Advanced Nursing, 23*, 1162-1167.

Wocial, L. D. (1993). Advocacy in action. *Neonatal Network: Journal of Neonatal Nursing, 12*(5), 43-48.

Wurzbach, M. E. (1996). Comfort and nurses' moral choices. *Journal of Advanced Nursing, 24*, 260-264.

Yoder, L. (1990). Mentoring: A concept analysis. *Nursing Administration Quarterly, 15*(1), 9-19.

Younger, J. G. (1991). A theory of mastery. *Advances in Nursing Science, 14*(1), 76–89.

Zauszniewski, J. A. (1995). Learned resourcefulness: A conceptual analysis. *Issues in Mental Health Nursing, 16*, 13–31.

Index

Note: Page numbers in *italics* refer to figures; those followed by t refer to tables.

ISBN 0-7216-8243-X

90038